Comprehensive Men's Mental Health

T0139637

Although research shows that there is a silent crisis in men's mental health, there remains surprisingly little literature on the subject. This important textbook provides up-to-date, practical and evidence-based information on how mental health issues affect men, and the way treatments should be offered to them. Key opinion leaders from across the globe have been brought together to offer much-needed understanding about the socio-politico-economic context of men's lives today, as well as ethnic and cultural effects and genetic, epigenetic and gene–environment interaction. Clinically focused chapters cover topics such as suicide and self-harm, violence, sociopathy and substance misuse in men; depression, anxiety and related disorders; and psychotic and cognitive disorders. The book uses a lifespan approach to assessment and treatment, accounting for age and developmental phase. An invaluable source of information for clinical specialists and trainees in psychiatry, psychology and mental health nursing, as well as social workers and occupational therapists.

David Castle is Professor of Psychiatry at St Vincent's Health and the University of Melbourne in Australia.

David Coghill is the Chair of Developmental Mental Health and Professor of Child and Adolescent Psychiatry in the departments of Paediatrics and Psychiatry at the University of Melbourne in Australia.

Comprehensive Men's Mental Health

Edited by

David Castle
University of Melbourne

David Coghill
University of Melbourne

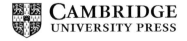
CAMBRIDGE
UNIVERSITY PRESS

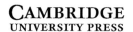

University Printing House, Cambridge CB2 8BS, United Kingdom

One Liberty Plaza, 20th Floor, New York, NY 10006, USA

477 Williamstown Road, Port Melbourne, VIC 3207, Australia

314–321, 3rd Floor, Plot 3, Splendor Forum, Jasola District Centre, New Delhi – 110025, India

79 Anson Road, #06–04/06, Singapore 079906

Cambridge University Press is part of the University of Cambridge.

It furthers the University's mission by disseminating knowledge in the pursuit of education, learning, and research at the highest international levels of excellence.

www.cambridge.org
Information on this title: www.cambridge.org/9781108740425
DOI: 10.1017/9781108646765

© Cambridge University Press 2021

First published 2021

Printed in the United Kingdom by TJ Books Limited, Padstow Cornwall

A catalogue record for this publication is available from the British Library.

Library of Congress Cataloging-in-Publication Data
Names: Castle, David, editor. | Coghill, David, editor.
Title: Comprehensive men's mental health / edited by David Castle, Chair of Psychiatry, University of Melbourne, David Coghill, Chair of Developmental Mental Health, University of Melbourne.
Description: Cambridge ; New York : Cambridge University Press, 2021. | Includes bibliographical references and index.
Identifiers: LCCN 2020036361 (print) | LCCN 2020036362 (ebook) | ISBN 9781108740425 (paperback) | ISBN 9781108646765 (epub)
Subjects: LCSH: Men–Mental health. | Men–Psychology. | Sex differences.
Classification: LCC RC451.4.M45 C66 2021 (print) | LCC RC451.4.M45 (ebook) | DDC 616.890081–dc23

LC record available at https://lccn.loc.gov/2020036361
LC ebook record available at https://lccn.loc.gov/2020036362

ISBN 978-1-108-74042-5 Paperback

Contents

Contributors

Osvaldo P. Almeida
Professor of Geriatric Psychiatry, Western Australian Centre for Health & Ageing, Medical School, University of Western Australia, Perth, Australia

Dinesh Bhugra CBE
Professor Emeritus, Institute of Psychiatry, Psychology and Neuroscience, King's College London, London, United Kingdom

Lucy Blake
Registrar, South London and Maudsley NHS Foundation Trust, London, United Kingdom

Yvonne Bonomo
Associate Professor, Department of Medicine, University of Melbourne, Director Department of Addiction Medicine, St Vincent's Hospital and Head of Women's Alcohol and Drug Service, Royal Women's Hospital, Melbourne, Australia

David Castle
Professor, Department of Psychiatry, St Vincent's Hospital and The University of Melbourne, Melbourne, Australia

Terence W. H. Chong
Senior Research Fellow in Psychiatry of Old Age, Department of Psychiatry, University of Melbourne and St Vincent's Hospital Melbourne, Australia

David Coghill
Chair of Developmental Mental Health, University of Melbourne, Melbourne, Australia

Kimberlie Dean
Chair of Forensic Mental Health and Acting Head of School of Psychiatry, University of New South Wales; and Clinical Academic Forensic Psychiatrist, Justice Health and Forensic Mental Health Network, Sydney, Australia

Karen-Leigh Edward
CEO, Her Heart; Adjunct Professor, Swinburne University of Technology, Australia; and Adjunct Professor, University of Huddersfield, United Kingdom

Joel Peter Eigen
Charles A. Dana Professor of Sociology, Emeritus, Franklin and Marshall College, Lancaster, Pennsylvania, USA

Jaco Erasmus
Clinical Lead, Gender Clinic, Monash Health, Melbourne, Australia

Ian Paul Everall
Executive Dean, Institute of Psychiatry, Psychology and Neuroscience, King's College London and South London and Maudsley NHS Foundation Trust, London, United Kingdom

Richard Fletcher
Associate Professor, Family Action Centre, Brain and Mental Health Priority Research Centre Faculty of Health and Medicine The University of Newcastle, Newcastle, Australia

David Forbes
Director, Phoenix Australia: Centre for Posttraumatic Mental Health and Department of Psychiatry, The University of Melbourne, Melbourne, Australia

Rupert Goodman
Research Assistant, Department of Psychiatry, University of Cape Town, Cape Town, South Africa

Guy Goodwin
Emeritus Professor, University Department of Psychiatry, University of Oxford, Oxford, United Kingdom

Scott Griffiths
Lecturer, Melbourne School of Psychological
Sciences, The University of Melbourne, Melbourne,
Australia

Philip Hazell
Conjoint Professor, Specialty of Psychiatry, The
University of Sydney School of Medicine, Sydney,
Australia

Joe Herbert
Emeritus Professor of Neuroscience, John van Geest
Centre for Brain Repair, Department of Clinical
Neurosciences, University of Cambridge, Cambridge,
United Kingdom

Diego Hidalgo-Mazzei
Consultant Psychiatrist and Postdoctoral Researcher,
Bipolar and Depressive Disorders Unit, Department
of Psychiatry and Psychology, Neurosciences
Institute, Hospital Clínic de Barcelona, University of
Barcelona, Barcelona, Spain; and Visiting Researcher,
Centre for Affective Disorders, Institute of Psychiatry,
Psychology and Neuroscience, King´s College
London, London, United Kingdom

Louise M. Howard
Professor in Women's Mental Health, Section of
Women's Mental Health, King's College London,
Institute of Psychiatry, Psychology and Neuroscience,
London, United Kingdom

Matthew Kelly
Student, Department of Psychology,
Institute of Psychiatry, Psychology and Neuroscience,
Kings College London, United Kingdom

David W. Kissane AC
Professor and Chair of Palliative Medicine Research,
The University of Notre Dame Australia, and
The Cunningham Centre for Palliative Care Research,
St Vincent's Hospital, Sydney;
Emeritus Professor of Psychiatry,
Department of Psychiatry, Monash University, and
Department of Oncology, Cabrini Health,
Melbourne, Australia

Daria Korobanova
Senior Research Officer, Justice Health and Forensic
Mental Health Network; and Conjoint Lecturer,
School of Psychiatry, University of New South Wales,
Sydney, Australia

Nicola T. Lautenschlager
Director of Academic Unit for Psychiatry of Old Age,
Department of Psychiatry, University of Melbourne
and NorthWestern Mental Health, Royal Melbourne
Hospital, Melbourne, Australia

J. Buckley Lennox
Research Officer, Department of Addiction Medicine,
St Vincent's Hospital, Melbourne, Australia

Christine Lochner
Professor, Department of Psychiatry,
Stellenbosch University, Stellenbosch,
South Africa

Deirdre MacManus
Clinical Reader in Forensic Psychiatry, Department
of Forensic and Neurodevelopmental Science,
Institute of Psychiatry Psychology and
Neuroscience, King's College London, London,
United Kingdom

Stuart B. Murray
Associate Professor, Department of Psychiatry and
Behavioral Sciences, University of Southern
California, California, USA

Erica Neill
Research Fellow, Department of Psychiatry, Faculty
of Medicine, Dentistry and Health, University of
Melbourne, Melbourne, Australia

David J. Pedder
Clinical Specialist, Phoenix Australia: Centre for
Posttraumatic Mental Health and Department of
Psychiatry, The University of Melbourne,
Melbourne, Australia

Harriet Quigley
Registrar, South London and Maudsley NHS
Foundation Trust, London, United Kingdom

Alyssa M. Sbisa
Research Fellow, Phoenix Australia: Centre for
Posttraumatic Mental Health and Department of
Psychiatry, The University of Melbourne,
Melbourne, Australia

Chantal F. Ski
Professor and Director, Integrated Care
Academy, University of Suffolk, Ipswich,
United Kingdom

Dan J. Stein
Professor, Department of Psychiatry, University of Cape Town, Cape Town, South Africa

Anna F. Taylor
Researcher, Forensic and Neurodevelopmental Sciences Department, King's College London, Institute of Psychiatry, Psychology and Neuroscience, London, United Kingdom

Sonia Terhaag
Research Fellow, Phoenix Australia: Centre for Posttraumatic Mental Health and Department of Psychiatry, The University of Melbourne, Melbourne, Australia

Renee Testa
Lecturer, Monash University School of Psychological Sciences, Monash University, Clayton, Australia; Senior Clinical Neuropsychologist, Department of Mental Health, Royal Children's Hospital, Melbourne, Australia

David R. Thompson
Professor, School of Nursing and Midwifery, Queen's University Belfast, Belfast, United Kingdom

Bruce Tonge
Emeritus Professor, Monash University Centre for Developmental Psychiatry and Psychology, Monash Medical Centre, Melbourne, Australia

Allan H. Young
Professor, Department of Psychological Medicine, Institute of Psychiatry, Psychology and Neuroscience, King's College London and South London and Maudsley NHS Foundation Trust, Bethlem Royal Hospital, Beckenham, Kent, United Kingdom.

Taylan Yukselen
Registrar, South London and Maudsley NHS Foundation Trust, London, United Kingdom

Preface

This book provides a comprehensive, up-to-date, and evidence-based review of men's mental health. It starts by considering the developmental context and neuro-developmental disorders, including autism spectrum disorders, attention deficit disorder, and schizophrenia (Section 1). These chapters are fronted with a chapter considering the development of the male brain and implications for mental health in males, and augmented by a chapter on adolescent development in males.

Section 2 addresses body image, sexuality, and anxiety disorders in males. The socio-politico-economic context of men's lives today as well as ethnic and cultural effects are covered, followed by chapters specifically on gender dysphoria and body image disorders in males; and anxiety and post-traumatic syndromes as they affect and manifest in males.

The particular issues affecting mood in males are the subject of Section 3, with consideration of suicide and suicide prevention in young men; postnatal depression in men; and broader issues of depression and bipolar disorder as they affect males. Implications for treatment are specifically addressed.

The impact of alcohol and illicit drugs on men as well as issues pertaining to domestic violence and criminality in males are covered in Section 4. Chapter 15 looks at how males with a mental illness are dealt with by the justice system, with recommendations for better, gender-informed care.

Section 5 deals with the overlap between physical and mental health in males, with a focus on HIV, cardiovascular disease, and cancers. Section 6 provides an overview of special considerations in dementia in men, and an integrative chapter on mental health of males in later life.

We trust that the breadth of topics covered and the mix of research and clinical perspectives will make this book of interest to a broad readership.

As editors, we were delighted and gratified by the positive response we had from highly esteemed chapter contributors from around the globe, and express our gratitude to them for their fine contributions. We thank also Cambridge University Press for their support and encouragement in producing this volume.

Chapter

1

Human Brain Development
Implications for Maladies of the Male Mind

David Coghill

As you work through the chapters in this book it will become very clear that since the beginning of the 'decade of the brain' in 1990 we have made considerable progress in understanding how the brain works and the way that it develops across the lifespan. We have also made significant progress in understanding the genetic and environmental factors that contribute to the development of mental health problems. We still, however, struggle to develop new and innovative treatments and therapies and in our understanding of what works for whom in what circumstances – more recently labelled precision or personalized medicine. There are, of course, many factors that contribute to this lack of concrete progress. Psychiatric disorders are complex and heterogeneous across several levels of analysis: phenotypically, with co-morbidity being the rule rather than the exception; aetiologically, with a complex genetic architecture based on different types of genetic variants and gene–environment interplay and diverse brain alterations. Also, as there is no stable, agreed-upon, and biologically valid construct for any of the recognized psychiatric disorders, the current taxonomy provides an unclear basis for informed biological research. Attempts to define biologically homogeneous subtypes ('biotypes') or pathophysiological dimensions of psychiatric disorders are under way but have yet to deliver (Feczko et al., 2019). From another angle, enormous scientific challenges are still presented by the complexity of the brain's architecture and physiology, our far from complete understanding of how these change across development, and the relationships between structure and function and between cognition and behaviour/symptoms. These continue to present enormous scientific challenges.

Sex is an often unrecognized but essential variable in this whole picture. There are sex differences in prevalence for most psychiatric disorders. Being male is a significant risk for the development of neurodevelopmental and neuropsychiatric disorders (e.g. schizophrenia, attention deficit hyperactivity disorder

(ADHD), autism spectrum disorder (ASD), Tourette's disorder, and intellectual disability (ID)). While being female appears to afford some degree of protection against these common disorders, it increases risk, at least after puberty, for depression and eating disorders. A discussion of these sex differences forms the core of this book. In this opening chapter we focus on sex differences in brain development. While our understanding of these differences is far from complete, the hope is that, in time, knowledge of the biological origins and functional consequences of these risk and protective factors will generate novel therapeutic targets and approaches for prevention and intervention.

We focus on two main lines of evidence that arise from human neuroimaging studies on the one hand and animal models on the other. Animal studies are particularly important in this context not only because they deliver several advantages in experimental design that are not possible in human studies but also because it is possible in animal models to separate sex from gender. In humans, gender is a complex construct that is based on a combination of our own and societal perception of our sex (see Chapter 7).

Interestingly it is only in the last 60 years that it has been accepted that the brain plays an important role in determining sex differences in human behaviours. Up until this time it was generally accepted that it was the somatic characteristics and differences between males and females (i.e. their differing genitalia and secondary sexual characteristics) that led to their characteristic sexual behaviours. This idea was convincingly challenged in 1959 when Phoenix and colleagues published a seminal study demonstrating that, when pregnant guinea pigs were treated with testosterone, their female offspring – when adults – showed a copulatory pattern of males despite not having a penis (Phoenix et al., 1959).

Sex differences between male and female embryos can be detected as soon as the second day following conception, by which time male embryos (in humans and rodents) are seen to have more cells and a higher metabolic rate (Burgoyne et al., 1995; Ray et al., 1995). A pivotal event in human sexual differentiation occurs at around six weeks post-conception when, in males, the *Sry* gene on the Y chromosome interacts with gene products from the X chromosome and other autosomal gene products to stimulate the primordial fetal gonad to develop into testes (Koopman, 1999). In the absence of these factors the fetus is programmed to develop into a female. The testicular hormones, including testosterone, start to be produced by the testes between 12 and 16 weeks post-conception and they then trigger the processes that lead to masculinization and defeminization of the male fetus.

Dimensions of Sex Differences in Behaviour and Brain Development

Before addressing the various causal agents that impact on sex differences in brain development it is worth considering the various dimensions along which these differences are realized. Joel and McCarthy (2017) proposed four helpful and non-mutually exclusive dimensions:

1. Direct versus indirect: this refers to whether the impact of the causal agent is direct (e.g. hormonal genetic – XX, YY) or indirect (e.g. as a consequence of stress or rearing practices).

2. Persistent versus transient: sometimes sex differences (manifest often as behavioural differences) appear only under certain circumstances and/or may disappear under others (e.g. sex differences in rough and tumble play that disappear during and after puberty).

3. Context-independent versus context-dependent: for example, stress-related sex differences in behaviour. In many species there is an interaction between age/stage of development and stress response whereby males show a greater response to stress at some ages while females respond more strongly at others.

4. Dimorphic versus continuous: sexually dimorphic brain differences are more commonly seen in non-mammalian species. For example, the neural circuitry controlling singing in songbirds is highly dimorphic with the nuclei responsible for generating complex courtship songs present only

in males. In mammals, sex differences are more often seen when an end point varies along a continuum and where the mean value is significantly different for males versus females. As there is often considerable overlap between the end points this means that despite there being a significant difference at the group level it is not possible to predict sex for any one individual based on their score.

A fifth important dimension that has been added is the concept of convergence versus divergence (McCarthy, 2016). Again the clearest examples are seen in animal studies. Performance on an eye-blink conditioning task, which taps into learning and memory processes, is strongly influenced by stress. Although there are no sex differences in task performance in a stress-free environment, males and females respond to stress differently. Under stressful conditions male performance improves, while female performance deteriorates (although only at a particular stage of the oestrus cycle) (Shors, 2016). Convergence has also been demonstrated in animal models both at the behavioural and cellular levels. For example, the males of a particular species of vole have a separate and additional neural circuit to females that drives them to show parenting behaviour. The assumption is that this is required because the males do not experience pregnancy or lactation, which are thought to be associated with the neural circuits required for parenting (De Vries, 2004). At a cellular level – for reasons that remain unknown – the control of synaptic potentiation and inhibition via glutamate and GABA in some species of rodents is achieved via distinct cellular pathways in the hippocampus (Barraclough and Gorski, 1961; Oberlander and Woolley, 2016). Here the end result is no sex difference in function, but this is achieved differently in males and females.

A further important factor in understanding sex differences in the brain and its development (highlighted by McCarthy, 2016) is that when you understand the mechanism by which sex differences in one brain region are established you understand *only* how differences in that region have been established. There is no general template or set of principles that can be applied across the brain. Each region has its own profile and set of influences. This is key to understanding the patterns of sex differences across the brain, which, as highlighted in the section 'Sex

Differences in Brain Structure', resemble a patchwork of relative maleness and femaleness in any one individual with considerable inter-individual (as well as intra-individual) variability.

We will now consider some of the mechanisms by which sex differences in the brain are brought about before highlighting some of the differences that have been described.

Direct Genetic Effects on Sex Differences in the Brain

The recognition that some sex differences are initiated before male sex hormones are produced highlights the potential for the X and Y chromosomes to impact directly on sexual differentiation either through their own gene products or through regulation of the transcription of autosomal genes. This process has been investigated using clever experimental designs by Arnold and colleagues (De Vries et al., 2002). They were able to remove the *Sry* gene from the Y chromosome and replace it with an autosome. This allowed XX female experimental mice to develop testes and XY experimental animals to develop ovaries. The initial studies, which focused on more traditional sexual behaviours and the underlying neural architecture supporting these, found few differences between experimental and wild-type animals. However, later in the programme when they started to look at emotional, cognitive, and motivational outcomes, many differences were noted. Direct gene effects were found for habit formation, aggression, parenting, weight gain, and more (Arnold, 2012; Arnold et al., 2004).

Despite widespread anticipation it has not yet been possible to identify the specific genes on the X and Y chromosome that are responsible for these differences. Indeed, it now seems that it may not always be the presence or absence of the specific genes but the number of X chromosomes that is the key factor. The X chromosome contains many important genes and is particularly enriched in genes associated with brain development and cognitive functioning (Zechner et al., 2001). In order to keep the dose of X chromosomes relatively even between males and females, one of the X chromosomes is inactivated in females. However, it is now recognized that this inactivation is incomplete and that around 15% of the genes on the X chromosome are capable of biallelic expression in women (Berletch et al., 2010). It

has also become clear that there is a cost associated with inactivating the second X and that this creates what has been termed a 'heterochromatic sink' that sucks up valuable resources that could otherwise be used to regulate gene expression of the autosomes (Arnold et al., 2016). Studies with extreme individuals (e.g. XXY, Kleinfelter syndrome, or XYY males and others) have also allowed investigation as to whether the number of X or Y chromosomes makes a difference to development. Rather surprisingly the effects of increasing numbers of either X or Y chromosomes on brain development appear to be similar. For example those people with a greater number of either X or Y have increasing distortions in the size and shape of the striatum, pallidum, and thalamus (Reardon et al., 2016). These studies do, however, emphasize the potential for the sex chromosomes to impact on brain structure.

Hormonal Effects on Sex Differences in the Brain

Notwithstanding these direct effects, most sex differences in the brain are programmed by one of two pathways (McCarthy, 2016):

1. By gonadal steroids during a developmentally critical period. In primates (including human) this critical period starts when testosterone first surges in the male testes – around the beginning of the second trimester – and ends by the developmental period during which females lose their sensitivity to exogenous steroids and cannot be masculinized. The timing of this offset appears to be different for different outcomes and is earlier for reproductive vs non-reproductive end points; or

2. Although many of the important changes in sexual development occur during the critical period of fetal development, puberty is clearly a key later stage during which there are further key changes in the hormonal milieu that differ in males and females and impact on brain development (see also Chapter 4). Puberty starts around the age of 6–8 years with adrenarche during which there is a sharp rise in the levels of adrenal hormones associated with the development of axillary and pubertal hair. This is followed by gonadarche, a separate process, that typically starts between 9 and 14 years in males and slightly earlier in females. Specialist hypothalamic neurones are activated and start to

secrete gonadotrophin-releasing hormone (GnRH), which then stimulate increased secretion of luteinizing hormone (LH) and follicle-stimulating hormone (FSH) from the pituitary gland. These then trigger increased production of testosterone in males and oestrogens in females.

As with the gonads, the brain is programmed to develop into the female phenotype. In adult males across species the regular but pulsatile secretion of leutinizing hormones results in continuous testosterone production and the associated continual interest in mating and the associated behaviours of male-to-male competition and mate guarding. The hormonal milieu of adult males and females is, however, much more nuanced than simply high testosterone vs fluctuating oestrogens and progesterone. Males also make oestrogens, particularly in the brain where the enzyme that converts testosterone to oestradiol is found in high levels. The brain can also create its own oestradiol through de novo steroidogenesis.

The effects of oestrogen and testosterone and their active metabolites on the brain are mediated through several distinct pathways. Testosterone is metabolized to dihydrotestosterone (DHT) and then oestradiol. Both DHT and oestradiol bind to specific receptors in the nucleus affecting the transcription of multiple genes. Oestrogen can promote neurogenesis and synaptic growth via stimulation of GABAergic neurons and also have a much more rapid effect through binding to membrane-bound receptors and second-messenger systems. The rate of conversion of testosterone to oestradiol is affected by fluctuating glutamate levels.

Epigenetic and Environmental Impacts on Brain Development

We have already highlighted that stress is an important environmental determinant of sex differences in brain development. It is likely that while some of these effects occur through a direct impact on hormone production, some are due to epigenetic effects determined by an impact on the enzymes that regulate DNA methylation and expression. A key difference between these epigenetic effects and the direct hormonal effects is that the epigenetic effects are often much longer lasting and sometimes permanent. An example from the animal literature is the discovery that in male rodent DNA methylation is down-regulated by steroid hormones decreasing gene expression and resulting in masculinization. In females these genes must be continually repressed to prevent masculinization (Nugent et al., 2015).

Sex Differences in Brain Structure

Total Brain Volume

There are now many studies that have demonstrated sex differences in brain structure. Taken together, post-mortem studies and in vivo imaging studies of children, adolescents, and adults consistently demonstrate a total brain volume in males 9–12% greater than that for females (Lenroot and Giedd, 2010). It is also clear that these overall differences are not accounted for by body size in either children or adults. While some studies have reported that the grey matter–white matter ratio (GM–WM) is smaller in males than in females, these differences are minimal when overall brain sizes are accounted for. The complexity of the relationship between cortical morphometry and brain size is further demonstrated by a study that investigated the relationships between total brain volume and a range of cortical features such as thickness, surface area, and gyrification (Im et al., 2008). That study found that increases in grey matter volume were driven by increased surface area rather than cortical thickening and that increased brain size was associated with marked increases in folding of the cortical surface. Interestingly and importantly there were no other sex differences found in this study once sex differences in total brain volume were accounted for (Pakkenberg and Gundersen, 1997).

Regional Differences

In addition to the differences in total brain volume, sex differences have been demonstrated in several specific brain regions in adolescents and adults (see Lenroot and Giedd, 2010, for a detailed review). Many of these are seen in regions with higher densities of sex steroid receptors. The sex steroids can act both directly and indirectly. Several dopaminergic and serotonergic neurons have been demonstrated to be sensitive to changes in sex steroids. This is particularly interesting because dopaminergic neurotransmission has been implicated in schizophrenia and ADHD and serotonergic neurotransmission in depression, all of which show marked sex differences in prevalence.

Other regions with high levels of sex steroid receptors include the frontal cortex, posterior parietal cortex, motor and somatosensory cortex. There does appear to be an association between these regions and those for which sex differences in architecture have been most consistently found. When total brain volume is accounted for the orbitofrontal and paralimbic brain regions and the caudate have been reported to be smaller in males, while the fronto-medial cortex, hypothalamus, amygdala, and angular gyrus have been shown to be proportionately larger in men (Lenroot and Giedd, 2010).

In a key study for the field, Neufang and colleagues looked at the relationships between sex steroid levels and brain structure (Neufang et al., 2009). In boys, a region of the amygdala was larger. Apart from higher levels of serum testosterone in older males, there were no differences in sex steroid levels in their sample. They also found that grey matter intensity in the amygdala was predicted by testosterone levels in both males and females. In a whole brain regression analysis, testosterone was positively associated with increased grey matter density in right-sided diencephalic structures in males, and negatively correlated with parietal GM volume in males. Peper and colleagues investigated the effects of puberty on brain development in a large cohort of Dutch twins. They found that total grey matter volume correlated negatively with oestradiol levels in females and positively with testosterone in males (Peper et al., 2009).

Sex Differences in Connectivity

Studies have started to appear that use diffusion tensor imaging (DTI) to investigate sex differences in brain white matter. In general, studies across adolescence suggest increasing white matter as adolescence progresses. The literature on sex differences in DTI-based measures shows functional anisotropy (FA) values in bilateral frontal regions, the right arcuate fasciculus, and left parietal and parieto-occipital regions in males (Clayden et al., 2012; Herting et al., 2012; Hsu et al., 2008), while in females FA is increased in the corpus callosum (Kanaan et al., 2012). Interestingly correlations of FA with age differ between brain regions in males and females; for example, left frontal lobe FA is positively correlated with age in boys, but negatively correlated with age in girls (Schmithorst et al., 2008). Taken together it would appear that the structural

properties and development of white matter are not uniform throughout the brain or across males and females.

A more recent use of DTI has been to examine what has been termed the 'structural connectome' through measures indexing the patterns and strength of brain connectivity both locally and globally. The hope is that the identification of network properties such as communities or the communication backbone can advance our understanding of how complex behaviours emerge from the integration of segregated neuronal clusters (Schwarz et al., 2008). Gur and Gur evaluated sex differences in the structural connectome to elucidate sex differences in the Philadelphia Neurodevelopmental Cohort (PNC) and found stronger intra-hemispheric connectivity bilaterally in males and stronger inter-hemispheric connectivity in females (Ingalhalikar et al., 2014). This fits well with the previous DTI findings.

Cortical Morphometry

Post-mortem studies in adults have consistently found sex differences in the cortical cytoarchitecture. These have been summarized by Lenroot and Geidd (2010) and include: higher neuronal densities in granular cortical layers in females; higher overall neuronal densities and numbers in males; and more neuropil in females without overall differences in cortical thickness. A greater number of neurons in the brain and a thicker cortex have also been reported in males regardless of overall body size (Pakkenberg and Gundersen, 1997) as well as higher synaptic density in males throughout the cortex (Alonso-Nanclares et al., 2008). Results of neuroimaging studies that have commented on sex differences in cortical thickness are mixed. Some found no sex differences in cortical thickness after covarying for total brain volume (Nopoulos et al., 2000; O'Donnell et al., 2005; Salat et al., 2004). Some have found a trend towards greater thickness in males (Salat et al., 2004), while others have found that after taking differences in overall brain volume into account the cortex was thicker in females.

Sex Differences in Developmental Trajectories

There is now an extensive literature showing that adolescence is associated with changes in brain structure, including reduced grey matter volume and increased white matter volume, which have also been related to sex differences (Lenroot and Giedd, 2010).

The pioneering longitudinal studies of brain development conducted by the Child Psychiatry branch at the US National Institute for Mental Health (NIMH) that were initiated in 1989 and that continue through to today have clearly demonstrated the importance of considering not just static differences in brain development but also the developmental trajectories of these differences. By doing so it has been possible to develop size-by-age curves that describe different developmental trajectories for males and females and demonstrate that these curves differ across different brain regions (Lenroot et al., 2007). Thus, total brain size development followed an inverted U-shaped curve for both males and females but with different timings for peak total brain size that were on average four years earlier for females (10.5 years) compared to males (14.5 years). Other grey matter brain regions also showed a similar inverted U-shaped trajectory and also peaked earlier in females. White matter volumes continued to increase for both males and females across the age range covered by the study (3–27 years). In both this sample and that from an independent study (De Bellis et al., 2001) white matter development in males was more rapid than in females and this resulted in greater white matter volumes for males at any particular age than for females. When volumes were corrected for total brain size many of these apparent sex differences were no longer significant. There were, however, still differences in grey matter in the frontal lobes and white matter in the corpus callosum, both of which were bigger in females (Lenroot et al., 2007). In males the lateral ventricles were larger (Lenroot et al., 2007). Data from an earlier analysis of the NIMH cohort also demonstrated several sex differences across adolescence. Geidd and colleagues found that during adolescence there was a more rapid increase in amygdala size in males and in the hippocampus in females (Giedd et al., 1997).

Notwithstanding its seminal importance, one drawback of the NIMH data is that the lack of information about hormonal status makes it difficult to distinguish between age and hormonal effects. There is currently very limited data available that can start to separate age from hormonal effects and it is too early to draw any clear conclusions.

Sex Differences in Behaviour Linked to Brain Function

Cognitive testing has the potential to act as a window into the brain and its development. It is now generally accepted that specific cognitive domains exhibit different developmental patterns. Executive control, for example, continues to develop well into the third decade of life (Conklin et al., 2007; Pickering, 2001) while lower order cognitive domains (e.g. low executive-demand spatial and verbal memory) reach adult levels before puberty in many individuals (Coghill, 2010). One problem with much of the available data is a lack of specificity for many tasks between cognitive functioning and neural substrate. Most of the cognitive measures currently employed to describe developmental changes were developed for clinical purposes and are administered using paper-and-pencil formats, which precludes their use in neuroimaging studies. Equally importantly, most of the tasks are broadly defined and load heavily on the 'g factor', which makes it difficult to separate different cognitive processes and separate accuracy from speed (Salthouse, 2004). While there are computerized cognitive batteries that have been developed from a neuroscience perspective (e.g. The Cambridge Automated Neuropsychological Testing Assessment Battery; Morris et al., 1987) and for which the neural substrates have been well defined, these tasks have not generally been applied in large-scale developmental studies from childhood to adulthood; and the literature is especially limited in the application of an identical neurocognitive test battery across a population ranging from childhood through puberty and young adulthood.

Those data that do exist suggest sex differences in cognitive performance, which by extrapolation supports the notion of underlying differences in brain function. Males have been demonstrated to perform better than females on spatial (e.g. Voyer et al., 1995) and motor tasks (e.g. Moreno-Briseno et al., 2010), with females performing better than males on some verbal and memory tasks (e.g. Hedges and Nowell, 1995) as well as measures of social cognition (e.g. Gur et al., 2010). However, for the reasons described above the developmental course of sex differences in brain–behaviour relationships, especially in adolescence and across neurobehavioral domains, remain to be fully elucidated, particularly with longitudinal studies.

The Impact of Sex Differences in Brain Development on Psychiatric Disorders

As was noted at the start of this chapter, and as is discussed in detail throughout the rest of this book, there are sex differences in the prevalence, presentation, and course of many psychiatric disorders, and while it is now clear that these must, at least in part, reflect sex differences in brain structure and function, the precise mechanisms linking the two remain uncertain. Several early onset neuropsychiatric disorders such as autism spectrum disorder (ASD), attention deficit hyperactivity disorder (ADHD), as well as disorders such as schizophrenia and Tourette's syndrome, which 'onset' later in life but have been associated with early differences that can be measured before the actual onset of the disorder, are all more frequent in males and associated with differences in brain structure and function from very early in life. Although it seems almost certain that these differences arise during fetal development, the balance between direct genetic and hormonal (or indeed gene x environment interactions and/or epigenetic) influences is not yet clear. It is also not clear whether males are more vulnerable to these disorders or whether females are 'protected': a subtle but important difference. For depressive disorders, where the sex differences in prevalence do not appear until later in development, around puberty, it would be reasonable to speculate that hormonal changes around puberty and perhaps environmentally induced epigenetic factors are more important. These concepts and constructs are expanded on by the authors of subsequent chapters, all experts in their specific fields.

References

Alonso-Nanclares, L., Gonzalez-Soriano, J., Rodriguez, J. R., and Defelipe, J. 2008. Gender differences in human cortical synaptic density. *Proc Natl Acad Sci USA*, 105, 14615-9.

Arnold, A. P. 2012. The end of gonad-centric sex determination in mammals. *Trends Genet*, 28, 55–61.

Arnold, A. P., Reue, K., Eghbali, M., Vilain, E., Chen, X., Ghahramani, N., Itoh, Y., Li, J., Link, J. C., Ngun, T., and Williams-Burris, S. M. 2016. The importance of having two X chromosomes. *Philos Trans R Soc Lond B Biol Sci*, 371, doi: 10.1098/rstb.2015.0113.

Arnold, A. P., Xu, J., Grisham, W., Chen, X., Kim, Y. H., and Itoh, Y. 2004. Minireview: Sex chromosomes and brain sexual differentiation. *Endocrinology*, 145, 1057–62.

Barraclough, C. A. and Gorski, R. A. 1961. Evidence that the hypothalamus is responsible for androgen-induced sterility in the female rat. *Endocrinology*, 68, 68–79.

Berletch, J. B., Yang, F., and Disteche, C. M. 2010. Escape from X inactivation in mice and humans. *Genome Biol*, 11, 213.

Burgoyne, P. S., Thornhill, A. R., Boudrean, S. K., Darling, S. M., Bishop, C. E., and Evans, E. P. 1995. The genetic basis of XX–XY differences present before gonadal sex differentiation in the mouse. *Philos Trans R Soc Lond B Biol Sci*, 350, 253–60, 260–1.

Clayden, J. D., Jentschke, S., Munoz, M., Cooper, J. M., Chadwick, M. J., Banks, T., Clark, C. A., and Vargha-Khadem, F. 2012. Normative development of white matter tracts: similarities and differences in relation to age, gender, and intelligence. *Cereb Cortex*, 22, 1738–47.

Coghill, D. 2010. Heterogeneity in ADHD. MD thesis, University of Dundee.

Conklin, H. M., Luciana, M., Hooper, C. J., and Yarger, R. S. 2007. Working memory performance in typically developing children and adolescents: behavioral evidence of protracted frontal lobe development. *Dev Neuropsychol*, 31, 103–28.

De Bellis, M. D., Keshavan, M. S., Beers, S. R., Hall, J., Frustaci, K.,

Masalehdan, A., Noll, J., and Boring, A. M. 2001. Sex differences in brain maturation during childhood and adolescence. *Cereb Cortex*, 11, 552–7.

De Vries, G. J. 2004. Minireview: Sex differences in adult and developing brains: compensation, compensation, compensation. *Endocrinology*, 145, 1063–8.

De Vries, G. J., Rissman, E. F., Simerly, R. B., Yang, L. Y., Scordalakes, E. M., Auger, C. J., Swain, A., Lovell-Badge, R., Burgoyne, P. S., and Arnold, A. P. 2002. A model system for study of sex chromosome effects on sexually dimorphic neural and behavioral traits. *J Neurosci*, 22, 9005–14.

Feczko, E., Miranda-Dominguez, O., Marr, M., Graham, A. M., Nigg, J. T., and Fair, D. A. 2019. The heterogeneity problem: approaches to identify psychiatric subtypes. *Trends Cogn Sci*, 23, 584–601.

Giedd, J. N., Castellanos, F. X., Rajapakse, J. C., Vaituzis, A. C., and Rapoport, J. L. 1997. Sexual dimorphism of the developing human brain. *Prog Neuropsychopharmacol Biol Psychiatry*, 21, 1185–201.

Gur, R. C., Richard, J., Hughett, P., Calkins, M. E., Macy, L., Bilker, W. B., Brensinger, C., and Gur, R. E. 2010. A cognitive neuroscience-based computerized battery for efficient measurement of individual differences: standardization and initial construct validation. *J Neurosci Methods*, 187, 254–62.

Hedges, L. V. and Nowell, A. 1995. Sex differences in mental test scores, variability, and numbers of high-scoring individuals. *Science*, 269, 41–5.

Herting, M. M., Maxwell, E. C., Irvine, C., and Nagel, B. J. 2012. The impact of sex, puberty, and hormones on white matter microstructure in adolescents. *Cereb Cortex*, 22, 1979–92.

Hsu, J. L., Leemans, A., Bai, C. H., Lee, C. H., Tsai, Y. F., Chiu, H. C., and Chen, W. H. 2008. Gender differences and age-related white matter changes of the human brain: a diffusion tensor imaging study. *Neuroimage*, 39, 566–77.

Im, K., Lee, J. M., Lyttelton, O., Kim, S. H., Evans, A. C., and Kim, S. I. 2008. Brain size and cortical structure in the adult human brain. *Cereb Cortex*, 18, 2181–91.

Ingalhikar, M., Smith, A., Parker, D., Satterthwaite, T. D., Elliott, M. A., Ruparel, K., Hakonarson, H., Gur, R. E., Gur, R. C., and Verma, R. 2014. Sex differences in the structural connectome of the human brain. *Proc Natl Acad Sci USA*, 111, 823–8.

Joel, D. and Mccarthy, M. M. 2017. Incorporating sex as a biological variable in neuropsychiatric research: where are we now and where should we be? *Neuropsychopharmacology*, 42, 379–85.

Kanaan, R. A., Allin, M., Picchioni, M., Barker, G. J., Daly, E., Shergill, S. S., Woolley, J., and Mcguire, P. K. 2012. Gender differences in white matter microstructure. *PLoS One*, 7, e38272.

Koopman, P. 1999. Sry and Sox9: mammalian testis-determining genes. *Cell Mol Life Sci*, 55, 839–56.

Lenroot, R. K. and Giedd, J. N. 2010. Sex differences in the adolescent brain. *Brain Cogn*, 72, 46–55.

Lenroot, R. K., Gogtay, N., Greenstein, D. K., Wells, E. M., Wallace, G. L., Clasen, L. S., Blumenthal, J. D., Lerch, J., Zijdenbos, A. P., Evans, A. C., Thompson, P. M., and Giedd, J. N. 2007. Sexual dimorphism of brain developmental trajectories during childhood and adolescence. *Neuroimage*, 36, 1065–73.

Mccarthy, M. M. 2016. Sex differences in the developing brain as a source of inherent risk. *Dialogues Clin Neurosci*, 18, 361–72.

Moreno-Briseno, P., Diaz, R., Campos-Romo, A., and Fernandez-Ruiz, J. 2010. Sex-related differences in motor learning and performance. *Behav Brain Funct*, 6, 74.

Morris, R. C., Evendon, J. L., Sahakian, B. J., and Robbins, T. W. 1987. Computer-aided assessment of dementia: comparative studies of neuropsychological deficits in Alzheimer-type dementia and Parkinson's disease. In: S. M. Stahl, S. D. Iversen, and E. D. Goodman (eds) *Cognitive Neurochemistry*. Oxford: Oxford University Press.

Neufang, S., Specht, K., Hausmann, M., Gunturkun, O., Herpertz-Dahlmann, B., Fink, G. R., and Konrad, K. 2009. Sex differences and the impact of steroid hormones on the developing human brain. *Cereb Cortex*, 19, 464–73.

Nopoulos, P., Flaum, M., O'Leary, D., and Andreasen, N. C. 2000. Sexual dimorphism in the human brain: evaluation of tissue volume, tissue composition and surface anatomy using magnetic resonance imaging. *Psychiatry Res*, 98, 1–13.

Nugent, B. M., Wright, C. L., Shetty, A. C., Hodes, G. E., Lenz, K. M., Mahurkar, A., Russo, S. J., Devine, S. E., and Mccarthy, M. M. 2015. Brain feminization requires active repression of masculinization via DNA methylation. *Nat Neurosci*, 18, 690–7.

Oberlander, J. G. and Woolley, C. S. 2016. 17beta-estradiol acutely potentiates glutamatergic synaptic transmission in the hippocampus through distinct mechanisms in males and females. *J Neurosci*, 36, 2677–90.

O'Donnell, S., Noseworthy, M. D., Levine, B., and Dennis, M. 2005. Cortical thickness of the frontopolar area in typically developing children and adolescents. *Neuroimage*, 24, 948–54.

Pakkenberg, B. and Gundersen, H. J. 1997. Neocortical neuron number in humans: effect of sex and age. *J Comp Neurol*, 384, 312–20.

Peper, J. S., Brouwer, R. M., Schnack, H. G., Van Baal, G. C., Van Leeuwen, M., Van Den Berg, S. M., Delemarre-Van De Waal, H. A., Boomsma, D. I., Kahn, R. S., and Hulshoff Pol, H. E. 2009. Sex steroids and brain structure in pubertal boys and girls. *Psychoneuroendocrinology*, 34, 332–42.

Phoenix, C. H., Goy, R. W., Gerall, A. A., and Young, W. C. 1959. Organizing action of prenatally administered testosterone propionate on the tissues mediating mating behavior in the female guinea pig. *Endocrinology*, 65, 369–82.

Pickering, S. J. 2001. The development of visuo-spatial working memory. *Memory*, 9, 423–32.

Ray, P. F., Conaghan, J., Winston, R. M., and Handyside, A. H. 1995. Increased number of cells and metabolic activity in male human preimplantation embryos following in vitro fertilization. *J Reprod Fertil*, 104, 165–71.

Reardon, P. K., Clasen, L., Giedd, J. N., Blumenthal, J., Lerch, J. P., Chakravarty, M. M., and Raznahan, A. 2016. An allometric analysis of sex and sex chromosome dosage effects on subcortical anatomy in humans. *J Neurosci*, 36, 2438–48.

Salat, D. H., Buckner, R. L., Snyder, A. Z., Greve, D. N.,

Desikan, R. S., Busa, E., Morris, J. C., Dale, A. M., and Fischl, B. 2004. Thinning of the cerebral cortex in aging. *Cereb Cortex*, 14, 721–30.

Salthouse, T. A. 2004. Localizing age-related individual differences in a hierarchical structure. *Intelligence*, 32.

Schmithorst, V. J., Holland, S. K., and Dardzinski, B. J. 2008. Developmental differences in white matter architecture between boys and girls. *Hum Brain Mapp*, 29, 696–710.

Schwarz, A. J., Gozzi, A., and Bifone, A. 2008. Community structure and modularity in networks of correlated brain activity. *Magn Reson Imaging*, 26, 914–20.

Shors, T. J. 2016. A trip down memory lane about sex differences in the brain. *Philos Trans R Soc Lond B Biol Sci*, 371, doi: 10.1098/rstb.2015.0124.

Voyer, D., Voyer, S., and Bryden, M. P. 1995. Magnitude of sex differences in spatial abilities: a meta-analysis and consideration of critical variables. *Psychol Bull*, 117, 250–70.

Zechner, U., Wilda, M., Kehrer-Sawatzki, H., Vogel, W., Fundele, R., and Hameister, H. 2001. A high density of X-linked genes for general cognitive ability: a run-away process shaping human evolution? *Trends Genet*, 17, 697–701.

Chapter

2

Autism Spectrum Disorder in Males
Considerations for Outcomes and Intervention

Renee Testa and Bruce Tonge

In this chapter we present an overview of autism spectrum disorder (ASD) and describe the differences in prevalence, co-morbidity, and clinical presentation between males and females. We then discuss factors to consider in the assessment of males in the autism spectrum across the lifespan. We complete our discussion with an overview of outcomes in adulthood, and potential ways to progress and improve the trajectories of this clinical group. It is important to note that given the significantly higher prevalence rate of males to females in ASD, the majority of studies have an overwhelming proportion of males, regardless of whether they focused upon gender differences.

Autism spectrum disorder (ASD) are a highly heterogenous group of neurodevelopmental conditions with a prevalence of 1–3% (Idring et al., 2012). The higher male than female prevalence within ASD is well established, with reported ratios of 3–5:1 (Fombonne et al., 2011; Schaafsma and Pfaff, 2014; Lai et al., 2015; Loomes et al., 2017); however, some population studies have reported a lower ratio (Idring et al., 2012). The cause of this male predominance is not yet established, but is thought to be a result of genetic, epigenetic, and environmental factors (Newschaffer et al., 2007; Baron-Cohen et al., 2011; Hallmayer et al., 2011; May et al., 2019). A consistent finding in the literature is the significant variability in the presentation of children, adolescents, and adults within the autistic spectrum (Lai et al., 2011). This led to the identification of categorical subgroups, such as high-functioning autism and asperger disorder, in addition to descriptors of multiple clinical phenotypes. Phenotypic and behavioural variability is reportedly greatest within cognitively higher-functioning individuals without intellectual disability. It is within this subgroup that the male predominance is reportedly greatest, when compared to lower-functioning ASD individuals (Lai

et al., 2011, 2015). A 1.9:1 male-to-female ratio was reported in individuals with intellectual disability, while a 5.75:1 male-to-female ratio was found in higher-functioning individuals (Fombonne, 2003, 2005, 2009). A female protective factor has been considered a cause in the high ratio of males in ASD (Robinson et al., 2013; Zhang, Li, et al., 2020). Difficulty identifying females within the higher-functioning ASD population is also thought to contribute; it is proposed that females are better able to 'mask' or compensate for their social difficulties (Hiller et al., 2014). Indeed, Sutherland et al. (2017) found that parents report that females with ASD try to hide their difficulties, presenting with autistic behaviours that are more subtle and less disruptive than behaviours exhibited by males. This has caused uncertainty in the accuracy of the gender ratio in ASD and highlighted the limitations of previous research that overwhelmingly includes a larger sample population of males compared to females.

Multiple and interacting aetiological mechanisms, including genetic (Hu et al., 2014), epigenetic (Shulha et al., 2012; Loke et al., 2015), and environmental factors (Juul-Dam et al., 2001) likely contribute to the variety of presentations of individuals with ASD. Genetic contributions have been found to be most significant, with concordance rates amongst monozygotic twins reaching 60% and 30% for dizygotic twins (Bailey et al., 1995; Frazier et al., 2014) and of the 'broader autism phenotype' in relatives of affected individuals (Bolton et al., 1994; Sasson et al., 2013). Further, the discordant rates in males and females also strongly suggest a genetic basis (Werling and Geschwind, 2013). A number of non-genetic risk factors have been associated with ASD, as shown in Box 2.1. These risk factors have been found to be of low magnitude, suggesting they may only have a small causative role in the development of ASD (Guinchat et al., 2012).

Box 2.1 Non-genetic risk factors for ASD

- Prenatal:
  - o   advanced maternal and paternal age
  - o   bleeding during pregnancy
  - o   certain medications
  - o   maternal diabetes

- Perinatal:
  - o   preterm birth
  - o   breech position
  - o   planned caesarean birth

- Neonatal:
  - o   small for gestational age
  - o   low Apgar scores
  - o   neonatal encephalopathy
  - o   hyperbilirubinemia
  - o   birth defects

Classification Systems

The DSM-IV classification of ASD was focused upon differences between individuals with ASD to define clinical subgroups (American Psychiatric Association, 2000). It presented a categorical system detailing groups within the spectrum, including autistic disorder, asperger disorder (AD), and Pervasive Developmental Disorder Not Otherwise Specified (PDD-NOS). In contrast, the DSM-5 (American Psychiatric Association, 2013) moved away from describing clinical phenotypes to a dimensional classification of autistic spectrum disorder. It describes a dyad of impairments that are core to the disorder and similar across individuals: first, social communication deficits, and second, routine/ritualistic behavioural impairments and sensory sensitivities (RRBI). As such, all previously diagnosed individuals (i.e., AD, AS, and PDD-NOS) were reclassified within a single diagnostic group of ASD. Previously identified differences between subgroups within cognitive, language, and motor domains were not considered for diagnostic purposes. Gender differences were also not recognized, with the removal of asperger syndrome, seen to be reserved for a subgroup of high-functioning males with no delay in language development (Lai et al., 2013). A further change in DSM-5 is the classification of ASD according to the severity of impairment

separately for each dyad of symptoms, specifying three levels of support: in need of, support, or substantial support, or very substantial support. In recognition of the variability in ASD, DSM-5 also prescribes the addition of specifiers regarding the level and profile of cognitive ability, language ability, medical/genetic conditions, any co-morbid psychopathology such as anxiety, and family/socio/cultural considerations be specified together with the core ASD symptoms and severity ratings.

While progression to the dimensional approach in DSM-5 eliminates the previous confusion in diagnosing subtypes, the removal of defined subtypes and classification of all individuals within the single diagnostic category increases the phenotypic heterogeneity included under this diagnostic label. The variability in the expression and combination of social communication and RRBI symptomatology, both between individuals with ASD and within individuals over the lifetime, raises concerns that the DSM-5 classification system minimizes potentially important differences between individuals.

Clinical Assessment and Diagnosis of ASD

There are many challenges within the diagnostic field of ASD. At present there is no psychological, behavioural, or biological instrument or test that allows for a definitive diagnosis. Given the complexity of the ASD phenotype, practice guidelines recommend a multidisciplinary assessment to characterize the broad areas of functioning and specifiers implicated in the disorder.

Informant report regarding developmental history and current functioning, as well as direct behavioural observation, and administration of semi-structured assessment tools all form important components of the ASD diagnostic process (Filipek et al., 1999, 2000; Ozonoff et al., 2005; Falkmer et al., 2013). A detailed account of the child or adolescent's early developmental progression and symptom presentation, in addition to direct observation and interaction with the child, is required. Given that parental report can be biased or not provide enough information, gathering data from multiple settings and sources is imperative (such as school, teacher, tutor, home environment, two parents). Children with autism are very sensitive to their environment as well as the structure or support they are provided with during assessment.

Therefore, they can behave and exhibit vastly different behaviours across different settings. In addition to this, the assessment of cognitive, language, and adaptive skills in order to define any scatter of abilities or the presence of developmental delay and language impairments is necessary. This may be carried out by a team of clinicians but is required to ensure that the presenting behaviours are not consistent or co-morbid with another neurodevelopmental condition. Many ASD-type behaviours are not specific and therefore a comprehensive and wide-ranging assessment needs to occur to rule out alternative aetiologies (Constantino and Charman, 2012). In adulthood, the gathering of early developmental history is invaluable. Assessment of the family and socio/cultural context and current functioning in both the home and work environment is necessary, and reports from a significant other, family member, friend, or work colleague can help to identify and describe the individual's behaviour.

There are a growing number of specific measures that purport to evaluate the ASD clinical phenotype, including screening questionnaires, caregiver interviews, and structured observation assessments completed by a trained clinician (Oien et al., 2018; Autism Mental Status Exam). These assessments are generally designed to allow the clinician to determine a cut-off score to indicate whether ASD criteria are likely to be met. Measurements are directed at identifying specific behaviours characteristic of ASD according to a diagnostic system such as DSM-5, which differentiate them from neurotypical age-related peers. The most widely used and validated assessment tools are the ADI-R (Lord et al., 1994) and ADOS-2 (Lord et al., 2012). Administration of these measures together is considered best practice with reference to the clinical application of a 'gold standard' diagnostic classification system such as the DSM-5 (American Psychiatric Association, 2013) or the ICD 11 (World Health Organization, 2018) criteria for ASD (Filipek et al., 1999, 2000; Ozonoff et al., 2005; Falkmer et al., 2013). The ADOS is a direct observational assessment, while the ADI-R is a caregiver interview capturing current behaviour and early development. Both tools purport to evaluate functioning within core ASD symptom domains and provide diagnostic algorithms to support clinical assessment and treatment decision-making. A key challenge in using standardized assessment tools for ASD diagnosis is ensuring that symptomatology is reliably evaluated across the full range of the autism spectrum. Symptomatology varies according to age, gender, cognition, and language functioning (Gotham et al., 2007, 2008; Hus and Lord, 2013). In particular, sensitivity and specificity of the ADOS diagnostic algorithms is lowest for higher-functioning, verbal children, adolescents, and adults (Gotham et al., 2007, 2008). In view of the wide phenotypic differences, different assessment methods for the two subgroups of ASD may be required to reliably characterize symptomatology. Behaviours may be more subtle and complex in high-functioning ASD, making it more difficult to detect impairment in these individuals in a small number of assessment sessions and only one setting.

A significant obstacle to the reliability and validity of autism assessments is that they are not regarded as gender specific or sensitive, and poorly account for phenotypic variations and socio/cultural contexts in which children, adolescents, and adults present over the lifespan. This is relevant, given that gender differences in social development have been found to change across early childhood (Barbu et al., 2011; and see Chapter 1). Males in early childhood exhibit more solitary play than their female counterparts who are more advanced in their social and play skills. However, in early primary school, males progress and match their female peers. Understanding these normative developmental trajectories is necessary in determining how gender-specific ASD symptomatology arises. Greater research into neurodevelopmental and socio/cultural maturation and styles of cognitive, social, emotional, and behavioural development across and within each gender is necessary (Rinehart et al., 2011). There is also concern that the manner in which assessment instruments were developed biased them towards the description of male behaviour, predicting better and easier identification of symptoms in males (Russell et al., 2011). A suggested lack of understanding of how females with higher-functioning ASD present might also contribute to under-identification (Lai et al., 2015). This has led Lai et al. (2015) to suggest that a normative curve of ASD traits should be developed for both genders, to assist in improving diagnostic accuracy. Indeed, males have been found to score higher and exhibit more significant ASD symptomatology than females on autism questionnaires (Baron-Cohen et al., 2001). Further, Oien et al. (2018) reported gender differences in symptomatology and behaviour, as assessed by available ASD measurements. Autism measurements therefore need to be better operationalized to reflect gender influences on clinical phenotype symptomatology (Lai and Szatmari, 2020).

Autism Spectrum over the Lifespan

A significant obstacle to the diagnosis of ASD is the wide-ranging spectrum of symptoms and changes that are present over the period from birth to adulthood. It has been reported that any individual can present with specific ASD-like behaviours over a lifetime, which may not be consistently evident. For example, repetitive behaviours of play observed in the early toddler years may not be seen from early childhood and may manifest as a circumscribed interest instead. Alternatively, some children may demonstrate no anxiety in relation to new events or social situations and exhibit an interest in peer friendships, but later demonstrate very specific routines of behaviour in their home environment that must be adhered to, otherwise significant anxiety-based behaviours are observed. The very specific nature of these ASD traits, which are dependent on the profile of the individual and their stage of development and age, mean that evaluation of the neurodevelopmental trajectories of ASD behaviours over time would be extremely informative for the assessment and diagnosis of ASD. If we were able to develop a profile of possible ASD behaviours exhibited in different subgroups of ASD individuals from birth to adulthood, we would be able to enquire more specifically about behaviours, characteristics, or traits that we could expect from each individual that may easily be overlooked. Indeed, in a prospective longitudinal study, Ozonoff and colleagues (Ozonoff et al., 2010) reported that children at high risk of developing ASD showed overt behavioural signs of ASD between 6 and 12 months of age, comprising reduced eye contact, social smiling, and social responsiveness. These differences were significant from their typically developing peers by 12–18 months.

The early identification and recognition of emerging autism-specific, and also gender-specific, behaviours has obvious implications for the early detection of children at risk. Greater understanding of the developmental trajectory of ASD between genders would assist the diagnostic process by informing clinicians of expected symptom presentation at different ages and would also help families by offering a clearer view of an affected individual's

expected development over time. For example, Simonoff et al. (2019) reported trajectories of cognition and ASD traits from early childhood to adulthood (12–23 years) in order to identify variables that may predict functioning level and change over time. The study noted improvements in intellectual functioning over time, but autism symptomatology was stable. Emotional and behavioural problems, social communication, and school setting were predictors of the level of ASD symptoms, with those attending mainstream school exhibiting fewer traits.

As previously discussed, a greater proportion of males with ASD are at the higher end of intellectual functioning, with prevalence of females and males more evenly distributed at the more cognitively impaired end of intellectual ability (Volkmar et al., 1993; Carter et al., 2007). As summarized in Box 2.2, the male ASD population also presents with better language functioning, but has a higher rate of sensory disturbances (Andersson et al., 2013; Oien et al., 2018). Social communication deficits appear more prevalent in males (Lai et al., 2011), who have been found to be weaker in their ability to discriminate facial emotional responses and empathize. Males have also been reported to have a higher rate of repetitive, restrictive behaviours and interests and stereotypical play, and greater atypical motor behaviours (Lord et al., 1982; Szatmari et al., 2012; Hiller et al., 2014; Van Wijngaarden-Cremers et al., 2014). Male adolescents with ASD have been found to exhibit greater externalizing and hyperactive behaviours and need more educational support (Mandy et al., 2012; May, Cornish, and Rinehart, 2016). Younger males with ASD were also found to be more hyperactive than their female ASD peers (May et al., 2016). However, Margari et al. (2019) examined co-morbidity in a mixed gender group of higher-functioning autistic patients and found no gender differences in reported co-morbidities,

---

Box 2.2 Features of males vs. females with ASD (note not all studies concur: see text)

- Better language function
- Higher rate of sensory disturbances
- More social communication deficits
- More impaired facial recognition
- Higher rates of repetitive, restrictive behaviours
- More stereotypical play
- Greater atypical motor behaviours
- More hyperactivity

including Attention Deficit Hyperactivity Disorder (ADHD; see Chapter 3), anxiety disorders, depressive disorders, bipolar disorder, and Obsessive-Compulsive Disorder. Anorexia Nervosa was significantly higher in females.

Other studies have found no phenotypic gender differences, with Pilowsky et al. (1998) and Lai et al. (2011) reporting that the severity of core ASD behaviours, in addition to capacity for empathy, and other co-morbid conditions (such as obsessive-compulsive disorder) did not differ between males and females. Harrop and colleagues (Harrop et al., 2015, 2018; Duvekot et al., 2017) also found that there were no significant gender differences in symptoms of ASD. Andersson et al. (2013) came to similar conclusions. These various studies suggest that reported gender differences may have been overestimated.

One possible cause of the discrepant research is the lack of normative comparison groups in studies investigating gender differences in autism, which creates uncertainty as to whether the reported gender differentiation is also found in the general population (Hull et al., 2017). Indeed, Hull et al.'s (2017) meta-analysis of comparisons of behavioural and cognitive features in males and females with and without an autism spectrum condition diagnosis found that core traits were comparable. Interestingly, expected gender differences in play, internalizing, and externalizing behaviours, and empathizing seen in a typically developing group was also identified in the ASD group. This supports the development of gender-specific phenotypes that replicate traditional normative gender differences (Harrop et al., 2017). This notion was also supported by May et al. (2016), who found a greater proportion of repetitive motor movements, deficits in communication, and inattention in both normal and ASD male samples when compared to their female counterparts. Therefore, the inclusion of neurotypical age-matched controls is necessary in longitudinal studies of ASD in order to better understand gender differences in ASD symptomatology (Van Wijngaarden-Cremers et al., 2014; Harrop et al., 2015).

Vocational, Behavioural, and Psychological Outcomes of Males with ASD

Individuals with ASD experience at least two-to-three times higher rates of behavioural and emotional difficulties than typically developing peers (Volker et al., 2010; Romero, Aguilar, et al., 2016; Mansour et al., 2017), or peers with Intellectual Disability (Tonge and Einfeld, 2003). Within ASD, higher-functioning individuals are particularly at risk (Witwer and Lecavalier, 2010). In high-functioning ASD, the estimated frequency of at least one co-morbid psychiatric disorder ranges from 74% (Mattila et al., 2010) to over 90% (Mukaddes, 2010; Kusaka, 2014), meaning that it is not unexpected for a child to experience psychiatric problems in addition to core ASD symptomatology. The most commonly occurring co-morbid conditions include behavioural disorders (e.g., ADHD, conduct disorder, and oppositional defiant disorder), anxiety disorders, mood disorders, and tic disorders (Mattila et al., 2010; Mukaddes et al., 2010; Kusaka et al., 2014) (see Box 2.3). The prevalence of anxiety and depression increases throughout adolescence in ASD, as greater self-awareness develops for some. Social communication and interaction also increase in complexity, and greater independence is expected, creating increased stress (White et al., 2009). The high prevalence of these co-morbid conditions suggests that psychiatric symptomatology separate to the core symptoms of ASD, such as anxiety and depression, may form part of the broader phenotype in this vulnerable population. The literature on any association between ASD and schizophrenia is contradictory with estimates of prevalence of schizophrenia in individuals with ASD varying widely from lower, to equal, to 50%. A recent comprehensive systematic review and meta-analysis of the literature has concluded that having an ASD does confer an increased risk of an association with schizophrenia. Zheng et al. (2018) found in their meta-analysis a 3.55 times increased risk of schizophrenia compared to controls and the systematic

> **Box 2.3 Psychiatric co-morbidities in males with ASD**
>
> - ADHD
> - Tic disorder
> - Conduct disorder
> - Oppositional defiant disorder
> - Anxiety disorders
> - Depressive disorders
> - Schizotypal traits
> - Schizophrenia
> - Substance use disorder

review revealed a prevalence of between 3.4 and 52%. It is not known how much of this risk is related to genetic factors, environmental factors such as stress, substance use, or an association with other co-morbid childhood neurodevelopmental disorders such as schizotypal disorder. For example youth with ASD often manifest more severe schizotypal traits compared to typically developing controls (Barneveld et al., 2011).

Co-morbid mood, anxiety, and behavioural disorders are associated with poorer functioning in ASD (Mattila et al., 2010). Behavioural and emotional difficulties can impact social relationships and daily functioning (Meyer et al., 2006; Faridi and Khosrowabadi, 2017; Pisula et al., 2017; de Giambattista et al., 2019). Behavioural and emotional difficulties can also make diagnosis more complex in ASD. For example, it can be difficult to discern whether withdrawn behaviour and limited interest in, or initiation of, social interaction is representative of core ASD symptomatology or a reflection of anxiety and depression. Moreover, behavioural and emotional difficulties can adversely impact responsiveness to treatments (Ogundele, 2018). Therefore, the assessment of any co-morbid psychopathology is an essential part of diagnostic assessment, treatment planning, and clinical management.

Depression and anxiety are prevalent in adults with ASD, with a higher prevalence reported in those without an intellectual disability (Rai et al., 2018; Arnold, Foley, Hwang, et al., 2019; Nimmo-Smith et al., 2020). Lasgaard et al. (2010) reported a high occurrence of loneliness in a group of adolescent boys with ASD. Further, despite the ongoing behavioural and psychological challenges experienced by adults with ASD, a population study in the UK did not find an over-representation of individuals with ASD within the criminal justice system (King and Murphy, 2014).

Long-term outcomes for children and adolescents with ASD transitioning to adulthood require further research. The findings of previous longitudinal investigations have been inconsistent (Magiati et al., 2014) with studies reporting stable, deteriorating, or improving outcomes in social, cognition, and language skills and behaviour. Howlin et al. (2004) followed the trajectory of children with ASD from early childhood (range 3–15 years) to adulthood (range 21–48 years). The majority of adults presented with ongoing language and cognitive difficulties, in addition to persistent stereotypical behaviours. Most remained dependent on the care of their families or support workers; a lack of close friendships and permanent employment was also reported. Overall, around half had a poor or very poor outcome. Higher intellectual functioning was a predictor of better outcomes (Gray et al., 2014; Howlin, 2014), but gender differences were not examined. Similarly, a longitudinal study of males (ASD vs developmental receptive language disorder) from childhood (7–8 years) to adulthood (23–24 years) highlighted the persisting pervasive social and communication impairments experienced in ASD (Mawhood et al., 2000). Gray et al. (2014) also reported in their longitudinal study that adults with ASD have poor social functioning, including reduced community participation and fewer employment opportunities.

Caregivers experience a high burden of care, stress, and a high prevalence of mental health conditions (particularly anxiety and depression and, for males, substance/alcohol abuse), a reduced quality of life, and interrupted employment (Ingersoll et al., 2011; Fewster et al., 2019; Ten Hoopen et al., 2020). The severity of the symptoms of autism and associated emotional and behavioural problems is also associated with reduced quality of parent–child interaction (Hobson et al., 2016). Parenting education and skills programs are effective in providing persisting benefit by reducing burden, improving parental mental health, and reducing problematic child behaviours (Tonge et al., 2014). However, there is a relative lack of provision of an evidence-based parenting skills program in early intervention services and for the families of older children and youth with ASD (B. Tonge et al., 2014; Sofronoff et al., 2018).

How Can We Improve Outcomes for Males with ASD?

Traditional forms of intervention for ASD include psychopharmacology as well as psychosocial and cognitive-behavioural therapies. Best practice is dependent on the individuals' needs and circumstances, with no generalized method being able to be applied (Syriopoulou-Delli et al., 2019). This leads to inconsistency in what treatments are offered, dependent on the treating clinician and access to services.

Interventions in the childhood period aim to prevent the development of poor social, emotional, educational, and functional outcomes (Estes et al., 2015; Studer et al., 2017). Implementing change and education in the early primary school or even preschool period can empower the child to develop a set of skills to provide better understanding of their social and emotional environments (Reichow and Wolery, 2009). This skill set emerges in early childhood in typically developing children (Nix et al., 2013); therefore, intervention at this early developmental stage to progress these foundation skills – including the ability to identify and recognize emotional states in self and others – is imperative. Initiating interventions when gaps in development are observed or noted, and not when significant problems arise, is the optimal time to ameliorate the difficulties that they will experience (Mottron, 2017; Christensen et al., 2019).

Treatment or intervention plans require a good understanding of the individual, including age (developmental and chronological), gender, neurocognitive profile, ASD symptomatology, comorbidities, and the familial and educational environment in which they are placed. Based upon this analysis, interventions should be devised and matched to the specific areas of needs that the individual is currently experiencing (Pellicano et al., 2014). A multifactorial approach is likely required, given the interplay between the domains affected in ASD. For example, language intervention to improve receptive and expressive skills should be delivered in conjunction with intervention to progress social interaction and reciprocity. Interventions also need to consider access to services and the motivation of the individual (and caregivers) to engage (Bejarano-Martin et al., 2019).

Early systematic assessment is required to identify those preschool and young children who are at risk, in order to implement required interventions (Kantzer et al., 2013). Early intervention for children with ASD can significantly improve language and play skills. It can also assist children with significant co-morbid disorders (e.g. ADHD, cognitive and language delay, epilepsy) that increase the disability experienced by the child and burden on the family (Ben-Itzchak and Zachor, 2007; Tonge et al., 2014).

A plethora of interventions have been promoted to treat ASD, from evidence-based and established treatments to unestablished interventions lacking any systematic evidence. The US National Autism Center has published a comprehensive report reviewing the ASD intervention literature for children and young people through to 22 years (National Autism Center, 2015). The review recommends fourteen established treatments that mainly comprise cognitive, language-based behavioural interventions using modelling, visual schedules, behavioural scripts, pivotal response training, natural teaching strategies, parent education, and skills training programs.

Interventions aimed at improving behavioural and emotional regulation may be best targeted to ameliorate the mental health burden on individuals with ASD (Cai et al., 2018). Difficulties in the regulation of emotions can be seen in young children, particularly in males with autism, who exhibit a greater degree of externalizing and acting out behaviours. This is seen throughout later childhood and adolescence, where greater prevalence of oppositional defiant disorder and conduct disorder can be found in males with ASD (Gadow et al., 2008). Deficits in emotional regulation are thought to underlie some of the complex presentation of emotional and behavioural difficulties in individuals with ASD, who are found to use a greater proportion of maladaptive emotion regulation strategies (Weiss et al., 2014; Samson et al., 2015).

In consideration of this, focusing on the application of early intervention in the recognition, understanding, and problem solving of different emotional states may be able to offset later developing difficulties identified in males, as earlier discussed. A focus on social skill training is a frequently chosen target of intervention in ASD; however, findings suggest that social skill group intervention does not significantly improve emotional recognition or greatly improve quality of life (Reichow et al., 2013). A Cochrane review of social skill group intervention suggested that some improvement of social competence in children and adolescents with ASD (with average or above-average IQ) was evident, but the robustness and generalizability of these findings were limited (Reichow et al., 2013). There is some evidence of therapeutic benefit for social communication and emotion recognition programs such as the Cool Kids ASD intervention (Bischof et al., 2018), Social Thinking (Crooke and Winner, 2016), and the Secret Agent Society (Beaumont, 2015), which have been tailored for use across a range of ages from childhood to adulthood. These programs are targeted at improving social and emotional understanding of everyday situations, in conjunction with developing strategies to manage stress, reduce anxiety, and improve mood. This dual approach may hold greater efficacy given the association between social and emotional difficulties in ASD and that better understanding of the link between these two domains may improve overall outcomes for ASD individuals.

Interventions also need consider the individual's neurocognitive functioning (i.e. cognitive, language, attention, executive) (Craig et al., 2016; Friedman and Sterling, 2019; Torske et al., 2020). In youth with ASD and lower intellectual functioning, executive functioning was associated with social and communicative functioning (Bertollo and Yerys, 2019). Gardiner and Iarocci (2018) also reported that in children with ASD, adaptive everyday functioning was related to executive, self-regulation skills. A poorer ability to be flexible and inhibit and control behavioural and emotional responses was related to depressive symptomatology. Given these findings, it would be important that the core cognitive ASD symptomatology of each individual is considered in the selection of interventions, and areas of weakness supported. If not, interventions may not be as efficacious due to weaknesses present in their neuropsychological profiles. This may also be the cause of variability in outcomes following the attendance to therapeutic services.

In regard to adulthood, significant barriers to developing good clinical services and mental health interventions for autistic adults are identified. The main barriers are a lack of clinician's knowledge and experience; poor competence; and low confidence in working within this population (Maddox et al., 2020). In general, there is a scarcity of mental health services for adults with neurodevelopmental conditions, with adults being refused assistance when their diagnosis is revealed (Maddox and Gaus, 2019). In the USA and the UK about 25% of adults with an ASD are unemployed or have no organized daily program (Howlin, 2014; Roux, 2017). This gap in services training and education needs to be addressed if the poor mental health outcomes within ASD are to be improved.

Pharmacotherapy

There is no compelling evidence to support the use of pharmacological treatments of the core symptoms of ASD, but pharmacotherapy may be effective in the treatment of co-morbid psychopathology such as disruptive behaviour, ADHD, depression, anxiety, and OCD when indicated (Sung et al., 2014). Paradoxically, research into drug treatments for psychopathology co-morbid with ASD has

focused on young people and not adults and has not considered gender differences in response. There is some evidence that antipsychotics such as risperidone and aripiprazole can reduce irritable, disruptive, and aggressive behaviours, including for adults with ASD (McDougle et al., 1998; Magiati et al., 2016). However, troublesome metabolic and neurological side effects can occur and this needs to be built into the decision-making about the use of such medications. Melatonin has been demonstrated to be beneficial for sleep disturbance in ASD (Doyen et al., 2011). Children with ASD and co-morbid ADHD respond variably and less predictably to stimulant medication than for those with only ADHD; and troublesome side effects are more likely (Siegel and Beaulieu, 2012). Antidepressants such as selective serotonin reuptake inhibitors (SSRIs) – particularly fluoxetine – as well as certain tricyclic antidepressants (TCAs) are used for the treatment of co-morbid depression, anxiety, and OCD, based on the evidence for their respective efficacy in general population studies (see other chapters in this book for details). Side effects might be more prominent in people with ASD (Taylor, 2015). The use of these drugs in individuals with ASD, of all ages, should be viewed as individual treatment trials. Behaviour and side-effect checklists, pre- and post-drug prescription, should be used to monitor response.

Conclusions

The specific individual ASD symptom profiles and cognitive, language, health, mental health, and socio/cultural contexts of both male and female children, adolescents, and adults with ASD need to be accounted for when developing intervention programs and services. Despite the inconsistent findings in the literature when examining outcomes in males with ASD, a significant increase in mental health conditions, including depression, anxiety, and behavioural disorders, has been consistently reported, and these co-morbidities are associated with poorer social, vocational, and quality-of-life outcomes. A major obstacle to improving outcomes is a lack of understanding of the clinical phenotypes of ASD in both males and females, in addition to a lack of validated and reliable research in intervention programs, particularly for older adolescents and adults with ASD (Tachibana et al., 2017).

References

American Psychiatric Association. 2000. *Diagnostic and Statistical Manual of Mental Disorders*. 4th ed. Washington, DC: American Psychiatric Association.

2013. *Diagnostic and Statistical Manual of Mental Disorders: DSM-5*. 5th ed. Arlington, VA: American Psychiatric Association.

Andersson, G. W., Gillberg, C., and Miniscalco, C. 2013. Pre-school children with suspected autism spectrum disorders: do girls and boys have the same profiles? *Research in Developmental Disabilities*, 34(1), 413–22. doi:10.1016/j.ridd.2012.08.025

Arnold, S., Foley, K. R., Hwang, Y. I. J., Richdale, A. L., Uljarevic, M., Lawson, L. P., Cai, R. Y., Falkmer, T., Falkmer, M., Lennox, N. G., Urbanowicz, A., and Trollor, J. 2019. Cohort profile: the Australian Longitudinal Study of Adults with Autism (ALSAA). *BMJ Open*, 9(12), e030798. doi:10.1136/bmjopen-2019-030798

Bailey, A., Le Couteur, A., Gottesman, I., Bolton, P., Simonoff, E., Yuzda, E., and Rutter, M. 1995. Autism as a strongly genetic disorder: evidence from a British twin study. *Psychological Medicine*, 25(1), 63–77. doi:10.1017/s0033291700028099

Barbu, S., Cabanes, G., and Le Maner-Idrissi, G. 2011. Boys and girls on the playground: sex differences in social development are not stable across early childhood. *PloS One*, 6 (1), e16407. doi:10.1371/journal. pone.0016407

Barneveld, P. S., Pieterse, J., de Sonneville, L., van Rijn, S., Lahuis, B., van Engeland, H., and Swaab, H. 2011. Overlap of autistic and schizotypal traits in adolescents with autism spectrum disorders. *Schizophrenia Research*, 126(1–3), 231–6. doi:10.1016/j. schres.2010.09.004

Baron-Cohen, S., Lombardo, M. V., Auyeung, B., Ashwin, E.,

Chakrabarti, B., and Knickmeyer, R. 2011. Why are autism spectrum conditions more prevalent in males? *PLoS Biology*, 9(6), e1001081. doi:10.1371/journal.pbio.1001081

Baron-Cohen, S., Wheelwright, S., Skinner, R., Martin, J., and Clubley, E. 2001. The autism-spectrum quotient (AQ): evidence from asperger syndrome/high-functioning autism, males and females, scientists and mathematicians. *Journal of Autism and Developmental Disorders*, 31(1), 5–17. doi:10.1023/a:1005653411471

Beaumont, R. 2015. The Secret Agent Society social-emotional skills training program for children with autism spectrum disorders. *The Australian Clinical Psychologist*, 1, 27–29.

Bejarano-Martin, A., Canal-Bedia, R., Magan-Maganto, M., Fernandez-Alvarez, C., Cilleros-Martin, M. V., Sanchez-Gomez, M. C., Garcia-Primo, P., Rose-Sweeney, M., Boilson, A., Linertova, R., Roeyers, H., Van der Paelt, S., Schendel, D., Warberg, C., Cramer, S., Narzisi, A., Muratori, F., Scattoni, M. L., Moilanen, I., Yliherva, A., Saemundsen, E., Loa Jonsdottir, S., Efrim-Budisteanu, M., Arghir, A., Papuc, S. M., Vicente, A., Rasga, C., Roge, B., Guillon, Q., Baduel, S., Kafka, J. X., Poustka, L., Kothgassner, O. D., Kawa, R., Pisula, E., Sellers, T., and Posada de la Paz, M. 2019. Early detection, diagnosis and intervention services for young children with Autism Spectrum Disorder in the European Union (ASDEU): family and professional perspectives. *Journal of Autism and Developmental Disorders*. doi:10.1007/s10803-019-04253-0

Ben-Itzchak, E. and Zachor, D. A. 2007. The effects of intellectual functioning and autism severity on outcome of early behavioral intervention for children with autism. *Research in Developmental Disabilities*, 28(3), 287–303. doi:10.1016/j.ridd.2006.03.002

Bertollo, J. R. and Yerys, B. E. 2019. More than IQ: executive function explains adaptive behavior above and beyond nonverbal IQ in youth with autism and lower IQ. *Am J Intellect Dev Disabil*, 124(3), 191–205. doi:10.1352/1944-7558-124.3.191

Bischof, N. L., Rapee, R. M., Hudry, K., and Bayer, J. K. 2018. Acceptability and caregiver-reported outcomes for young children with autism spectrum disorder whose parents attended a preventative population-based intervention for anxiety: a pilot study. *Autism Research*, 11(8), 1166–74. doi:10.1002/aur.1963

Bolton, P., Macdonald, H., Pickles, A., Rios, P., Goode, S., Crowson, M., Bailey, A., and Rutter, M. 1994. A case-control family history study of autism. *Journal of Child Psychology and Psychiatry and Allied Disciplines*, 35(5), 877–900. doi:10.1111/j.1469-7610.1994. tb02300.x

Cai, R. Y., Richdale, A. L., Uljarevic, M., Dissanayake, C., and Samson, A. C. 2018. Emotion regulation in autism spectrum disorder: Where we are and where we need to go. *Autism Research*, 11(7), 962–78. doi:10.1002/aur.1968

Carter, A. S., Black, D. O., Tewani, S., Connolly, C. E., Kadlec, M. B., and Tager-Flusberg, H. 2007. Sex differences in toddlers with autism spectrum disorders. *Journal of Autism and Developmental Disorders*, 37(1), 86–97. doi:10.1007/s10803-006-0331-7

Christensen, Deborah L., Maenner, Matthew J., Bilder, Deborah, Constantino, John N., Daniels, Julie, Durkin, Maureen S., Fitzgerald, Robert T., Kurzius-Spencer, Margaret, Pettygrove, Sydney D., Robinson, Cordelia, Shenouda, Josephine, White, Tiffany, Zahorodny, Walter, Pazol, Karen, and Dietz, Patricia. 2019. Prevalence and characteristics of autism spectrum disorder among children aged 4 Years – Early Autism and Developmental Disabilities

Monitoring Network, seven sites, United States, 2010, 2012, and 2014. *Morbidity and mortality weekly report. Surveillance summaries (Washington, DC: 2002)*, 68(2), 1–19. doi:10.15585/mmwr.ss6802a1

Constantino, J. N. and Charman, T. 2012. Gender bias, female resilience, and the sex ratio in autism. *Journal of the American Academy of Child and Adolescent Psychiatry*, 51(8), 756–8. doi:10.1016/j. jaac.2012.05.017

Craig, F., Margari, F., Legrottaglie, A. R., Palumbi, R., de Giambattista, C., and Margari, L. 2016. A review of executive function deficits in autism spectrum disorder and attention-deficit/hyperactivity disorder. *Neuropsychiatric Disease and Treatment*, 12, 1191–1202. doi:10.2147/ndt.S104620

Crooke, P. J. and Winner, M. G. 2016. Social Thinking(R) Methodology. evidence-based or empirically supported? A response to Leaf et al. *Behav Anal Pract*, 9(4), 403–8. doi:10.1007/s40617-016-0151-y

de Giambattista, Concetta, Ventura, Patrizia, Trerotoli, Paolo, Margari, Mariella, Palumbi, Roberto, and Margari, Lucia. 2019. Subtyping the autism spectrum disorder: comparison of children with high functioning autism and asperger syndrome. *Journal of Autism and Developmental Disorders*, 49(1), 138–50. doi:10.1007/s10803-018-3689-4

Doyen, C., Mighiu, D., Kaye, K., Colineaux, C., Beaumanoir, C., Mouraeff, Y., Rieu, C., Paubel, P., and Contejean, Y. 2011. Melatonin in children with autistic spectrum disorders: recent and practical data. *European Child and Adolescent Psychiatry*, 20(5), 231–9. doi:10.1007/s00787-011-0162-8

Duvekot, J., van der Ende, J., Verhulst, F. C., Slappendel, G., van Daalen, E., Maras, A., and Greaves-Lord, K. 2017. Factors influencing the probability of a diagnosis of autism spectrum disorder in girls versus boys. *Autism*, 21(6), 646–58. doi:10.1177/1362361316672178

Estes, Annette, Munson, Jeffrey, Rogers, Sally J., Greenson, Jessica, Winter, Jamie, and Dawson, Geraldine. 2015. Long-term outcomes of early intervention in 6-year-old children with autism spectrum disorder. *Journal of the American Academy of Child and Adolescent Psychiatry*, 54(7), 580–7. doi:10.1016/j.jaac.2015.04.005

Falkmer, T., Anderson, K., Falkmer, M., and Horlin, C. 2013. Diagnostic procedures in autism spectrum disorders: a systematic literature review. *European Child and Adolescent Psychiatry*, 22(6), 329–40. doi:10.1007/s00787-013-0375-0

Faridi, Farnaz and Khosrowabadi, Reza. 2017. Behavioral, cognitive and neural markers of asperger syndrome. *Basic and Clinical Neuroscience*, 8(5), 349–59. doi:10.18869/nirp.bcn.8.5.349

Fewster, D. L., Govender, P., and Uys, C. J. 2019. Quality of life interventions for primary caregivers of children with autism spectrum disorder: a scoping review. *J Child Adolesc Ment Health*, 31(2), 139–59. doi:10.2989/17280583.2019.1659146

Filipek, P. A., Accardo, P. J., Ashwal, S., Baranek, G. T., Cook, E. H., Jr, Dawson, G., Gordon, B., Gravel, J. S., Johnson, C. P., Kallen, R. J., Levy, S. E., Minshew, N. J., Ozonoff, S., Prizant, B. M., Rapin, I., Rogers, S. J., Stone, W. L., Teplin, S. W., Tuchman, R. F., and Volkmar, F. R. 2000. Practice parameter: screening and diagnosis of autism: report of the Quality Standards Subcommittee of the American Academy of Neurology and the Child Neurology Society. *Neurology*, 55(4), 468–79. doi:10.1212/wnl.55.4.468

Filipek, P. A., Accardo, P. J., Baranek, G. T., Cook, E. H., Jr., Dawson, G., Gordon, B., Gravel, J. S., Johnson, C. P., Kallen, R. J., Levy, S. E., Minshew, N. J., Ozonoff, S., Prizant, B. M., Rapin, I., Rogers, S. J., Stone, W. L., Teplin, S., Tuchman, R. F., and Volkmar, F. R. 1999. The screening and diagnosis of autistic spectrum disorders. *Journal of Autism and Developmental Disorders*, 29(6), 439–84. doi:10.1023/a:1021943802493

Fombonne, E. 2003. Epidemiological surveys of autism and other pervasive developmental disorders: an update. *Journal of Autism and Developmental Disorders*, 33(4), 365–82. doi:10.1023/a:1025054610557

Fombonne, E. 2005. Epidemiology of autistic disorder and other pervasive developmental disorders. *Journal of Clinical Psychiatry*, 66 Suppl 10, 3–8.

2009. Epidemiology of pervasive developmental disorders. *Pediatric Research*, 65(6), 591–8. doi:10.1203/PDR.0b013e31819e7203

Fombonne, E., Quirke, S., and Hagen, A. 2011. Epidemiology of pervasive developmental disorders. In: A. Geschwind, A. Amaral, and G. Dawson (eds) *Autism Spectrum Disorders*. Oxford: Oxford University Press.

Frazier, T. W., Georgiades, S., Bishop, S. L., and Hardan, A. Y. 2014. Behavioral and cognitive characteristics of females and males with autism in the Simons Simplex Collection. *Journal of the American Academy of Child and Adolescent Psychiatry*, 53(3), 329–40.e321–3. doi:10.1016/j.jaac.2013.12.004

Friedman, L. and Sterling, A. 2019. A review of language, executive function, and intervention in autism spectrum disorder. *Seminars in Speech and Language*, 40(4), 291–304. doi:10.1055/s-0039-1692964

Gadow, K. D., Devincent, C. J., and Drabick, D. A. 2008. Oppositional defiant disorder as a clinical phenotype in children with autism spectrum disorder. *Journal of Autism and Developmental*

Disorders, 38(7), 1302–10. doi:10.1007/s10803-007-0516-8

Gardiner, E. and Iarocci, G. 2018. Everyday executive function predicts adaptive and internalizing behavior among children with and without autism spectrum disorder. *Autism Research*, 11(2), 284–95. doi:10.1002/aur.1877

Gotham, K., Risi, S., Dawson, G., Tager-Flusberg, H., Joseph, R., Carter, A., Hepburn, S., McMahon, W., Rodier, P., Hyman, S. L., Sigman, M., Rogers, S., Landa, R., Spence, M. A., Osann, K., Flodman, P., Volkmar, F., Hollander, E., Buxbaum, J., Pickles, A., and Lord, C. 2008. A replication of the Autism Diagnostic Observation Schedule (ADOS) revised algorithms. *Journal of the American Academy of Child and Adolescent Psychiatry*, 47(6), 642–51. doi:10.1097/CHI.0b013e31816bffb7

Gotham, K., Risi, S., Pickles, A., and Lord, C. 2007. The Autism Diagnostic Observation Schedule: revised algorithms for improved diagnostic validity. *Journal of Autism and Developmental Disorders*, 37(4), 613–27. doi:10.1007/s10803-006-0280-1

Gray, K. M., Keating, C. M., Taffe, J. R., Brereton, A. V., Einfeld, S. L., Reardon, T. C., and Tonge, B. J. 2014. Adult outcomes in autism: community inclusion and living skills. *Journal of Autism and Developmental Disorders*, 44(12), 3006–15. doi:10.1007/s10803-014-2159-x

Guinchat, V., Thorsen, P., Laurent, C., Cans, C., Bodeau, N., and Cohen, D. 2012. Pre-, peri- and neonatal risk factors for autism. *Acta Obstetricia et Gynecologica Scandinavica*, 91(3), 287–300. doi:10.1111/j.1600-0412.2011.01325.x

Hallmayer, J., Cleveland, S., Torres, A., Phillips, J., Cohen, B., Torigoe, T., Miller, J., Fedele, A., Collins, J., Smith, K., Lotspeich, L., Croen, L. A., Ozonoff, S., Lajonchere, C., Grether, J. K., and Risch, N. 2011.

Genetic heritability and shared environmental factors among twin pairs with autism. *Archives of General Psychiatry*, 68(11), 1095–1102. doi:10.1001/archgenpsychiatry.2011.76

Harrop, C., Green, J., and Hudry, K. 2017. Play complexity and toy engagement in preschoolers with autism spectrum disorder: Do girls and boys differ? *Autism*, 21(1), 37–50. doi:10.1177/1362361315622410

Harrop, C., Gulsrud, A., and Kasari, C. 2015. Does gender moderate core deficits in ASD? An investigation into restricted and repetitive behaviors in girls and boys with ASD. *Journal of Autism and Developmental Disorders*, 45(11), 3644–55. doi:10.1007/s10803-015-2511-9

Harrop, C., Jones, D., Zheng, S., Nowell, S., Boyd, B. A., and Sasson, N. 2018. Circumscribed interests and attention in autism: the role of biological sex. *Journal of Autism and Developmental Disorders*, 48 (10), 3449–59. doi:10.1007/s10803-018-3612-z

Hiller, R. M., Young, R. L., and Weber, N. 2014. Sex differences in autism spectrum disorder based on DSM-5 criteria: evidence from clinician and teacher reporting. *Journal of Abnormal Child Psychology*, 42(8), 1381–93. doi:10.1007/s10802-014-9881-x

Hobson, J. A., Tarver, L., Beurkens, N., and Hobson, R. P. 2016. The relation between severity of autism and caregiver–child interaction: a study in the context of relationship development intervention. *Journal of Abnormal Child Psychology*, 44 (4), 745–55. doi:10.1007/s10802-015-0067-y

Howlin, P. 2014. Outcomes in adults with autism spectrum disorders. In: R. Paul F. R. Volkmar, S. J. Rogers, and K. A. Pelphrey (eds) *Handbook of autism and pervasive developmental disorders: Vol.1 Diagnosis, development, and brain

mechanisms*. 4th ed. Hoboken, NJ: Wiley, pp. 97–116.

Howlin, P., Goode, S., Hutton, J., and Rutter, M. 2004. Adult outcome for children with autism. *Journal of Child Psychology and Psychiatry and Allied Disciplines*, 45(2), 212–29. doi:10.1111/j.1469-7610.2004.00215.x

Hu, W. F., Chahrour, M. H., and Walsh, C. A. 2014. The diverse genetic landscape of neurodevelopmental disorders. *Annu Rev Genomics Hum Genet*, 15, 195–213. doi:10.1146/annurev-genom-090413-025600

Hull, L., Mandy, W., and Petrides, K. V. 2017. Behavioural and cognitive sex/gender differences in autism spectrum condition and typically developing males and females. *Autism*, 21(6), 706–27. doi:10.1177/1362361316669087

Hus, V. and Lord, C. 2013. Effects of child characteristics on the Autism Diagnostic Interview-Revised: implications for use of scores as a measure of ASD severity. *Journal of Autism and Developmental Disorders*, 43(2), 371–81. doi:10.1007/s10803-012-1576-y

Idring, S., Rai, D., Dal, H., Dalman, C., Sturm, H., Zander, E., Lee, B. K., Serlachius, E., and Magnusson, C. 2012. Autism spectrum disorders in the Stockholm Youth Cohort: design, prevalence and validity. *PloS One*, 7(7), e41280. doi:10.1371/journal.pone.0041280

Ingersoll, B., Meyer, K., and Becker, M. W. 2011. Increased rates of depressed mood in mothers of children with ASD associated with the presence of the broader autism phenotype. *Autism Research*, 4(2), 143–8. doi:10.1002/aur.170

Juul-Dam, N., Townsend, J., and Courchesne, E. 2001. Prenatal, perinatal, and neonatal factors in autism, pervasive developmental disorder-not otherwise specified, and the general population. *Pediatrics*, 107(4), E63. doi:10.1542/peds.107.4.e63

Kantzer, A. K., Fernell, E., Gillberg, C., and Miniscalco, C. 2013. Autism in community pre-schoolers: developmental profiles. *Research in Developmental Disabilities*, 34(9), 2900–2908. doi:10.1016/j.ridd.2013.06.016

King, C. and Murphy, G. H. 2014. A systematic review of people with autism spectrum disorder and the criminal justice system. *Journal of Autism and Developmental Disorders*, 44(11), 2717–33. doi:10.1007/s10803-014-2046-5

Kusaka, H., Miyawaki, D., Nakai, Y., Okamoto, H., Futoo, E., Goto, A., Okada, Y., and Inoue, K. 2014. Psychiatric comorbidity in children with high-functioning pervasive developmental disorder. *Osaka City Medical Journal*, 60(1), 1–10.

Lai, M. C., Lombardo, M. V., Auyeung, B., Chakrabarti, B., and Baron-Cohen, S. 2015. Sex/gender differences and autism: setting the scene for future research. *Journal of the American Academy of Child and Adolescent Psychiatry*, 54(1), 11–24. doi:10.1016/j.jaac.2014.10.003

Lai, M. C., Lombardo, M. V., Chakrabarti, B., and Baron-Cohen, S. 2013. Subgrouping the autism 'spectrum': reflections on DSM-5. *PLoS Biology*, 11(4), e1001544. doi:10.1371/journal.pbio.1001544

Lai, M. C., Lombardo, M. V., Pasco, G., Ruigrok, A. N., Wheelwright, S. J., Sadek, S. A., Chakrabarti, B., and Baron-Cohen, S. 2011. A behavioral comparison of male and female adults with high functioning autism spectrum conditions. *PloS One*, 6 (6), e20835. doi:10.1371/journal.pone.0020835

Lai, M. C. and Szatmari, P. 2020. Sex and gender impacts on the behavioural presentation and recognition of autism. *Curr Opin Psychiatry*, 33(2), 117–23. doi:10.1097/yco.0000000000000575

Lasgaard, M., Nielsen, A., Eriksen, M. E., and Goossens, L. 2010. Loneliness and social support in adolescent boys with autism

spectrum disorders. *Journal of Autism and Developmental Disorders*, 40(2), 218–26. doi:10.1007/s10803-009-0851-z

Loke, Y. J., Hannan, A. J., and Craig, J. M. 2015. The role of epigenetic change in autism spectrum disorders. *Frontiers in Neurology*, 6, 107. doi:10.3389/fneur.2015.00107

Loomes, R., Hull, L., and Mandy, W. P. L. 2017. What is the male-to-female ratio in autism spectrum disorder? A systematic review and meta-analysis. *Journal of the American Academy of Child and Adolescent Psychiatry*, 56(6), 466–74. doi:10.1016/j.jaac.2017.03.013

Lord, C., Rutter, M., DiLavore, P. C., Risi, S., Gotham, K., and Bishop, S. L. 2012. *Autism Diagnostic Observation Schedule*. 2nd ed. Torrance, CA: Western Psychological Services.

Lord, C., Rutter, M., and Le Couteur, A. 1994. Autism Diagnostic Interview-Revised: a revised version of a diagnostic interview for caregivers of individuals with possible pervasive developmental disorders. *Journal of Autism and Developmental Disorders*, 24(5), 659–85. doi:10.1007/bf02172145

Lord, C., Schopler, E., and Revicki, D. 1982. Sex differences in autism. *Journal of Autism and Developmental Disorders*, 12(4), 317–30. doi:10.1007/bf01538320

Maddox, B. B., Crabbe, S., Beidas, R. S., Brookman-Frazee, L., Cannuscio, C. C., Miller, J. S., Nicolaidis, C., and Mandell, D. S. 2020. 'I wouldn't know where to start': perspectives from clinicians, agency leaders, and autistic adults on improving community mental health services for autistic adults. *Autism*, 24(4), 919–30. doi:10.1177/1362361319882227

Maddox, B. B. and Gaus, V. L. 2019. Community mental health services for autistic adults: good news and bad news. *Autism Adulthood*, 1(1), 15–19. doi:10.1089/aut.2018.0006

Magiati, I., Ong, C., Lim, X. Y., Tan, J. W., Ong, A. Y., Patrycia, F., Fung, D. S., Sung, M., Poon, K. K., and Howlin, P. 2016. Anxiety symptoms in young people with autism spectrum disorder attending special schools: associations with gender, adaptive functioning and autism symptomatology. *Autism*, 20(3), 306–20. doi:10.1177/1362361315577519

Magiati, I., Tay, X. W., and Howlin, P. 2014. Cognitive, language, social and behavioural outcomes in adults with autism spectrum disorders: a systematic review of longitudinal follow-up studies in adulthood. *Clinical Psychology Review*, 34(1), 73–86. doi:10.1016/j.cpr.2013.11.002

Mandy, W., Chilvers, R., Chowdhury, U., Salter, G., Seigal, A., and Skuse, D. 2012. Sex differences in autism spectrum disorder: evidence from a large sample of children and adolescents. *Journal of Autism and Developmental Disorders*, 42(7), 1304–13. doi:10.1007/s10803-011-1356-0

Mansour, R., Dovi, A. T., Lane, D. M., Loveland, K. A., and Pearson, D. A. 2017. ADHD severity as it relates to comorbid psychiatric symptomatology in children with Autism Spectrum Disorders (ASD). *Research in Developmental Disabilities*, 60, 52–64. doi:10.1016/j.ridd.2016.11.009

Margari, L., Palumbi, R., Peschechera, A., Craig, F., de Giambattista, C., Ventura, P., and Margari, F. 2019. Sex-gender comparisons in comorbidities of children and adolescents with high-functioning autism spectrum disorder. *Front Psychiatry*, 10, 159. doi:10.3389/fpsyt.2019.00159

Mattila, M. L., Hurtig, T., Haapsamo, H., Jussila, K., Kuusikko-Gauffin, S., Kielinen, M., Linna, S. L., Ebeling, H., Bloigu, R., Joskitt, L., Pauls, D. L., and Moilanen, I. 2010. Comorbid psychiatric disorders associated with asperger syndrome/high-functioning autism: a community- and clinic-based study. *Journal of Autism and Developmental Disorders*, 40(9), 1080–93. doi:10.1007/s10803-010-0958-2

Mawhood, L., Howlin, P., and Rutter, M. 2000. Autism and developmental receptive language disorder – a comparative follow-up in early adult life. I: Cognitive and language outcomes. *Journal of Child Psychology and Psychiatry and Allied Disciplines*, 41(5), 547–59. doi:10.1111/1469-7610.00642

May, T., Adesina, I., McGillivray, J., and Rinehart, N. J. 2019. Sex differences in neurodevelopmental disorders. *Current Opinion in Neurology*, 32(4), 622–6. doi:10.1097/wco.0000000000000714

May, T., Cornish, K., and Rinehart, N. J. 2016. Gender profiles of behavioral attention in children with autism spectrum disorder. *J Atten Disord*, 20(7), 627–35. doi:10.1177/1087054712455502

McDougle, C. J., Holmes, J. P., Carlson, D. C., Pelton, G. H., Cohen, D. J., and Price, L. H. 1998. A double-blind, placebo-controlled study of risperidone in adults with autistic disorder and other pervasive developmental disorders. *Archives of General Psychiatry*, 55(7), 633–41. doi:10.1001/archpsyc.55.7.633

Meyer, Jessica A., Mundy, Peter C., Van Hecke, Amy Vaughan, and Durocher, Jennifer Stella. 2006. Social attribution processes and comorbid psychiatric symptoms in children with asperger syndrome. *Autism: The International Journal of Research and Practice*, 10(4), 383–402. doi:10.1177/1362361306064435

Mottron, Laurent. 2017. Should we change targets and methods of early intervention in autism, in favor of a strengths-based education? *European Child and Adolescent Psychiatry*, 26(7), 815–25. doi:10.1007/s00787-017-0955-5

Mukaddes, N. M., Herguner, S., and Tanidir, C. 2010. Psychiatric disorders in individuals with high-functioning autism and asperger's disorder: similarities and differences. *World Journal of Biological Psychiatry*, 11(8), 964–71. doi:10.3109/15622975.2010.507785

National Autism Center. 2015. Findings and Conclusions: National Standards Project. Phase 2. Retrieved from www.nationalautismcenter.org/national-standards-project/phase-2/, Randolph, MA: National Autism Center.

Newschaffer, C. J., Croen, L. A., Daniels, J., Giarelli, E., Grether, J. K., Levy, S. E., Mandell, D. S., Miller, L. A., Pinto-Martin, J., Reaven, J., Reynolds, A. M., Rice, C. E., Schendel, D., and Windham, G. C. 2007. The epidemiology of autism spectrum disorders. *Annual Review of Public Health*, 28, 235–58. doi:10.1146/annurev.publhealth.28.021406.144007

Nimmo-Smith, V., Heuvelman, H., Dalman, C., Lundberg, M., Idring, S., Carpenter, P., Magnusson, C., and Rai, D. 2020. Anxiety disorders in adults with autism spectrum disorder: a population-based study. *Journal of Autism and Developmental Disorders*, 50(1), 308–18. doi:10.1007/s10803-019-04234-3

Nix, Robert L., Bierman, Karen L., Domitrovich, Celene E., and Gill, Sukhdeep. 2013. Promoting children's social-emotional skills in preschool can enhance academic and behavioral functioning in kindergarten: findings from Head Start REDI. *Early Education and Development*, 24(7). doi:10.1080/10409289.2013.825565

Ogundele, Michael O. 2018. Behavioural and emotional disorders in childhood: A brief overview for paediatricians. *World Journal of Clinical Pediatrics*, 7(1), 9–26. doi:10.5409/wjcp.v7.i1.9

Oien, R. A., Vambheim, S. M., Hart, L., Nordahl-Hansen, A., Erickson, C., Wink, L., Eisemann, M. R., Shic, F.,

Volkmar, F. R., and Grodberg, D. 2018. Sex-differences in children referred for assessment: an exploratory analysis of the Autism Mental Status Exam (AMSE). *Journal of Autism and Developmental Disorders*, 48(7), 2286–92. doi:10.1007/s10803-018-3488-y

Ozonoff, S., Goodlin-Jones, B. L., and Solomon, M. 2005. Evidence-based assessment of autism spectrum disorders in children and adolescents. *Journal of Clinical Child and Adolescent Psychology*, 34 (3), 523–40. doi:10.1207/s15374424jccp3403_8

Ozonoff, S., Iosif, A. M., Baguio, F., Cook, I. C., Hill, M. M., Hutman, T., Rogers, S. J., Rozga, A., Sangha, S., Sigman, M., Steinfeld, M. B., and Young, G. S. 2010. A prospective study of the emergence of early behavioral signs of autism. *Journal of the American Academy of Child and Adolescent Psychiatry*, 49(3), 256–66.e251–2.

Pellicano, Elizabeth, Dinsmore, Adam, and Charman, Tony. 2014. What should autism research focus upon? Community views and priorities from the United Kingdom. *Autism: The International Journal of Research and Practice*, 18(7), 756–70. doi:10.1177/1362361314529627

Pilowsky, T., Yirmiya, N., Shulman, C., and Dover, R. 1998. The Autism Diagnostic Interview-Revised and the Childhood Autism Rating Scale: differences between diagnostic systems and comparison between genders. *Journal of Autism and Developmental Disorders*, 28(2), 143–51. doi:10.1023/a:1026092632466

Pisula, Ewa, Pudło, Monika, Słowińska, Monika, Kawa, Rafał, Strząska, Magdalena, Banasiak, Anna, and Wolańczyk, Tomasz. 2017. Behavioral and emotional problems in high-functioning girls and boys with autism spectrum disorders: Parents' reports and adolescents' self-reports. *Autism: The*

International Journal of Research and Practice, 21(6), 738–48. doi:10.1177/1362361316675119

Rai, Dheeraj, Culpin, Iryna, Heuvelman, Hein, Magnusson, Cecilia M. K., Carpenter, Peter, Jones, Hannah J., Emond, Alan M., Zammit, Stanley, Golding, Jean, and Pearson, Rebecca M. 2018. Association of autistic traits with depression from childhood to age 18 years. *JAMA Psychiatry*, 75(8), 835–43. doi:10.1001/jamapsychiatry.2018.1323

Reichow, B., Steiner, A. M., and Volkmar, F. 2013. Cochrane review: social skills groups for people aged 6 to 21 with autism spectrum disorders (ASD). *Evidence-Based Child Health*, 8(2), 266–315. doi:10.1002/ebch.1903

Reichow, B. and Wolery, M. 2009. Comprehensive synthesis of early intensive behavioral interventions for young children with autism based on the UCLA young autism project model. *Journal of Autism and Developmental Disorders*, 39(1), 23–41. doi:10.1007/s10803-008-0596-0

Rinehart, N. J., Cornish, K. M., and Tonge, B. J. 2011. Gender differences in neurodevelopmental disorders: autism and fragile x syndrome. *Current Topics in Behavioral Neurosciences*, 8, 209–29. doi:10.1007/7854_2010_96

Robinson, E. B., Lichtenstein, P., Anckarsater, H., Happe, F., and Ronald, A. 2013. Examining and interpreting the female protective effect against autistic behavior. *Proceedings of the National Academy of Sciences of the United States of America*, 110(13), 5258–62. doi:10.1073/pnas.1211070110

Romero, Marina, Aguilar, Juan Manuel, Del-Rey-Mejías, Ángel, Mayoral, Fermín, Rapado, Marta, Peciña, Marta, Barbancho, Miguel Ángel, Ruiz-Veguilla, Miguel, and Lara, José Pablo. 2016. Psychiatric comorbidities in autism spectrum disorder: a comparative study between DSM-IV-TR and DSM-5 diagnosis. *International Journal of Clinical and Health Psychology*, 16 (3), 266–75. doi:10.1016/j.ijchp.2016.03.001

Roux, A. M., Shattuck, P. T., Rast, J. E., and Anderson, K. A. 2017. National Autism Indicators Report: Developmental Disability Services and Outcomes in Adulthood. Retrieved from https://drexel.edu/autismoutcomes/publications-and-reports/publications/National-Autism-Indicators-Report-Developmental-Disability-Services-and-Outcomes-in-Adulthood/

Russell, G., Steer, C., and Golding, J. 2011. Social and demographic factors that influence the diagnosis of autistic spectrum disorders. *Social Psychiatry and Psychiatric Epidemiology*, 46(12), 1283–93. doi:10.1007/s00127-010-0294-z

Samson, A. C., Hardan, A. Y., Podell, R. W., Phillips, J. M., and Gross, J. J. 2015. Emotion regulation in children and adolescents with autism spectrum disorder. *Autism Research*, 8(1), 9–18. doi:10.1002/aur.1387

Sasson, N. J., Lam, K. S., Parlier, M., Daniels, J. L., and Piven, J. 2013. Autism and the broad autism phenotype: familial patterns and intergenerational transmission. *Journal of Neurodevelopmental Disorders*, 5(1), 11. doi:10.1186/1866-1955-5-11

Schaafsma, S. M. and Pfaff, D. W. 2014. Etiologies underlying sex differences in Autism Spectrum Disorders. *Frontiers in Neuroendocrinology*, 35(3), 255–71. doi:10.1016/j.yfrne.2014.03.006

Shulha, H. P., Cheung, I., Whittle, C., Wang, J., Virgil, D., Lin, C. L., Guo, Y., Lessard, A., Akbarian, S., and Weng, Z. 2012. Epigenetic signatures of autism: trimethylated H3K4 landscapes in prefrontal neurons. *Archives of General Psychiatry*, 69(3), 314–24. doi:10.1001/archgenpsychiatry.2011.151

Siegel, M. and Beaulieu, A. A. 2012. Psychotropic medications in children with autism spectrum disorders: a systematic review and synthesis for evidence-based practice. *Journal of Autism and Developmental Disorders*, 42(8), 1592–605. doi:10.1007/s10803-011-1399-2

Simonoff, E., Kent, R., Stringer, D., Lord, C., Briskman, J., Lukito, S., Pickles, A., Charman, T., and Baird, G. 2019. Trajectories in symptoms of autism and cognitive ability in autism from childhood to adult life: findings from a longitudinal epidemiological cohort. *Journal of the American Academy of Child and Adolescent Psychiatry*. doi:10.1016/j.jaac.2019.11.020

Sofronoff, K., Gray, K. M., Einfeld, S. l., & Tonge, B. J. 2018. Supporting families of children with a disability. In: M. R. Sanders and T. G. Mazzucchelli (eds.) *The Power of Positive Parenting*. Oxford: Oxford University Press, chapter 41, pp. 442–456.

Studer, Nadja, Gundelfinger, Ronnie, Schenker, Tanja, and Steinhausen, Hans-Christoph. 2017. Implementation of early intensive behavioural intervention for children with autism in Switzerland. *BMC Psychiatry*, 17(1), 34–34. doi:10.1186/s12888-017-1195-4

Sung, Min, Chin, Chee Hon, Lim, Choon Guan, Liew, Hwee Sen Alvin, Lim, Chau Sian, Kashala, Espérance, and Weng, Shih-Jen. 2014. What's in the pipeline? Drugs in development for autism spectrum disorder. *Neuropsychiatric Disease and Treatment*, 10, 371–81. doi:10.2147/NDT.S39516

Sutherland, R., Hodge, A., Bruck, S., Costley, D., and Klieve, H. 2017. Parent-reported differences between school-aged girls and boys on the autism spectrum. *Autism*, 21(6), 785–94. doi:10.1177/1362361316668653

Syriopoulou-Delli, C. K., Polychronopoulou, S. A., Kolaitis,

G. A., and Antoniou, A. G. 2019. Views of teachers on anxiety symptoms in students with autism spectrum disorder. *Journal of Autism and Developmental Disorders*, 49(2), 704–20. doi:10.1007/s10803-018-3752-1

Szatmari, P., Liu, X. Q., Goldberg, J., Zwaigenbaum, L., Paterson, A. D., Woodbury-Smith, M., Georgiades, S., Duku, E., and Thompson, A. 2012. Sex differences in repetitive stereotyped behaviors in autism: implications for genetic liability. *American Journal of Medical Genetics. Part B: Neuropsychiatric Genetics*, 159b(1), 5–12. doi:10.1002/ajmg.b.31238

Tachibana, Y., Miyazaki, C., Ota, E., Mori, R., Hwang, Y., Kobayashi, E., Terasaka, A., Tang, J., and Kamio, Y. 2017. A systematic review and meta-analysis of comprehensive interventions for pre-school children with autism spectrum disorder (ASD). *PloS One*, 12(12), e0186502. doi:10.1371/journal.pone.0186502

Taylor, D.; Paton, C., and Kapur, K. 2015. Autism spectrum disorders. In: *The Maudsley Prescribing Guidelines in Psychiatry*. 12th ed. Oxford: Wiley Blackwell.

Ten Hoopen, L. W., de Nijs, P. F. A., Duvekot, J., Greaves-Lord, K., Hillegers, M. H. J., Brouwer, W. B. F., and Hakkaart-van Roijen, L. 2020. Children with an autism spectrum disorder and their caregivers: capturing health-related and care-related quality of life. *Journal of Autism and Developmental Disorders*, 50(1), 263–77. doi:10.1007/s10803-019-04249-w

Tonge, B., Brereton, A., Kiomall, M., Mackinnon, A., and Rinehart, N. J. 2014. A randomised group comparison controlled trial of 'preschoolers with autism': a parent education and skills training

intervention for young children with autistic disorder. *Autism*, 18 (2), 166–77. doi:10.1177/1362361312458186

Tonge, B. and Einfeld, S. L. 2003. Psychopathology and intellectual disability: the Australian child to adult longitudinal study. In: L. M. Glidden (ed.) *International Review of Research in Mental Retardation*. 1st ed. San Diego, CA: Academic Press, vol. 26, pp. 61–91.

Tonge, B. J., Bull, K., Brereton, A., and Wilson, R. 2014. A review of evidence-based early intervention for behavioural problems in children with autism spectrum disorder: the core components of effective programs, child-focused interventions and comprehensive treatment models. *Curr Opin Psychiatry*, 27(2), 158–65. doi:10.1097/yco.0000000000000043

Torske, T., Naerland, T., Bettella, F., Bjella, T., Malt, E., Hoyland, A. L., Stenberg, N., Oie, M. G., and Andreassen, O. A. 2020. Autism spectrum disorder polygenic scores are associated with every day executive function in children admitted for clinical assessment. *Autism Research*, 13(2), 207–20. doi:10.1002/aur.2207

Van Wijngaarden-Cremers, P. J., van Eeten, E., Groen, W. B., Van Deurzen, P. A., Oosterling, I. J., and Van der Gaag, R. J. 2014. Gender and age differences in the core triad of impairments in autism spectrum disorders: a systematic review and meta-analysis. *Journal of Autism and Developmental Disorders*, 44(3), 627–35. doi:10.1007/s10803-013-1913-9

Volker, M. A., Lopata, C., Smerbeck, A. M., Knoll, V. A., Thomeer, M. L., Toomey, J. A., and Rodgers, J. D. 2010. BASC-2 PRS profiles for students with high-functioning autism spectrum disorders. *Journal of Autism and Developmental*

Disorders, 40(2), 188–99. doi:10.1007/s10803-009-0849-6

Volkmar, F. R., Szatmari, P., and Sparrow, S. S. 1993. Sex differences in pervasive developmental disorders. *Journal of Autism and Developmental Disorders*, 23(4), 579–91. doi:10.1007/bf01046103

Weiss, J. A., Thomson, K., and Chan, L. 2014. A systematic literature review of emotion regulation measurement in individuals with autism spectrum disorder. *Autism Research*, 7(6), 629–48. doi:10.1002/aur.1426

Werling, D. M., and Geschwind, D. H. 2013. Sex differences in autism spectrum disorders. *Current Opinion in Neurology*, 26(2), 146–53. doi:10.1097/WCO.0b013e32835ee548

White, S. W., Oswald, D., Ollendick, T., and Scahill, L. 2009. Anxiety in children and adolescents with autism spectrum disorders. *Clinical Psychology Review*, 29(3), 216–29. doi:10.1016/j.cpr.2009.01.003

Witwer, Andrea N., and Lecavalier, Luc. 2010. Validity of comorbid psychiatric disorders in youngsters with autism spectrum disorders. *Journal of Developmental and Physical Disabilities*, 22(4), 367–80. doi:10.1007/s10882-010-9194-0

Zhang, Y., Li, N., Li, C., Zhang, Z., Teng, H., Wang, Y., Zhao, T., Shi, L., Zhang, K., Xia, K., Li, J., and Sun, Z. 2020. Genetic evidence of gender difference in autism spectrum disorder supports the female-protective effect. *Transl Psychiatry*, 10(1), 4. doi:10.1038/s41398-020-0699-8

Zheng, Z., Zheng, P., and Zou, X. 2018. Association between schizophrenia and autism spectrum disorder: a systematic review and meta-analysis. *Autism Research*, 11(8), 1110–19. doi:10.1002/aur.1977

Chapter

3

Attention Deficit Hyperactivity Disorder in Males

David Coghill

Unlike most of the disorders discussed in this book, attention deficit hyperactivity disorder (ADHD) is, in childhood at least, more common in males than in females. This is both an advantage and disadvantage when it comes to writing a chapter such as this. Whilst most of the research has been conducted in males, meaning that there is a lot to say, those studies that have included females with ADHD or attempted to contrast males and females have often been underpowered and delivered inconclusive findings. Also many of these studies have failed to include healthy comparison groups, making it difficult to know what is specific to ADHD and which differences are simply reflecting more general differences between the sexes.

In this chapter I will first present a broad overview of ADHD, briefly commenting on causality and theories for the observed sex differences, and I will discuss the course of ADHD and the common comorbidities and longer-term outcomes, highlighting where possible the evidence for sex differences. I will then discuss the management of ADHD and the importance of measuring outcomes in routine clinical practice.

Historical Context

Although the recognition of ADHD, and our understanding of it as a major cause of burden for those who suffer from it – their families and society in general – has increased considerably over the last twenty-five years, ADHD is not, as is sometimes assumed, a new disorder. The core concepts of ADHD were originally developed in the early nineteenth century, through the work of Benjamin Rush in the USA, Alexander Crichton in Scotland, and George Frederick Still in England, who all noted in their clinical work that some children and young people are more challenging to look after and have significant problems with self-control. They all also recognized that these difficulties were developmental

in nature and most often arose early in life (Taylor, 2011). From this time on the concepts were refined and built on by authors such as Kramer and Pollnow who introduced the term 'hyperkinetic syndrome', and Tredgold whose diagnosis of 'minimal brain dysfunction' overlapped considerably with ADHD. These new concepts started to bring together the ideas of motor dyscontrol with the concept of behavioural dysregulation. The discovery of the therapeutic actions of the psychostimulants and an acknowledgement that they improved not only hyperactivity but also aspects of impulsivity and inattention shaped the current clinical construct of ADHD, which has been supported through the development and analysis of systematic rating scales that demonstrated that this triad of behaviours does indeed cluster together and is often associated with impairments across a broad range of life situations. Further longitudinal studies showed that if untreated these difficulties tend to persist but that they do respond well to treatment, at least in the short term. Although ADHD can remit in adolescence or adulthood, this is not, as was traditionally assumed, inevitable and many children with ADHD will continue to have problems as adults. The proportion who do not remit remains unclear. In a classic analysis of US data Faraone and colleagues demonstrated that whilst relatively few of those with ADHD (around 15%) continued to meet full diagnostic criteria as adults, around two-thirds did continue to have significant ADHD-related impairments (Faraone et al., 2006). A more recent analysis of a Dutch clinical sample suggested a much higher rate of persistence of 86.5% (van Lieshout et al., 2016). A possible explanation for the difference in these two studies is that the ADHD in those receiving a diagnosis in the Netherlands, where at the time of the study rates of recognition of ADHD were quite low, was more severe than those included in the US sample (where rates of diagnosis were and remain much higher). This would suggest that the more severe the

ADHD in childhood the more likely it is to persist into adulthood. Whilst several recent studies have suggested that ADHD may arise de novo in adults, a comprehensive review of the current evidence, whilst not explicitly refuting this suggestion, has suggested that this finding may be a methodological artefact (Coghill et al., 2018). It is, however, clear that some of those with ADHD manage to cope with limited impairment during childhood and adolescence, particularly when they are well scaffolded by a supportive family and school, but then when moving to the more independent environments of college, university, work, or indeed unemployment can decompensate and present to clinical services. A careful history will usually uncover long-term symptoms and some impairment.

Whilst previous versions of the WHO's International Classification of Disease did not include ADHD as a diagnosis preferring the more restrictive 'hyperkinetic disorder', the most recent version (ICD-11) has for the first time included ADHD in a format that is very similar to the broader DSM-5 definition. This recognition that ADHD is a valid psychiatric disorder has been welcomed by most patients, their families, and their clinicians. As a part of their first comprehensive ADHD guideline development programme, the UK National Institute for Health and Care Excellence (NICE) conducted a major systematic review of the scientific evidence and concluded that the ADHD construct is indeed a valid way of describing a common and impairing mental health condition in children, adolescents, and adults (NICE, 2008). Nevertheless ADHD continues to be a controversial topic and there remain many educators, journalists, and politicians across the world who continue to question the validity of the diagnosis and express a view that it is more of a social construct that a medical condition, that it is over-diagnosed and that it should not be treated with medication. Whilst I believe that the evidence from multiple studies refutes these beliefs, there do remain several important unanswered questions about ADHD: Why is there so much variation in rates of diagnosis, not only between different countries but also within countries and within regions in those countries? Has the line between ADHD and not-ADHD been drawn at the right place? Does the lack of a valid and reliable biomarker invalidate the diagnosis? And as highlighted above, can ADHD start for the first time

in adulthood? Of course these questions can be asked about most psychiatric disorders but are often directed at ADHD, which remains controversial primarily because psychostimulants are the treatment of choice and because most of those currently treated are children.

Definitions of ADHD

As noted above ADHD is a clinical diagnosis where the core symptoms are inattention, hyperactivity, and impulsivity. These symptoms are required to be not just present but developmentally inappropriate, pervasive (across different situations such as home and school), and to be persistent over time. Current diagnostic rules also insist that onset is in childhood and that the core symptoms are associated with substantial impairments in social, academic, and/or occupational functioning. Both ICD and DSM now include an almost identical set of 18 symptoms (8 hyperactive/impulsive and 8 inattentive – see Box 3.1). Both systems now also recognized three presentations. In DSM these are operationally defined as: a predominantly inattentive presentation, which displays at least six (or more) symptoms of inattention, and less than six of hyperactivity/impulsivity, a predominantly hyperactive/impulsive presentation suffering from six (or more) symptoms of hyperactivity/impulsivity, and less than six of inattention, and a combined presentation, which meets both sets of criteria. These presentations took over from the previous description of 'subtypes' when it was realized that the stability over time across the different presentations was much less than previously assumed. The other criteria for DSM-5 are detailed in Box 3.2. Whilst there are still some differences between ICD and DSM, these are now much less than before and it seems likely that the two systems will now describe similar groups of individuals. The change in symptoms over time has been recognized in the most recent versions of DSM whereby the required symptoms for making a diagnosis in adults has been reduced from 6 to 5. ADHD describes a group of individuals who fall towards the end of the attention, hyperactivity, and impulsivity continua. The actual numbers of symptoms required for a diagnosis are somewhat arbitrary and whilst they do stand up to statistical analysis and are useful both clinically and for research, they are not based on empirical evidence and therefore should not be seen as being set in stone.

Box 3.1 Symptom domains for ADHD

Inattention

Often . . .

- fails to give close attention to details or makes careless mistakes in schoolwork, work, or during other activities (e.g. overlooks or misses details, work is inaccurate)
- has difficulty sustaining attention in tasks or play activities (e.g. has difficulty remaining focused during lectures, conversations, or lengthy reading)
- does not seem to listen when spoken to directly (e.g. mind seems elsewhere, even in the absence of any obvious distraction)
- does not follow through on instructions and fails to finish schoolwork, chores, or duties in the workplace (not due to oppositional behaviour or failure to understand instructions; e.g. starts tasks but quickly loses focus and is easily sidetracked)
- has difficulty organizing tasks and activities (e.g. difficulty managing sequential tasks; difficulty keeping materials and belongings in order; messy, disorganized work; has poor time management; fails to meet deadlines)
- avoids, dislikes, or is reluctant to engage in tasks that require sustained mental effort (e.g. schoolwork or homework; for older adolescents and adults, preparing reports, completing forms, reviewing lengthy papers)
- loses things necessary for tasks or activities (e.g. toys, school assignments, pencils, books, tools, school materials, pencils, books, tools, wallets, keys, paperwork, spectacles, mobile telephones)
- easily distracted by extraneous stimuli (for older adolescents and adults, may include unrelated thoughts)
- forgetful in daily activities (e.g. doing chores, running errands; for older adolescents and adults, returning calls, paying bills, keeping appointments)

Hyperactivity

Often . . .

- fidgets with or taps hands or feet or squirms in seat
- leaves seat in situations in which remaining seated is expected (e. g. leaves his or her place in the classroom, in the office or other workplace, or in other situations that require remaining in place)
- runs about or climbs in situations where it is inappropriate (in adolescents or adults, may be limited to feeling restless)
- unable to play or engage in leisure activities quietly
- 'on the go' or acting as if 'driven by a motor' (e.g. is unable to be or uncomfortable being still for extended time, as in restaurants, meetings; may be experienced by others as being restless or difficult to keep up with (DSM-5); exhibits a persistent pattern of excessive motor activity that is not substantially modified by social context or demands (ICD-10)
- talks excessively (DSM-5)

Impulsivity

Often. . .

- talks excessively without appropriate response to social constraints (ICD-10)
- blurts out answers before questions have been completed (e.g. completes people's sentences; cannot wait for turn in conversation)
- has difficulty waiting his or her turn (e.g. while waiting in line)
- interrupts or intrudes on others (e.g. butts into conversations, games, or activities; may start using other people's things without receiving permission; for adolescents and adults, may intrude into or take over what others are doing)

Most specialists would agree that it is reasonable in routine clinical practice to make a clinical diagnosis in individuals whose symptom count falls just short of the required number as long as those symptoms that are present are clearly present and significantly impairing. Although the dimensional nature of ADHD has been put forward as a reason to question the validity of the diagnosis, it is no different in this respect to many physical health problems such as hypertension and obesity.

Box 3.2 DSM-5 diagnostic criteria for ADHD

A. Either 1 or 2[#]

    1. Six (or more) symptoms of inattention have persisted for at least six months to a degree that is maladaptive and inconsistent with developmental level[*]

    2. Six (or more) symptoms of hyperactivity/impulsivity have persisted for at least six months to a degree that is maladaptive and inconsistent with developmental level[*]

B. Several hyperactive/impulsive or inattentive symptoms were present before 12 years of age

C. Several inattentive or hyperactive/impulsive symptoms are present in two or more settings (e.g. at school/work or at home)

D. There must be clear evidence of clinically significant interference in social, academic, or occupational functioning

E. The symptoms do not occur exclusively during the course of schizophrenia or other psychotic disorder, and are not better accounted for by another mental disorder (e.g. mood disorder, anxiety disorder, dissociative disorder, or personality disorder)

[#] The symptoms are not only a manifestation of oppositional behaviour, defiance, hostility, or inability to understand task or instructions.

[*] For older adolescents and adults (age 17 and older) at least five symptoms are required.

Epidemiology

The differences between countries in the rate of diagnosis of ADHD has generated considerable controversy. However, Polanczyk and colleagues demonstrated that, when operational definitions of ADHD are used, the differences between countries are small and those differences that are seen in epidemiological studies are mainly the consequence of methodological issues (Polanczyk et al., 2007). These include: the use of differing diagnostic criteria from different versions of ICD and DSM; the source of the diagnostic information and how information from different informants is combined (e.g. parents *and* teachers vs parent *or* teachers); whether or not impairment was required for a diagnosis to be made. Once these were accounted for the estimates for different regions did not differ from each other. Based on the findings from 102 studies the overall prevalence for children and adolescents was 5.3% – children 6.5%, adolescents 2.7% (Polanczyk et al., 2007). Despite a consistency between countries and regions with respect the epidemiological prevalence, there are considerable differences in administrative prevalence between and within countries – how often a diagnosis is made in clinical practice. Rates of diagnosis are much higher in the USA, where 9.4% of children 2–17 years of age had been diagnosed with ADHD, according to a parent report in 2016 (Danielson et al., 2018), whilst in Scotland the rate was around 0.6% in 2012 (Healthcare Improvement Scotland, 2012).

Whilst some other developed countries have rates of around 2.5% and a few regions within countries have diagnosis rates of around 5%, there are none with rates approaching those of the USA, and many, such as China, where rates of diagnosis of ADHD are considerably lower than those for even Scotland, despite a clear indication that ADHD is as common in China as it is in the West (Jin et al., 2013). When compared to the epidemiological prevalence these rates suggest under-diagnosis and treatment in much of the developed world, and the clear possibility of over-diagnosis in the USA, rates of diagnosis in low-to-middle-income countries are consistently lower than those in developed countries. A similar picture emerges when one looks at treatment rates. A recent cross-national study of prescribing rates for ADHD demonstrated considerable variation between countries, with rates of prescribing for those between 3 and 18 years of age of: USA 6.7%; Canada 1.8%; Australia 1.4%; UK 0.6%; Northern Europe 1.9%; western/southern Europe 0.7% and Asia-Pacific 0.9% (Raman et al., 2018). Rates of diagnosis and treatment have been rising in many of the countries/regions over the past twenty years, although this increase has slowed or stopped in many western countries over the past five years (e.g. Holden et al., 2013). This upward trend has led several commentators to raise concerns that rates of ADHD are increasing. However, in a further meta-regression analysis Polanczyk and colleagues found no evidence for an increase in the number of children in the community who meet criteria for ADHD in the past thirty years (Polanczyk et al., 2014). It is therefore likely that in most countries the increase in diagnosis of ADHD reflects an increase in recognition from a previously low baseline, although the situation in the USA is likely to be different.

Whilst the estimates for prevalence of ADHD in children and adolescents seem reasonably solid, those for adults continue to vary significantly. A meta-analysis of available studies in adults reported a prevalence rate of 2.5% (95% CI 2.1–3.1) (Simon et al., 2009). The first population study of ADHD in young adults using the DSM-5 criteria found a prevalence of 3.6% (95% CI 2.9–4.1) (Matte et al., 2015).

Sex Differences in Prevalence

Sex has a significant impact on the prevalence of ADHD and, interestingly, this effect seems to change across development. In childhood and adolescence there is a very clear male preponderance. However, this is considerably larger in clinical samples, where the male-to-female sex ratio is often quoted as between 9:1 and 4:1, than population samples where the figures are around 2.5:1. In population samples (Faraone et al., 2015; Polanczyk et al., 2007), whilst males are significantly more likely to meet diagnostic criteria for all of the ADHD presentations, the difference between the sexes is greater for combined ADHD presentation, and lower for the inattentive ADHD presentation (Willcutt, 2012; Willcutt et al., 1999; Graetz et al., 2005; Dopfner et al., 2008). The sex ratio in clinical samples has reduced over time, which is likely to reflect an increased recognition of ADHD in girls rather than a change in prevalence in boys. With respect to the epidemiological differences in childhood and adolescence it has been demonstrated that males in general have higher variability in inattentiveness and hyperactivity-impulsivity than females, which could be one reason why more males meet criteria for ADHD (Greven et al., 2011). There are of course many other reasons that we will explore in more detail below. It is often stated that girls are more likely to present with inattention rather than hyperactivity-impulsiveness. Whilst it has been consistently demonstrated that males are more likely to present with hyperactivity-impulsivity than females (Nussbaum, 2012; Gershon, 2002; Arnett et al., 2015; Williamson and Johnston, 2015; Greven et al., 2011),

the situation for inattention is less clear with some studies reporting less inattentiveness for males, others more, and yet others finding no difference (Novik et al., 2006; Gomez, 2013; Staller and Faraone, 2006; Rucklidge, 2010; Fedele et al., 2012). Clinically this is very important as it is often assumed that the predominant problem for boys with ADHD is their overactivity and impulsiveness (which are of course significant issues), but clearly we need to be fully aware of their inattention. Interestingly one study found that as children boys had more inattention than girls but that in adolescence the pattern was reversed (Kan et al., 2013).

In adults the literature is more consistent and shows that, irrespective of the sampling frame, the prevalence of ADHD is much more similar for males and females (Williamson and Johnston, 2015; Faraone et al., 2015; Matte et al., 2015). The reason for this shift in the male–female balance is less clear. Whilst this would for example suggest that if ADHD by definition starts early in life then it would seem to be less likely to persist in males than females, there are few strong studies that address this question, and the findings of those that do are contradictory. Longitudinal single-sex studies suggest a persistence of ADHD of around 30–60% for males and 60% for females, whilst retrospective self-reports studies in adults of both sexes report a persistence around 35–55% with no difference between the sexes (Williamson and Johnston, 2015). Before addressing the reasons for sex differences in ADHD and for the different patterns of recognition, it will be helpful to think about the impairments associated with ADHD as well as common co-morbidities and the different patterns seen in males and females.

Impairments

Impairment is an essential part of the diagnostic criteria for ADHD as it is for most psychiatric diagnoses. It is therefore inevitable that in addition to high rates of psychiatric co-morbidity and substance use disorders (see below) both clinical and population-based samples are associated with a wide range of impairments (Box 3.3). These impact not only on the individual with ADHD but all of those around them, and impose a significant cost on society in general (Holden et al., 2013; Quintero et al., 2018). There is a suggestion in the literature that females with ADHD may be more impaired relative to males.

Box 3.3   Common impairments in ADHD

Educational failure: underachievement or erratic performance; increased rates of suspension and exclusion; lower rates of graduation; less likely to proceed to tertiary education; lower total years of education

Poor employment history: lower number of full-time jobs; more likely to have been fired from employment; higher rates of absenteeism and lower productivity; jobs often not commensurate with their intelligence and educational background; less likely to be promoted; even when employed in an appropriate job this comes at great emotional cost and without much success and is experienced as underachievement. When severe, adults with ADHD are not able to retain themselves in any kind of employment

Family life: high rates of family stress and expressed emotion; emotional dysregulation may be a particular source of difficulty with family relationships; disorganization and forgetfulness may be disruptive of family life; increased rates of parental divorce and separation

Relationships: reduced capacity for intimacy; often isolated with fewer friends; but younger age at first sexual intercourse; higher numbers of sexual partners and increased rates of teenage pregnancy; often unaware of the ways in which their ADHD-caused behaviour patterns have contributed to relationship failures

Activities of daily living (ADL): even high-functioning individuals with ADHD may have difficulties with ADL, such as shopping, cleaning, dressing, or managing money. There is a dissociation between what one can do and what one actually does. This is often interpreted as laziness when in reality it relates more to cognitive impairments in areas such as memory, set shifting, attention, inhibition, delay aversion, and decision making

Other common impairments: increased risk of accidents in general and specifically traffic accidents, both as a pedestrian and a driver; increased driving offences; financial difficulties; high rates of criminal offences and incarceration

Females diagnosed with ADHD are reported to have lower self-esteem, feel less effective, and be more affected by negative life events than males with ADHD (Rucklidge, 2010). They also report higher levels of impairment in home and social life, education, money management, and daily life activities (Fedele et al., 2012). As these studies were reporting on clinical samples it is possible that the higher rates of impairment represent a higher diagnostic threshold for females than males. Males were reported in one review to experience higher overall impairment, particularly at school (Staller and Faraone, 2006). However, this may also reflect under-diagnosis in girls. Across both sexes the combined presentation is associated with the greatest impairment. Interestingly in males the hyperactive-impulsive presentation is associated with higher impairment than the inattentive presentation, whilst in females the opposite seems to be true (Staller and Faraone, 2006). In adults a recent review suggests similar levels of impairment in men and women but that women report more functional impairment due to their symptoms (Williamson and Johnston, 2015). One interesting area of study is the impact of ADHD on criminality. Children with ADHD are at a higher risk of criminal convictions in adulthood (Dalsgaard et al., 2013).

Rates of criminal convictions in adults are significantly higher for both men (ADHD 36.6%: general population 8.9%) and women (ADHD 15.4%: general population 2.2%) (Lichtenstein et al., 2012). Thus whilst the absolute rates are much higher in men, the proportionate increase is higher for women (7 times) than men (4 times). Young males with ADHD make up around 30% of the population in youth prisons, which is a fivefold increase in the expected prevalence, and in adult prisons the rate for men is around 25%, which is a tenfold increase (Young et al., 2015). Many people do not realize that ADHD is also associated with a significant increase in mortality rates. Overall there is a twofold increase, but this rises to a fourfold increase for those whose ADHD was not diagnosed until they were over 18 years of age (Dalsgaard et al., 2015). The increased mortality is mainly due to deaths from unnatural causes, particularly accidents. These important data really emphasize the importance of early identification of ADHD.

The impact of ADHD on quality of life is now well documented, with the mean scores for quality of life often falling more than 2 standard deviations from the norm, which translates to being in the bottom one or two per cent of the population (Jonsson et al., 2017;

Danckaerts et al., 2010). Much of the quality of life data in children comes from proxy parent reports, but studies that directly assessed quality of life from children themselves also document significant impairment, albeit less than rated by their parents (Coghill and Hodgkins, 2016). These data also highlight that the impact of ADHD on quality of life is greater than is seen for insulin-dependent diabetes. The few data that have investigated the impact of sex on quality of life suggest the males and females are equally affected.

Co-morbidity

Co-morbidity is so common in ADHD that it should be expected and considered the norm (Yoshimasu et al., 2012). Figure 3.1 shows the profiles of co-morbidity from three separate clinical child samples from Europe (Steinhausen et al., 2006), Brazil (Souza et al., 2004), and the USA (MTA Cooperative Group 1999). Whilst there are differences in detail, they demonstrate consistently high levels of co-morbidity across a wide range of disorders. The overall pattern of co-morbidity remains high in adults. Perhaps the most informative data come from a population study from the USA that indicates substantially elevated

rates of co-morbid psychiatric disorders in adults with ADHD (Figure 3.2; Kessler et al., 2006). This study identified a high risk for antisocial personality disorder (up to ten times that of controls; about 20% of the cases) as well as elevated rates of mood disorder (two to six times), anxiety disorders (two to four times), and continued problems with various learning disorders. Both children and adults with ADHD also have high rates of executive function deficits in attention, behavioural inhibition, working memory, problem-solving ability, and planning, as well as emotional dysregulation difficulties (Hervey et al., 2004).

Rates of co-morbidity differ by sex. Males with ADHD are more likely to have co-morbid oppositional defiant disorder and conduct disorder, as well as autism, tics, and specific learning and developmental disorders (e.g. language, learning, and motor development). Compared to females with ADHD they are less likely to suffer from co-morbid internalizing problems (especially affective and anxiety disorders, and problems with emotion dysregulation) as well as eating disorders (Nussbaum, 2012; Rucklidge, 2010; Jensen and Steinhausen, 2015; Robison et al., 2008). Rates of substance misuse in children and adolescents with ADHD are twice that of the general population, and those with ADHD start to misuse substances earlier and find it harder to quit (Wilens, 2007). Rates in adults are even higher at around 4–6 times those in the general population. Again the pattern for the sexes changes over time. During childhood the rates of substance use disorders in ADHD are similar in males and females (Jensen and Steinhausen, 2015; Lee et al., 2011). In adults with ADHD, however, the rates are significantly higher for males for most substances (Rucklidge, 2010; Williamson and Johnston, 2015). The exception appears to be cigarette smoking, where females with ADHD are particularly vulnerable (Van Voorhees et al., 2012). One caveat on these findings on sex differences in co-morbidity is that few studies compared males or females with ADHD to a same-sexed group without ADHD. It is therefore not possible to separate the differences expected by sex from those attributable to ADHD.

From a clinical perspective it is important to remember that ADHD is vastly under-recognized in adults. Clinical experts will often comment that most if not all adults referred to them for diagnosis have already had extensive contact with psychiatric services and have usually received several diagnoses before their ADHD is recognized. There is still considerable

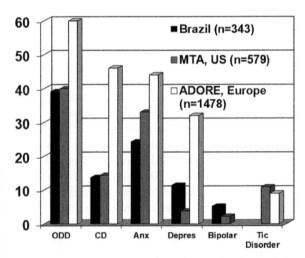

Figure 3.1 ADHD co-morbid profile in three studies: the MTA (MTA Cooperative Group, 1999), the ADORE (Steinhausen et al., 2006), and Souza et al. (2004; Brazil). Data are presented as percentages. In the Brazilian study, the co-morbid profile is described only for one site (Porto Alegre) and no information is reported for tic disorders. In the MTA, only ADHD-combined type is included and several restrictions were applied to enrol patients with severe mood disorders. No information is available for bipolar disorder in the ADORE study. ODD – oppositional defiant disorder; CD – conduct disorder; Anx – anxiety; Depres – depression. Reproduced from Coghill et al. (2008), with kind permission from Karger, Basel.

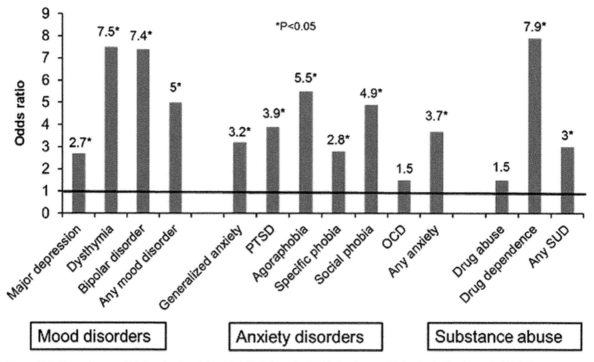

Figure 3.2 Rates of co-morbid disorders in adults with ADHD from the US National co-morbidity Study (Kessler et al., 2006). Data are presented as odds ratios.
*Significant at the level 0.05. ADHD: attention-deficit hyperactivity disorder; OCD: obsessive-compulsive disorder; PTSD: post-traumatic stress disorder; SUD: substance use disorder.

scepticism about adult ADHD and those seeking a diagnosis are often thought to be engaging in drug-seeking behaviours. Whilst this is certainly true for some, many will have either tried, unsuccessfully, to get help and support for their ADHD-related problems for many years or not recognized that their problems are treatable. It is important that clinicians recognize the impact of ADHD on individuals, their families, and society in general and that, as we will see later in this chapter, even in adulthood ADHD is an eminently treatable condition. Treating ADHD can often result in improvements in other disorders as well as reduction in impairment. It can also help an individual make use of other therapeutic supports that were too difficult to engage with before the ADHD was treated.

What Are the Causes of Sex Differences in ADHD?

Environmental and Genetic Causes

The findings from quantitative genetic studies comparing family members with different levels of genetic relatedness (e.g. monozygotic vs dizygotic twins) are inconsistent with respect to potential genetic and environmental influences on sex differences in ADHD. This is most likely due to the limited power of these, mostly small studies. However, the larger studies and meta-analyses have found little evidence to support a strong pattern of genetic and environmental influences on sex differences in ADHD or ADHD traits (Larsson et al., 2013; Nikolas and Burt, 2010).

Molecular genetic research on sex differences in ADHD has focused on sex chromosome genes (i.e. X- and Y-linked genes). These genes influence sex differences not only through their impact on hormonal pathways (particularly sex hormones) but also through an independent impact on brain development. There are several complementary theories of the way that the sex differences in ADHD may be linked to the sex chromosomes. One suggestion is a male-limited over-expression of Y-linked genes. There is some limited support for this in that males with additional Y genes (XYY or XXYY) are at increased risk for some of the motor problems observed in ADHD (Davies, 2014). Another potential functional link is that the sex-determining region on the Y-chromosome is expressed in particular in brain regions involved in motor control, reward, and attention, and has been shown to be involved in regulating dopamine function in the male brain (Loke et al., 2015). Whilst it has been speculated that X-linked imprinting may also increase male risk for ADHD, this remains largely speculative (Zayats et al., 2015; Davies, 2014).

Both under- and over-dosage of X-linked gene expression have also been implicated as contributing factors to sex differences in ADHD. Females with only one X-chromosome (XO; Turner syndrome) have higher rates of ADHD symptoms (Loke et al., 2015), which suggests that the additional X-chromosome may be protective against ADHD. Both males and females with an additional X chromosome (XXY, Klinefelter's syndrome, and XXX females) are at increased risk for ADHD-like symptoms (Davies, 2014). MAOA, which is an X-linked gene, meaning that males have only one allele that encodes for monoamine oxidase, is linked to an increased risk for ADHD, attention deficit, impulsivity, and co-morbid conduct disorder. This may explain part of the increased risk and the differential relationship between MAOA for males and females (Davies, 2014). Other genes that have been linked to ADHD and that have been shown to be sexually dimorphic include DRD4, DAT1, COMT, and DBH (Loke et al., 2015). Whilst the impact of these genes is likely to involve gene by environment interactions, there are as yet no strong data to inform us what these might be.

In summary, whilst there is some evidence to support a role for the sex chromosomes as causal factors in the sex differences found in ADHD, these remain speculative and are not yet supported by findings of the behavioural genetic studies.

Brain Development and Endocrine Factors

Another obvious mechanism for the sex differences in ADHD is through differences in hormonal levels, particularly differences in exposure to androgens and testosterone. Androgens have complex effects on brain development during gestation, early infancy, around puberty, and into adolescence (Davies, 2014; Waddell and McCarthy, 2012). Male and female brains mature at different rates (Durston et al., 2001); although the average brain volumes are larger

in males throughout development, volume trajectories peak much earlier in females. There are clear and replicated differences between the brains of both males and females with ADHD compared to healthy controls (Shaw et al., 2011) and these appear to reflect a dimensional tendency with those youth who have higher levels of hyperactivity-impulsivity, also having a slower rate of cortical thinning, and children with ADHD having the slowest rate of thinning. Several studies have identified sex differences in the patterns of structural differences in the brains of those with ADHD. In males with ADHD, reductions were found in the basal ganglia, premotor, and medial prefrontal cortex, while females with ADHD showed reductions in prefrontal cortex and lateral premotor grey matter (Mahone et al., 2011; Dirlikov et al., 2015). There also appear to be differences in white matter whereby boys with ADHD are more affected in areas associated with control of basic actions, while girls have more deviations in regions associated with higher-level control (Jacobson et al., 2015). Whilst male–female differences have also been demonstrated in several functional imaging and EEG studies, these data are sparse and it is too early to focus on them.

As androgens play a significant role in determining the sex differences seen in normal brain development, it is possible, perhaps even likely, that they also play an important part in the differences seen in ADHD. They have also been shown to have strong downstream effects on the receptor density, distribution, and activity of several of the neurotransmitter systems likely to be involved in ADHD. These include the dopaminergic, GABAergic, and glutamatergic systems and serotonin (Waddell and McCarthy, 2012; Gillies et al., 2014). Whilst there is some evidence to suggest a role for antenatal androgen exposure influencing the development of autism, direct evidence for effects in ADHD is still lacking. One study that hypothesized that female twins with a male co-twin would have higher rates of ADHD due to being exposed to higher levels of androgens during gestation than would be the case for a female twin with a female co-twin actually found the opposite to be true (Eriksson et al., 2016). Whilst a study of women with polycystic ovary syndrome (PCOS), which is associated with high androgen levels, did find that, whilst these women compared to healthy controls did in fact have higher levels of ADHD symptoms, there was no correlation between levels of hormone and ADHD symptoms (Herguner et al.,

2015). Taken together we are still a long way from identifying the biological factors that result in the increased rates of ADHD in males that are consistently found in child and adolescent samples.

Recognition and Referral

Notwithstanding the epidemiological evidence for increased rates of ADHD in males at the population level, these differences are inflated in clinical samples, suggesting that there are also differences in recognition, referral, and diagnosis. It is likely that this results from several additive factors acting at different points along the referral pathway. Perhaps the most obvious of these is a sampling bias that arises due to higher rates of hyperactive, impulsive, and overtly disruptive behaviours in boys in general and in those with ADHD in particular (Sassi, 2010; Gaub and Carlson, 1997). These behaviours are more likely to bring boys with ADHD to the attention of parents, teachers, and others in the community than a girl, who is more likely to be inattentive, sitting quietly distracted at the back of the class. On the other hand it may be the case that an initial focus on ADHD in boys biased the information used to create the clinical criteria for ADHD (Arnett et al., 2015), which were originally designed to describe the symptoms in boys aged 7 to 11 years (Laufer and Denhoff, 1957). Whilst this does not invalidate the ADHD diagnosis, it does question whether the current description is broad enough or accurate enough to properly identify girls with ADHD. Several authors have suggested that slightly lowering the number of symptoms required for ADHD diagnosis for girls, as has been done for adults, may result in a prevalence rate that is similar to that of boys (Hudziak et al., 2007; Rohde, 2008; Waschbusch and King, 2006). The DSM committee did consider sex-specific criteria for ADHD but in the end decided that there is not yet enough evidence to support such a significant change. However, it remains an important open question that has the potential to impact significantly on clinical practice.

Assessment and Clinical Management

Children and Adolescents

The key aspects of assessment and management of ADHD do not differ between the sexes. Whilst it is likely that assessment for males will focus more on externalizing symptoms and behaviours than on depression, anxiety, and trauma-related symptoms, these latter symptoms, whilst more common in females, are not uncommon in males and should be screened for in all cases. One of the essential points to keep in mind when assessing someone for ADHD is that this is a mental health assessment rather than an ADHD assessment. The aims are not only to assess whether or not patients meet the diagnostic criteria for ADHD but also to distinguish ADHD from other disorders and exclude other explanations for the presenting behaviours and then to assess whether patients are suffering from any co-morbid disorders (see Box 3.4 for a suggested approach to assessment in children and adolescents; Coghill, 2015). In order to fulfil these requirements the assessment needs to be comprehensive enough to develop a formulation that fully explains a person's strengths and difficulties. This process also requires skill, specialist training, and experience with a broad range of mental health and developmental disorders. It is therefore often best conducted jointly by members of a multidisciplinary team. Ideally such a team will include (or at least have good access to) mental health, paediatric, clinical psychology, and neuropsychological and occupational therapy skills, and have access to speech and language therapy, family/systemic therapy, physiotherapy, and educational skills. A good-quality full assessment takes time and cannot normally be completed in a single meeting. Whilst the full assessment should be seen as a whole it can also be broken down into several key 'tasks'.

The basis for assessment consists of a patient's history, observation of the patient's current behaviour, and the account of parents and teachers about the child's functioning in his or her places. It is not uncommon for there to be differences between informants (children, parents, and teachers) about their perceptions of the child's mental health. Children often do not reliably inform about their own behavioural symptoms and have low test–retest agreement for ADHD symptoms. They can, however, make invaluable comments about other aspects of their life and their inner worlds. Parents seem to be good informants with respect to ADHD symptoms but often are less accurate at describing emotional difficulties.

It is invaluable to also have the views of another person outside of the family. For children and adolescents this is usually a teacher. Sometimes teachers have a tendency to overestimate the presence of ADHD symptoms. This is especially the case for

Box 3.4 ADHD assessment (child and adolescent)

Clinicians involved	Child and Adolescent Mental Health Services (CAMHS) Developmental/behavioural paediatrics
Aims	To assess whether or not patient meets diagnostic criteria for ADHD To distinguish ADHD from other disorders and exclude other explanations for behaviours To assess whether patient is suffering from any co-morbid disorders
Recommended assessment	A full assessment should be conducted. This will require more than one meeting and should include: • Clinical interview with the parents • A separate interview with the child • Preschool, kindergarten, and school information • School observation if required • Physical evaluation and investigations • Intelligence/cognitive tests if there is a specific indication
Outcomes	Confirmation or exclusion of an ADHD diagnosis In cases where ADHD is confirmed there should also be confirmation or exclusion of any co-morbid disorders In cases where a diagnosis of ADHD is excluded there should be a formulation of an alternative explanation for the presentation

boys when there are other disruptive behavioural problems. At other times some teachers can minimize a child's difficulties as they want to avoid them being labelled as having ADHD. With adolescents, the value of the information given by teachers can be less consistent. Teens have several teachers, each of whom spends little time with each class, which can prevent them from knowing each student well enough to comment accurately. However, the process of diagnostic evaluation necessarily involves collection of data from each of these sources as each can provide complementary information. A detailed discussion of the assessment process is outside the scope of this chapter but can be found in several short (Coghill, 2015) and longer (Danckaerts and Coghill, 2018) texts.

Assessment of Adults

Assessment in adults follows a similar pattern to other adult mental health assessments. Many adult psychiatrists worry about their ability to conduct an ADHD assessment. However, the skills are the same required for the more familiar assessments conducted every day for other disorders. Just like other mental health disorders, ADHD is a clinical and behavioural phenotype and is best evaluated by clinical diagnostic interview, with supporting evidence from informants, such as parents or siblings, concerning childhood symptoms, or a partner for current symptoms and functional impairment. Unlike most other adult mental health disorders, the symptoms of ADHD do not usually reflect changes from the premorbid mental state. Rather, they more commonly present as enduring traits sustained throughout development. It is therefore important when assessing an adult for ADHD to ask about both current and retrospective behaviours and mental state, including a developmental history of the onset and development of the symptoms and impairments over time. The most characteristic clinical picture is of the onset of symptoms and impairment during early to middle childhood, with persistence of similar symptoms and impairments to the time of the assessment as an adult.

There are now reliable ADHD screening tools for adults. The best-known and most widely used is the Adult ADHD Self-Report Scale (ASRS), which has been updated and validated for DSM-5 (Ustun et al., 2017). The full version includes the full DSM 18-items reworded to reflect the DSM-5 definition for adults. There is an embedded short version consisting of a subset of only six items that has been shown to have good sensitivity and specificity when used in community surveys. Although sensitivity is high, specificity may be low in some groups, such as those with co-morbid disorders such as SUDs (van de Glind et al., 2013). Screening instruments and rating scales are helpful but should never be used on their own to establish the diagnosis as there will always be a proportion of cases either wrongly identified or missed. As in children, the diagnosis remains a clinical one and is established following a detailed clinical assessment. Currently many practicing clinicians were not trained to assess ADHD during their specialist training. It is therefore helpful that there are now several good semi-structured interviews that can help guide questioning until the script becomes internalized just like the other parts of the assessment. The two most widely used interviews used are the Conners Adult ADHD Diagnostic Interview for DSM-IV (CAADID) (Epstein et al., 2001), and the Diagnostic Interview for ADHD in Adults (DIVA), which has just been updated to reflect the changes in DSM-5 (Kooij, 2019; www.divacenter.eu). Parents and older siblings are useful informants when asking about symptoms during childhood and adolescence. Partners can be very helpful in providing information about current symptoms and behaviours.

Whilst it can, at first, be difficult to distinguish ADHD symptoms from those of other common mental health disorders, with experience this generally becomes no more or less complicated than those seen for other mental health conditions. One important issue for assessment in adults that has been highlighted by Asherson (2015) is that symptoms of ADHD can mimic symptoms of other disorders (Box 3.5). Notably, some of these symptoms that overlap with other conditions are not included as core symptoms of ADHD. They do, however, commonly accompany ADHD in adults. Examples are initial insomnia, restless sleep, emotional dysregulation, mental restlessness, and restless agitation. When making the assessment it is important to keep in mind that these overlaps are common and, even though you may more commonly

assign them to the other disorder, they are often related to ADHD. Asherson also points out that ADHD should be seen as a developmental risk factor for other disorders, including anxiety, depression, bipolar disorder, borderline and antisocial personality disorder, and alcohol and drug dependency. There are multiple mechanisms by which these risks are mediated, which include: shared genetic and environmental risk factors; increased exposure to risky environments for other disorders (e.g. repeated educational and social failures); increasing the impact of other risk factors (e.g. children with ADHD and the COMT genotype are more likely to develop antisocial behavioural problems, an effect that is not seen in the non-ADHD population). Whilst it is again beyond the scope of this chapter to give a full description of the assessment process for adults with ADHD, this information can readily be found in other texts (Kooij et al., 2018; Asherson, 2015).

Treatment and Management of ADHD

A full discussion of the treatment and management of ADHD is also outside the scope of this chapter. For children and adolescents the reader interested to know more is directed to Zuddas et al. (2018), Coghill and Danckaerts (2018), Dopfner (2015), and for adults Asherson (2015), and Asherson and J. A. (2018).

There is no strong evidence to support the use of different treatment strategies for males and females with ADHD. Whilst there is some limited evidence for slight differences in pharmacodynamic responses to psychostimulants between the sexes (Cornforth et al., 2010), these are relatively minor and do not impact on clinical practice in a meaningful way. Despite all the treatment guidelines for ADHD stressing the importance of high-quality psychoeducation

Box 3.5	Symptoms associated with ADHD that mimic other disorders
Disorder	**Symptoms**
Anxiety	Mental restlessness, ceaseless thoughts, restlessness, poor sleep, avoidance of situations (e.g. queues, social situations)
Depression	Initial insomnia and restless sleep, impulsive eating, low self-esteem, unstable moods, impatience and irritability, concentration problems
Borderline personality disorder	Chronic symptoms emerge from childhood/adolescence, impulsive behaviour, mood instability, angry outbursts, impaired social relationships
Bipolar disorder	Mood instability, motor restlessness, mental restlessness and distractible mind, distractibility and difficulty concentration, over-talkativeness

for both the patient and their families, this is not well operationalized and the effects of standardized measurement-based approaches are not well studied. However, it is very important that clinicians treating ADHD have a strong understanding of the disorder to be able to help patients make fully informed decisions about their care.

Although there were historical differences between the approach to treatment of ADHD in the USA and Europe, with the USA favouring medication as a first-line treatment whilst in Europe clinicians tended to start with a non-pharmacological treatment (parent training for children, cognitive behavioural approaches for adolescents and adults), this has started to change. Many of these changes arose after the publication of an influential systematic review that presented the findings from a series of meta-analyses that investigated the evidence for efficacy across a range of non-pharmacological treatments (Sonuga-Barke et al., 2013). This review concluded that, when blinded ratings were considered, whilst there was some evidence to support removal of artificial food colourings (effect size 0.42) and omega 3 fatty acids (effects size 0.16), there was no evidence to support an effect on core ADHD symptoms for restrictive elimination diets, cognitive training, neurofeedback, or, very surprisingly, parent training. Whilst parent training did not improve ADHD per se, subsequent analyses demonstrated that it does result in more positive and less negative parenting and improves oppositional behaviours (Daley et al., 2018). These findings have had a significant impact on attitudes and treatment guidelines in Europe. NICE, who in their 2008 guidelines were clear that parent training should be the first-line treatment for ADHD with medication reserved for those with the most problematic form of the condition, now recommend that if symptoms remained after psychoeducation and environmental adaptations, medication should be considered as a first-line treatment for all ADHD (NICE, 2018). This brings NICE much closer to the US guidelines than previously. Whilst not all guidelines have been quite as radical, it is generally accepted now that medication, usually psychostimulant medication, is an integral part of the treatment of most of those with ADHD.

The evidence for short-term efficacy of ADHD medications, at least in the short term, is strong, as evidenced by a recent network meta-analysis (Cortese et al., 2018). Whilst there is some variation in availability across the world, the main medications licensed for ADHD are methylphenidate, the amphetamines (dexamphetamine, and in the USA mixed amphetamine salts), the amphetamine prodrug lisdexamfetamine, and the non-stimulant medications atomoxetine and extended release guanfacine (as well as extended release clonidine in the USA). The stimulants and atomoxetine all block reuptake of dopamine and noradrenaline whilst guanfacine and clonidine are noradrenaline alpha2 agonists. The effect sizes in children with ADHD for the stimulants are amongst the largest for any medication (depending on how measured between 0.8 and 1.0), and whilst the non-stimulant medications are less efficacious (effect size around 0.7), they are still highly effective when compared to other psychiatric medications. The effect sizes for adults are lower (around 0.5–0.8 for the stimulants and 0.45 for atomoxetine) but still very respectable. The usual recommendation is to start with one of the psychostimulants (methylphenidate or an amphetamine derivative). It is not yet possible to predict who will respond to which psychostimulant so the choice is with the clinician guided by availability and cost. Around 70% of those with ADHD have a strong response to methylphenidate and 70% to an amphetamine with between 90% and 95% responding well to one or the other (Hodgkins et al., 2012). It is therefore always worth trying the other medication if the first has not been effective. For those with a partial response to a stimulant it is now possible in some countries to try adding guanfacine as an adjunctive treatment. This is safer than adding another stimulant or atomoxetine, both of which run the risk of increased adverse effects, and in particular increased blood pressure and heart rate. Where a stimulant is unsuitable, not tolerated, or refused, either atomoxetine or guanfacine are options. Their onset of action is not as quick as for the psychostimulants and it is important to warn the patient of this and indicate that effects will increase over time. In our clinic we suggest at least twelve weeks on the therapeutic dose (1.2 mg/kg up to 100 mg maximum) for atomoxetine and between four to six weeks at 3 mg/day for guanfacine. Although many patients benefit from medication, few doctors currently follow a structured protocol with routine evaluation of both positive and negative responses to treatment. A structured approach to titration is the best was to optimize initial treatment response and evidence is starting to emerge that continued routine use of measurement-based care based on rating scales, preferably delivered face to face in an interview format, can significantly improve both short- and long-term treatment outcomes (Coghill and Seth, 2015). This is exceedingly important as when a less structured approach is used, long-term outcomes are not as positive as would be predicted from the short-term efficacy data (Swanson et al., 2018).

Reduction of core ADHD symptoms is an important first step in the management of ADHD. However, on its own it is not usually sufficient. A holistic approach to management is always appropriate and requires consideration of a much broader range of symptoms and problems, including co-morbid disorders and substance use problems, other developmental disorders and disabilities, academic and work-related problems, parent–child, sibling, and spousal relationships and communication problems, peer relationship difficulties, and offending behaviours. The ultimate aim is to improve functioning and quality of life. Typically this will require a carefully coordinated multi-professional, multidisciplinary, and multiagency approach.

Conclusions

ADHD is a common and disabling disorder that will often persist into adulthood and can cause considerable life problems over the whole lifespan. ADHD is one of the few mental health problems that is more common in males than females, although the reasons for this are still not well understood. Outside the USA, ADHD is still under-recognized and under-treated. Although ADHD is very treatable, with very strong effect sizes for medications, long-term outcomes are currently poor with high rates of other psychiatric disorders, substance misuse, criminality, relationship problems, and mortality. Those with ADHD also have lower than expected academic and employment outcomes. It is likely that these poor outcomes could be improved by increased recognition and treatment protocols that aim to optimize treatment based on routine outcome measurement and monitoring of adverse effects.

References

Arnett, A. B., Pennington, B. F., Willcutt, E. G., Defries, J. C., and Olson, R. K. 2015. Sex differences in ADHD symptom severity. *J Child Psychol Psychiatry*, 56, 632–9.

Asherson, P. 2015. ADHD in Adults. In: Banaschewski, T., Zuddas, A., Asherson, P., Buitelaar, J., Coghill, D., Danckaerts, M., Dopfner, M., Rohde, L. A., Sonuga-Barke, E., and Taylor, E. (eds) *ADHD and Hyperkinetic Disorder*. Oxford: Oxford University Press.

Asherson, P. and J. A., R. Q. 2018. Treatment in adults ADHD. In: Banaschewski, T., Coghill, D., and Zuddas, A. (eds) *Oxford Textbook of ADHD*. Oxford: Oxford University Press.

Coghill, D. 2015. Assessment. In: Banaschewski, T., Zuddas, A., Asherson, P., Buitelaar, J., Coghill, D., Danckaerts, M., Dopfner, M., Rohde, L. A., Sonuga-Barke, E., and Taylor, E. (eds) *ADHD and Hyperkinetic Disorder*. 2 ed. Oxford: Oxford University Press.

Coghill, D., Asherson, P., Faraone, S. V., and Rohde, L. A. 2018. The age of onset of attention-deficit hyperactivity disorder. In: De Girolamo, G., Mcgorry, P. D., and Sartorius, N. (eds) *Age of Onset of Mental Disorders: Etiopathogenetic and Treatment Implications*. New York: Springer.

Coghill, D. and Danckaerts, M. 2018. Organizing and delivering treatment for ADHD. In: Banaschewski, T., Coghill, D., and Zuddas, A. (eds) *Oxford Textbook for ADHD*. Oxford: Oxford University Press.

Coghill, D. and Hodgkins, P. 2016. Health-related quality of life of children with attention-deficit/ hyperactivity disorder versus children with diabetes and healthy controls. *Eur Child Adolesc Psychiatry*, 25, 261–71.

Coghill, D., Rohde, L. A., and Banaschewski, T. 2008. Attention-deficit/hyperactivity disorder. In: T. Banaschewski and L. A. Rohde (eds.) *Biological Child Psychiatry Recent Trends and Developments*. Basel: Karger, pp. 1–20.

Coghill, D. and Seth, S. 2015. Effective management of attention-deficit/ hyperactivity disorder (ADHD) through structured re-assessment: the Dundee ADHD Clinical Care Pathway. *Child Adolesc Psychiatry Ment Health*, 9, 52.

Cornforth, C., Sonuga-Barke, E., and Coghill, D. 2010. Stimulant drug effects on attention deficit/ hyperactivity disorder: a review of the effects of age and sex of patients. *Curr Pharm Des*, 16, 2424-33.

Cortese, S., Adamo, N., Del Giovane, C., Mohr-Jensen, C., Hayes, A. J., Carucci, S., Atkinson, L. Z., Tessari, L., Banaschewski, T., Coghill, D., Hollis, C., Simonoff, E., Zuddas, A., Barbui, C., Purgato, M., Steinhausen, H. C., Shokraneh, F., Xia, J., and Cipriani, A. 2018. Comparative efficacy and tolerability of medications for attention-deficit hyperactivity disorder in children, adolescents, and adults: a systematic review and network meta-analysis. *Lancet Psychiatry*, 5, 727–38.

Daley, D., Van Der Oord, S., Ferrin, M., Cortese, S., Danckaerts, M., Doepfner, M., Van Den Hoofdakker, B. J., Coghill, D., Thompson, M., Asherson, P., Banaschewski, T., Brandeis, D., Buitelaar, J., Dittmann, R. W., Hollis, C., Holtmann, M., Konofal, E., Lecendreux, M., Rothenberger, A., Santosh, P., Simonoff, E., Soutullo, C., Steinhausen, H. C., Stringaris, A., Taylor, E., Wong, I. C. K., Zuddas, A., and Sonuga-Barke, E. J. 2018. Practitioner review: current best practice in the use of parent training and other behavioural interventions in the treatment of children and adolescents with attention deficit hyperactivity disorder. *J Child Psychol Psychiatry*, 59(9), 932–47.

Dalsgaard, S., Mortensen, P. B., Frydenberg, M., and Thomsen, P. H. 2013. Long-term criminal outcome of children with attention deficit hyperactivity disorder. *Crim Behav Ment Health*, 23, 86–98.

Dalsgaard, S., Ostergaard, S. D., Leckman, J. F., Mortensen, P. B., and Pedersen, M. G. 2015. Mortality in children, adolescents, and adults with attention deficit hyperactivity disorder: a nationwide cohort study. *Lancet*, 385, 2190–6.

Danckaerts, M. and Coghill, D. 2018. Children and adolescents: assessment in everyday clinical practice. In: Banaschewski, T., Coghill, D., and Zuddas, A. (eds) *Oxford Textbook of Attention Deficit Hyperactivity Disorder*. Oxford: Oxford University Press.

Danckaerts, M., Sonuga-Barke, E. J., Banaschewski, T., Buitelaar, J., Dopfner, M., Hollis, C., Santosh, P., Rothenberger, A., Sergeant, J., Steinhausen, H. C., Taylor, E., Zuddas, A., and Coghill, D. 2010. The quality of life of children with

attention deficit/hyperactivity disorder: a systematic review. *Eur Child Adolesc Psychiatry*, 19, 83–105.

Danielson, M. L., Bitsko, R. H., Ghandour, R. M., Holbrook, J. R., Kogan, M. D., and Blumberg, S. J. 2018. Prevalence of parent-reported ADHD diagnosis and associated treatment among U.S. children and adolescents, 2016. *J Clin Child Adolesc Psychol*, 47, 199–212.

Davies, W. 2014. Sex differences in Attention Deficit Hyperactivity Disorder: Candidate genetic and endocrine mechanisms. *Front Neuroendocrinol*, 35(3), 331–46.

Dirlikov, B., Shiels Rosch, K., Crocetti, D., Denckla, M. B., Mahone, E. M., and Mostofsky, S. H. 2015. Distinct frontal lobe morphology in girls and boys with ADHD. *Neuroimage Clin*, 7, 222–9.

Dopfner, M. 2015. Psychosocial and other non-pharmacological treatments. In: Banaschewski, T., Zuddas, A., Asherson, P., Buitelaar, J., Coghill, D., Danckaerts, M., Dopfner, M., Rohde, L. A., Sonuga-Barke, E., and Taylor, E. (eds) *ADHD and Hyperkinetic Disorder*. 2nd ed. Oxford: Oxford University Press.

Dopfner, M., Breuer, D., Wille, N., Erhart, M., and Ravens-Sieberer, U. 2008. How often do children meet ICD-10/DSM-IV criteria of attention deficit-/hyperactivity disorder and hyperkinetic disorder? Parent-based prevalence rates in a national sample – results of the BELLA study. *Eur Child Adolesc Psychiatry*, 17 Suppl 1, 59–70.

Durston, S., Hulshoff Pol, H. E., Casey, B. J., Giedd, J. N., Buitelaar, J. K., and Van Engeland, H. 2001. Anatomical MRI of the developing human brain: what have we learned? *J Am Acad Child Adolesc Psychiatry*, 40, 1012–20.

Epstein, J. N., Johnson, D. E., and Conners, C. K. 2001. *CAADID: Conners Adult ADHD Diagnstic Interview for DSM-IV*. Toronto: Multi Health Systems.

Eriksson, J. M., Lundstrom, S., Lichtenstein, P., Bejerot, S., and Eriksson, E. 2016. Effect of co-twin gender on neurodevelopmental symptoms: a twin register study. *Mol Autism*, 7, 8.

Faraone, S. V., Asherson, P., Banaschewski, T., Biederman, J., Buitelaar, J. K., Ramos-Quiroga, J. A., Rohde, L. A., Sonuga-Barke, E. J. S., Tannock, R., and Franke, B. 2015. Attention-deficit/hyperactivity disorder. *Nature Reviews Disease Primers*, 1, 15020.

Faraone, S. V., Biederman, J., and Mick, E. 2006. The age-dependent decline of attention deficit hyperactivity disorder: a meta-analysis of follow-up studies. *Psychol Med*, 36, 159–65.

Fedele, D. A., Lefler, E. K., Hartung, C. M., and Canu, W. H. 2012. Sex differences in the manifestation of ADHD in emerging adults. *J Atten Disord*, 16, 109–17.

Gaub, M. and Carlson, C. L. 1997. Gender differences in ADHD: a meta-analysis and critical review. *J Am Acad Child Adolesc Psychiatry*, 36, 1036–45.

Gershon, J. 2002. Meta-analysis gender differences ADHD. *J Atten Disord*, 5, 143–54.

Gillies, G. E., Virdee, K., Mcarthur, S., and Dalley, J. W. 2014. Sex-dependent diversity in ventral tegmental dopaminergic neurons and developmental programing: a molecular, cellular and behavioral analysis. *Neuroscience*, 282(special issue), 69–85.

Gomez, R. 2013. ADHD and Hyperkinetic Disorder Symptoms in Australian adults: descriptive scores, incidence rates, factor structure, and gender invariance. *J Atten Disord*, 20(4), 325–34.

Graetz, B. W., Sawyer, M. G., and Baghurst, P. 2005. Gender differences among children with DSM-IV ADHD in Australia. *J Am Acad Child Adolesc Psychiatry*, 44, 159–68.

Greven, C., Richards, J., and Buitelaar, J. 2018. Sex differences in ADHD. In: Banaschewski, T., Coghill, D., and Zuddas, A. (eds) *Oxford Textbook of ADHD*. Oxford: Oxford University press.

Greven, C. U., Rijsdijk, F. V., and Plomin, R. 2011. A twin study of ADHD symptoms in early adolescence: hyperactivity-impulsivity and inattentiveness show substantial genetic overlap but also genetic specificity. *J Abnorm Child Psychol*, 39, 265–75.

Healthcare Improvement Scotland. 2012. *Attention Deficit and Hyperkinetic Disorders: Services Over Scotland*. Edinburgh: NHS Scotland.

Herguner, S., Harmanci, H., and Toy, H. 2015. Attention deficit-hyperactivity disorder symptoms in women with polycystic ovary syndrome. *Int J Psychiatry Med*, 50, 317–25.

Hervey, A. S., Epstein, J. N., and Curry, J. F. 2004. Neuropsychology of adults with attention-deficit/hyperactivity disorder: a meta-analytic review. *Neuropsychology*, 18, 485–503.

Hodgkins, P., Shaw, M., Coghill, D., and Hechtman, L. 2012. Amfetamine and methylphenidate medications for attention-deficit/hyperactivity disorder: complementary treatment options. *Eur Child Adolesc Psychiatry*, 21, 477–92.

Holden, S. E., Jenkins-Jones, S., Poole, C. D., Morgan, C. L., Coghill, D., and Currie, C. J. 2013. The prevalence and incidence, resource use and financial costs of treating people with attention deficit/hyperactivity disorder (ADHD) in the United Kingdom (1998 to 2010). *Child Adolesc Psychiatry Ment Health*, 7, 34.

Hudziak, J. J., Achenbach, T. M., Althoff, R. R., and Pine, D. S. 2007. A dimensional approach to developmental psychopathology. *Int J Methods Psychiatr Res*, 16 Suppl 1, S16–S23.

Jacobson, L. A., Peterson, D. J., Rosch, K. S., Crocetti, D., Mori, S., and Mostofsky, S. H. 2015. Sex-based dissociation of white matter microstructure in children with attention-deficit/hyperactivity disorder. *J Am Acad Child Adolesc Psychiatry*, 54, 938–46.

Jensen, C. M. and Steinhausen, H. C. 2015. Comorbid mental disorders in children and adolescents with attention-deficit/hyperactivity disorder in a large nationwide study. *Atten Defic Hyperact Disord*, 7, 27–38.

Jin, W., Du, Y., Zhong, X., and Coghill, D. 2013. Prevalence and contributing factors to attention deficit hyperactivity disorder: A study of five- to fifteen-year-old children in Zhabei District, Shanghai. *Asia Pac Psychiatry*, 6(4), 397–404.

Jonsson, U., Alaie, I., Lofgren Wilteus, A., Zander, E., Marschik, P. B., Coghill, D., and Bolte, S. 2017. Annual research review: quality of life and childhood mental and behavioural disorders – a critical review of the research. *J Child Psychol Psychiatry*, 58, 439–69.

Kan, K. J., Dolan, C. V., Nivard, M. G., Middeldorp, C. M., Van Beijsterveldt, C. E., Willemsen, G., and Boomsma, D. I. 2013. Genetic and environmental stability in attention problems across the lifespan: evidence from the Netherlands twin register. *J Am Acad Child Adolesc Psychiatry*, 52, 12–25.

Kessler, R. C., Adler, L., Barkley, R., Biederman, J., Conners, C. K., Demler, O., Faraone, S. V., Greenhill, L. L., Howes, M. J., Secnik, K., Spencer, T., Ustun, T. B., Walters, E. E., and Zaslavsky, A. M. 2006. The prevalence and correlates of adult ADHD in the United States: results from the National Comorbidity Survey Replication. *Am J Psychiatry*, 163, 716–23.

Kooij, J. J. 2012. *Adult ADHD: Diagnostic Assessment and Treatment*. New York: Springer.

Kooij, S. 2019. DIVA 2.0 the structured Diagnostic Interview for Adult ADHD. www.divacenter.eu (accessed 13 September 2020).

Kooij, S., Asherson, P., and Rosler, M. 2018. ADHD in adults: assessment issues. In: Banaschewski, T., Coghill, D., and Zuddas, A. (eds) *Oxford Textbook of ADHD*. Oxford: Oxford University Press.

Larsson, H., Asherson, P., Chang, Z., Ljung, T., Friedrichs, B., Larsson, J. O., and Lichtenstein, P. 2013. Genetic and environmental influences on adult attention deficit hyperactivity disorder symptoms: a large Swedish population-based study of twins. *Psychol Med*, 43, 197–207.

Laufer, M. W. and Denhoff, E. 1957. Hyperkinetic behavior syndrome in children. *J Pediatr*, 50, 463–74.

Lee, S. S., Humphreys, K. L., Flory, K., Liu, R., and Glass, K. 2011. Prospective association of childhood attention-deficit/hyperactivity disorder (ADHD) and substance use and abuse/dependence: a meta-analytic review. *Clin Psychol Rev*, 31, 328–41.

Lichtenstein, P., Halldner, L., Zetterqvist, J., Sjolander, A., Serlachius, E., Fazel, S., Langstrom, N., and Larsson, H. 2012. Medication for attention deficit-hyperactivity disorder and criminality. *N Engl J Med*, 367, 2006–14.

Loke, H., Harley, V., and Lee, J. 2015. Biological factors underlying sex differences in neurological disorders. *Int J Biochem Cell Biol*, 65, 139–50.

Mahone, E. M., Ranta, M. E., Crocetti, D., O'Brien, J., Kaufmann, W. E., Denckla, M. B., and Mostofsky, S. H. 2011. Comprehensive examination of frontal regions in boys and girls with attention-deficit/hyperactivity disorder. *J Int Neuropsychol Soc*, 17, 1047–57.

Matte, B., Anselmi, L., Salum, G. A., Kieling, C., Goncalves, H., Menezes, A., Grevet, E. H., and Rohde, L. A. 2015. ADHD in DSM-5: a field trial in a large, representative sample of 18- to 19-year-old adults. *Psychol Med*, 45, 361–73.

MTA Cooperative Group 1999. A 14-month randomized clinical trial of treatment strategies for attention-deficit/hyperactivity disorder. Multimodal treatment study of children with ADHD. *Arch Gen Psychiatry*, 56, 1073–86.

NICE 2008. *Attention Deficit Hyperactivity Disorder Diagnosis and Management of ADHD in Children, Young People and Adults.* London: National Institute for Health and Clinical Excellence.

NICE 2018. *Attention Deficit Hyperactivity Disorder: Diagnosis and Management.* Nice Guideline 87. London: National Institute for Health and Clinical Excellence.

Nikolas, M. A. and Burt, S. A. 2010. Genetic and environmental influences on ADHD symptom dimensions of inattention and hyperactivity: a meta-analysis. *J Abnorm Psychol*, 119, 1–17.

Novik, T. S., Hervas, A., Ralston, S. J., Dalsgaard, S., Rodrigues Pereira, R., and Lorenzo, M. J. 2006. Influence of gender on attention-deficit/hyperactivity disorder in Europe – ADORE. *European Child and Adolescent Psychiatry*, 15 Suppl 1, 115–24.

Nussbaum, N. L. 2012. ADHD and female specific concerns: a review of the literature and clinical implications. *J Atten Disord*, 16, 87–100.

Polanczyk, G., de Lima, M. S., Horta, B. L., Biederman, J., and Rohde, L. A. 2007. The worldwide prevalence of ADHD: a systematic review and metaregression analysis. *Am J Psychiatry*, 164, 942–8.

Polanczyk, G. V., Willcutt, E. G., Salum, G. A., Kieling, C., and Rohde, L. A. 2014. ADHD prevalence estimates across three decades: an updated systematic review and meta-regression analysis. *Int J Epidemiol*, 43(2), 434–42.

Quintero, J., Ramos-Quiroga, J. A., Sebastian, J. S., Montanes, F., Fernandez-Jaen, A., Martinez-Raga, J., Giral, M. G., Graell, M., Mardomingo, M. J., Soutullo, C., Eiris, J., Tellez, M., Pamias, M., Correas, J., Sabate, J., Garcia-Orti, L., and Alda, J. A. 2018. Health care and societal costs of the management of children and adolescents with attention-deficit/hyperactivity disorder in Spain: a descriptive analysis. *BMC Psychiatry*, 18, 40.

Raman, S. R., Man, K. K. C., Bahmanyar, S., Berard, A., Bilder, S., Boukhris, T., Bushnell, G., Crystal, S., Furu, K., Kaoyang, Y. H., Karlstad, O., Kieler, H., Kubota, K., Lai, E. C., Martikainen, J. E., Maura, G., Moore, N., Montero, D., Nakamura, H., Neumann, A., Pate, V., Pottegard, A., Pratt, N. L., Roughead, E. E., Macias Saint-Gerons, D., Sturmer, T., Su, C. C., Zoega, H., Sturkenbroom, M., Chan, E. W., Coghill, D., Ip, P., and Wong, I. C. K. 2018. Trends in attention-deficit hyperactivity disorder medication use: a retrospective observational study using population-based databases. *Lancet Psychiatry*, 5, 824–35.

Robison, R. J., Reimherr, F. W., Marchant, B. K., Faraone, S. V., Adler, L. A., and West, S. A. 2008. Gender differences in 2 clinical trials of adults with attention-deficit/hyperactivity disorder: a retrospective data analysis. *J Clin Psychiatry*, 69, 213–21.

Rohde, L. A. 2008. Is there a need to reformulate attention deficit hyperactivity disorder criteria in future nosologic classifications? *Child Adolesc Psychiatr Clin N Am*, 17, 405–20.

Rucklidge, J. J. 2010. Gender differences in attention-deficit/hyperactivity disorder. *Psychiatr Clin North Am*, 33, 357–73.

Sassi, R. B. 2010. Attention-deficit hyperactivity disorder and gender. *Arch Womens Ment Health*, 13, 29–31.

Shaw, P., Gilliam, M., Liverpool, M., Weddle, C., Malek, M., Sharp, W., Greenstein, D., Evans, A., Rapoport, J., and Giedd, J. 2011. Cortical development in typically developing children with symptoms of hyperactivity and impulsivity: support for a dimensional view of attention deficit hyperactivity disorder. *Am J Psychiatry*, 168, 143–51.

Simon, V., Czobor, P., Balint, S., Meszaros, A., and Bitter, I. 2009. Prevalence and correlates of adult attention-deficit hyperactivity disorder: meta-analysis. *Br J Psychiatry*, 194, 204–11.

Sonuga-Barke, E. J., Brandeis, D., Cortese, S., Daley, D., Ferrin, M., Holtmann, M., Stevenson, J., Danckaerts, M., Van Der Oord, S., Dopfner, M., Dittmann, R. W., Simonoff, E., Zuddas, A., Banaschewski, T., Buitelaar, J., Coghill, D., Hollis, C., Konofal, E., Lecendreux, M., Wong, I. C., Sergeant, J., and European, A. G. G. 2013. Nonpharmacological interventions for ADHD: systematic review and meta-analyses of randomized controlled trials of dietary and psychological treatments. *Am J Psychiatry*, 170, 275–89.

Souza, I., Pinheiro, M. A., Denardin, D., Mattos, P., and Rohde, L. A. 2004. Attention-deficit/hyperactivity disorder and comorbidity in Brazil: comparisons between two referred samples. *Eur Child Adolesc Psychiatry*, 13, 243–8.

Staller, J. and Faraone, S. V. 2006. Attention-deficit hyperactivity disorder in girls: epidemiology and management. *CNS Drugs*, 20, 107–23.

Steinhausen, H. C., Novik, T. S., Baldursson, G., Curatolo, P., Lorenzo, M. J., Rodrigues Pereira, R., Ralston, S. J., and Rothenberger, A. 2006.

Co-existing psychiatric problems in ADHD in the ADORE cohort. *European Child and Adolescent Psychiatry*, 15 Suppl 1, I25–9.

Swanson, J. M., Arnold, L. E., Jensen, P., Hinshaw, S. P., Hechtman, L. T., Conners, C. K., Kraemer, H. C., Wigal, T., Vitiello, B., Elliot, G. R., Abikoff, H. B., Hoza, B., Newcorn, J. H., Wells, K., Lerner, M., Molina, B. S. G., Epstein, J. N., Owens, E. B., Waxmonsky, J., Murray, D. W., Sibley, M. H., Mitchell, J. T., Roy, A., Stehli, A., and Group, M. C. 2018. Long- term outcomes in the multimodal treatment study of children with ADHD (the MTA): from beginning to end. In: Banaschewski, T., Coghill, D., and Zuddas, A. (eds) *The Oxford Textbook of ADHD*. Oxford: Oxford University Press.

Taylor, E. 2011. Antecedents of ADHD: a historical account of diagnostic concepts. *Atten Defic Hyperact Disord*, 3, 69–75.

Ustun, B., Adler, L. A., Rudin, C., Faraone, S. V., Spencer, T. J., Berglund, P., Gruber, M. J., and Kessler, R. C. 2017. The World Health Organization Adult Attention-Deficit/Hyperactivity Disorder Self-Report Screening Scale for DSM-5. *JAMA Psychiatry*, 74, 520–6.

Van De Glind, G., Van Den Brink, W., Koeter, M. W., Carpentier, P. J., Van Emmerik-Van Oortmerssen, K., Kaye, S., Skutle, A., Bu, E. T., Franck, J., Konstenius, M., Moggi, F., Dom, G., Verspreet, S., Demetrovics, Z., Kapitany-Foveny, M., Fatseas, M., Auriacombe, M., Schillinger, A., Seitz, A., Johnson, B., Faraone, S. V., Ramos-Quiroga, J. A., Casas, M., Allsop, S., Carruthers, S., Barta, C., Schoevers, R. A., Group, I. R., and Levin, F. R. 2013. Validity of the Adult ADHD Self-Report Scale (ASRS) as a screener for adult ADHD in treatment seeking substance use disorder patients. *Drug Alcohol Depend*, 132, 587–96.

Van Lieshout, M., Luman, M., Twisk, J. W., Van Ewijk, H., Groenman, A. P., Thissen, A. J., Faraone, S. V., Heslenfeld, D. J., Hartman, C. A., Hoekstra, P. J., Franke, B., Buitelaar, J. K., Rommelse, N. N., and Oosterlaan, J. 2016. A 6-year follow-up of a large European cohort of children with attention-deficit/hyperactivity disorder-combined subtype: outcomes in late adolescence and young adulthood. *Eur Child Adolesc Psychiatry*, 25, 1007–17.

Van Voorhees, E. E., Mitchell, J. T., Mcclernon, F. J., Beckham, J. C., and Kollins, S. H. 2012. Sex, ADHD symptoms, and smoking outcomes: an integrative model. *Med Hypotheses*, 78, 585–93.

Waddell, J. and Mccarthy, M. M. 2012. Sexual differentiation of the brain and ADHD: what is a sex difference in prevalence telling us? *Curr Top Behav Neurosci*, 9, 341–60.

Waschbusch, D. A. and King, S. 2006. Should sex-specific norms be used to assess attention-deficit/hyperactivity disorder or oppositional defiant disorder? *J Consult Clin Psychol*, 74, 179–85.

Wilens, T. E. 2007. The nature of the relationship between attention-deficit/hyperactivity disorder and substance use. *J Clin Psychiatry*, 68 Suppl 11, 4–8.

Willcutt, E. G. 2012. The prevalence of DSM-IV attention-deficit/hyperactivity disorder: a meta-analytic review. *Neurotherapeutics*, 9, 490–9.

Willcutt, E. G., Pennington, B. F., Chhabildas, N. A., Friedman, M. C., and Alexander, J. 1999. Psychiatric comorbidity associated with DSM-IV ADHD in a nonreferred sample of twins. *J Am Acad Child Adolesc Psychiatry*, 38, 1355–62.

Williamson, D. and Johnston, C. 2015. Gender differences in adults with attention-deficit/hyperactivity disorder: A narrative review. *Clin Psychol Rev*, 40, 15–27.

Yoshimasu, K., Barbaresi, W. J., Colligan, R. C., Voigt, R. G., Killian, J. M., Weaver, A. L., and Katusic, S. K. 2012. Childhood ADHD is strongly associated with a broad range of psychiatric disorders during adolescence: a population-based birth cohort study. *J Child Psychol Psychiatry*, 53, 1036–43.

Young, S., Moss, D., Sedgwick, O., Fridman, M., and Hodgkins, P. 2015. A meta-analysis of the prevalence of attention deficit hyperactivity disorder in incarcerated populations. *Psychological Medicine*, 45, 247–58.

Zayats, T., Johansson, S., and Haavik, J. 2015. Expanding the toolbox of ADHD genetics. How can we make sense of parent of origin effects in ADHD and related behavioral phenotypes? *Behav Brain Funct*, 11, 33.

Zuddas, A., Banaschewski, T., Coghill, D., and Stein, M. A. 2018. ADHD treatment: psychostimulants. In: Banaschewski, T., Coghill, D., and Zuddas, A. (eds) *Oxford Textbook of Attention Deficit Hyperactivity Disorder*. Oxford: Oxford University Press.

Chapter

4

Puberty and Affective Mental Illness in Males

Joe Herbert

Puberty is the major neuroendocrine cataclysm in the postnatal life of males. But it succeeds another, similar one during prenatal life, and it is impossible to understand the phenomenon of puberty fully without considering the earlier event. While testosterone is a major contributor to both events, it is not the only one. Thus, this chapter first addresses the impact of testosterone on the developing brain, before a broader consideration of puberty in males and its associations with perturbations of identity and of anxiety and mood.

Testosterone Secretion in Utero

Around 6–8 weeks in human gestation, the *sry* gene on the Y chromosome induces the formation of a testis from the primordial germ cells. The new testes promptly begin to secrete testosterone, which then acts on the developing fetus. Its first action is on the internal and external genitalia, and this encourages a male-type form but also sensitizes these tissues to later testosterone. Its action on the developing brain may occur a little later, but is no less formative. Experimental studies suggest that this results in gender-differentiated nuclei in the hypothalamus (and maybe in other parts of the limbic system). These have been described in both animals and people (Hines, 2006). The time interval between the action of testosterone on the genitalia and the brain suggests that disturbance in the latter (but not the former) might underly a transgender situation after birth. Current information does not allow us to assign a specific function to these gender-differentiated nuclei in the brain; that is, whether they are concerned with sexual orientation, gender identity, or other forms of

gender-differentiated behaviour or function (Hines, 2011; see Box 4.1).

Box 4.1 Testosterone

Secreted by testes (major) but also by adrenals (important in females)

Prenatal secretion during first trimester. Induces sex differences in brain in rodents

Low levels at birth, but rapid, temporary, increase for about 4–6 months after birth

Third surge at puberty. Moderate circadian rhythm (the highest in the morning)

Maximum levels during adolescence and early adulthood. Slow, variable decline with age

Binds (90–95%) to sex hormone binding globulin (SHBG) in blood

Only free fraction can enter brain

Converted by tissues to both dihydrotestosterone (DHT) (5α-reductase) and oestrogen (aromatase). Important for cellular actions

Binds to androgen receptor (AR). Intro-cytoplasmic, large protein, many mutations. Some alter sensitivity

Primary action on reproduction: fertility and sexual motivation

Many other actions to facilitate successful reproduction include: muscular strength, increased risk appetite, aggressiveness, growth of biological weapons in some species (claws, horns, teeth, etc.)

AR expressed by brain, primarily (but not exclusively) in limbic system (amygdala hypothalamus, hippocampus, etc.)

Prepubertal castration prevents development of sexuality

Post-pubertal castration results in slow decline, may never reach baseline

Levels responsive to environmental events (success, defeat, etc.)

I am most grateful to my colleague and friend Ian Goodyer for his helpful comments on an earlier version. Figure 4.3 is based on his original.

Recent evidence suggests that the gender-differentiating action of testosterone may be an epigenetic one. Gene expression is inhibited by methylation at CpG islands. Testosterone may remove this block in a selection of genes, resulting in the development of a male-like neural phenotype. Persistence of the block results in a female-type profile (Matsuda et al., 2012; Nugent et al., 2015).

The Androgen Receptor

The essential role of testosterone is not the result solely of altered levels during development. The role of the androgen receptor (AR) is important. Only tissues that express this large protein will respond to testosterone (e.g. penis, prostate, muscles, limbic areas of the brain). Several hundred mutations have been described in the AR (Gottlieb et al., 2012). Many have little effect, but some render the AR unresponsive to testosterone so that all the tissues, including the brain, are unaware of its presence (Kosti et al., 2019). The result is a phenotypical female, though one carrying the XY configuration, without ovaries (but with testes) or a uterus (the internal female-type organs are removed by another secretion from the testes, the Mullerian-inhibitory factor (MIF)). These androgen-insensitive females (AIS) are psychologically indistinguishable from 'normal' females, and their external genitalia are female-like (though they have a short vagina; Hines et al., 2003). Puberty does not occur. There are other factors in addition to the AR regulating the response to testosterone: a substantial proportion of AIS females do not have an AR mutation (Melo et al., 2003).

Variations in AR are also significant in postnatal responses to testosterone (Vermeersch et al., 2010). There is a CAG repeat in the first exon of the AR gene; the number of repeats is individually variable and is inversely related to sensitivity to testosterone. Hence, the response to a given level of testosterone at puberty will vary according to the number of CAG repeats in the AR. This will influence, inter alia, the effect that rising levels of testosterone have on both somatic function and behaviour.

There is a second surge of testosterone postnatally until around 24 weeks. The function of this infantile exposure to testosterone is not well understood (Alexander, 2014), though there have been suggestions that it could influence later male-type social interactions, or the growth of the penis. Unlike the first, prenatal surge, this one has no established influence on puberty or its consequences (Box 4.1).

The Onset of Puberty

The long prepubertal period in humans is due to active inhibition of neurons containing the peptide kisspeptin in the arcuate nucleus of the hypothalamus (Ojeda and Lomniczi, 2014). Puberty follows removal of this inhibition by epigenetic methylation of repressor genes, and consequent activation of kisspeptin neurons (Cortes et al., 2015). The exact mechanism that determines the timing of this event is still somewhat mysterious, but body weight and the quality of nutrition are important contributors. There are numerous neural inputs to the hypothalamus from other areas of the brain (principally the limbic system) that can also influence puberty. Kisspeptin activates GnRH neurons to stimulate the gonadotrophin-secreting cells of the anterior pituitary via the pituitary portal system. This, in turn, activates the testes to secrete increasing amounts of testosterone, with the widespread physical and behavioural changes that mark progression to the adult reproductive state (Uenoyama et al., 2019) (see Figure 4.1).

Unlike the female, in whom menarche is a convenient marker of puberty, there is no equivalent in the male. Approximate estimates are made by staging pubic hair growth or penile development (Tanner stages), and more accurate ones by measuring testosterone levels in either blood or saliva. The two sets of data are not always congruent. Not all the organizing actions of testosterone on the brain takes place in utero. Testosterone secreted during puberty has long-lasting actions on the brain; for example, prepubertal castration prevents the development of all sexual behaviour, whereas this is not always the case for post-pubertal castration (a fact well known to the Ancient Romans; Wierenga et al., 2018).

Adrenarche

Testosterone is not the only hormone to alter during early life. Dehydroepiandrosterone (DHEA: some is sulphated to DHEAS) is secreted in high amounts by the fetal zone of the adrenal gland, which involutes after birth, and acts as a major source of steroidogenesis by the placenta. Postnatal levels are very low, but increase sharply (10–14 fold) at around 8 years (adrenarche). Adrenarche precedes and is independent of puberty, though information on the mechanisms

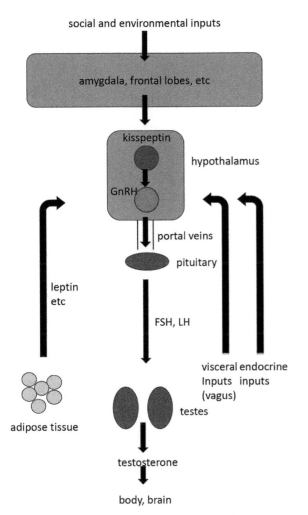

social and environmental inputs

amygdala, frontal lobes, etc

kisspeptin

hypothalamus

GnRH

portal veins

pituitary

leptin
etc

FSH, LH

adipose tissue

visceral endocrine
Inputs   inputs
(vagus)

testes

testosterone

body, brain

Figure 4.1 The mechanisms controlling the onset of puberty

> **Box 4.2   Dehydroepiandrosterone (DHEA)**
>
> Secreted from adrenal cortex innermost layer (zona reticularis)
>
> Major prenatal steroid: supplies placental steroidogenesis
>
> Mostly sulphated in plasma (DHEAS)
>
> Low levels at birth
>
> Rise at adrenarche (c. eight years)
>
> Highest blood level of any steroid
>
> Maximum levels in early 20s. Slightly higher in males
>
> Progressive decline with age. Individually variable
>
> No known receptor though may interact with sigma and GABA receptors
>
> Lowered during depression (and other illnesses)
>
> Moderates actions of glucocorticoids
>
> Stimulating action on immune system
>
> Moderates glucose metabolism (pentose shunt)
>
> Some formation within the brain
>
> Small conversion to androgens

regulating the timing of either is scanty. DHEA(S) comes from the zona reticularis of the adrenal gland, but how this is controlled is not well understood. ACTH has a minor effect on its levels. It is often called a 'weak androgen' or 'androgen precursor'. Although there is some conversion of DHEA to testosterone and other androgens, a major function is to moderate the action of cortisol, and thus have significant actions on the immune and inflammatory systems in both body and brain (Farooqi et al., 2019; Box 4.2). It is also largely responsible for the growth of pubic hair. Childhood DHEA(S) may influence the development of the brain, by encouraging plasticity and, through its known action on GABA-A and sigma receptors, influence emotions such as anxiety. It also has neuroprotective actions, moderating

toxic events (such as excess cortisol). However, it has to be acknowledged that the function of adrenarche, which is largely a primate phenomenon, is not yet well understood. DHEA(S) is also synthesized by the brain, and this contributes to its neural actions.

The activating actions of testosterone in males on behaviour during puberty thus takes place on a brain that has been organized by prior exposure to hormones, particularly testosterone, during earlier life (Berenbaum and Beltz, 2011). There will be individual variations in these formative, organizing events and those that occur later during puberty, and the behavioural outcome is an amalgam of both. These processes are further modulated by other agents, including genetic variation in AR, but also by other biological factors, many of which remain unclear. Added to these are experiential ones, such as those occurring during gestation, in early childhood, and during puberty itself. Puberty and its associated behaviours are therefore very individual sets of events (Berenbaum et al., 2015; Hodes and Epperson, 2019).

Adolescence

Adolescence as we know it is a relatively modern phenomenon. It has come about because of the progressive reduction in the age of puberty, which is largely, it is thought, one result of improved nutrition. The average age of male puberty in the nineteenth century was around 16–18 years, whereas now it is 12–14, a process that has continued during the twentieth century (Piekarski et al., 2017; Figure 4.2). This has opened a gap between maturation of the reproductive system and that of the brain, though whether there has been corresponding earlier development of the brain has not been established. The social and biological consequences of earlier puberty have been much discussed, particularly as an adaptive response to changing nutritional and family conditions (Hochberg and Belsky, 2013). Neuroimaging studies show that full maturation of the brain (particularly the frontal lobes) is not complete until the early 20s (later in boys than girls; Lenroot and Giedd, 2010). The interval between these two events is what is meant by adolescence. Pubertal testosterone acts on a brain that has yet to mature fully, and this can be held responsible for many of the behavioural features of adolescence.

Gender differences in behaviour are apparent long before puberty (for example, in patterns of play behaviour; Sandberg and Meyer-Bahlburg, 1994). How far these are the result of 'nature' (i.e. genetic or physiological factors during intra-uterine life) or 'nurture' (i.e. parental or cultural influence) has long been a topic of intense and largely fruitless debate. There is no question that the developing and infantile brain is highly susceptible to the determining actions of both. However, there is now ample evidence that genetic and other developmental events bias the environment and reaction to it that will occur later, and that this environment can influence the expression and action of genes through epigenetic mechanisms (Heim and Binder, 2012). Thus, these supposedly separate factors are actually different components of a single, complex developmental process that is responsible both for gender differences and individual patterns of neural function and behaviour.

Much of the range of behavioural characteristics of adolescence in boys can be attributed to the biological actions of testosterone (Box 4.1). In order to fulfil its primary function, enabling successful reproduction, testosterone has to activate a range of physical and behavioural features, since reproduction is a competitive and risky process (Herbert, 2017). These features include increased muscular strength (and, in other species, growth of teeth, claws, or antlers), heightened aggressiveness and competitiveness, increased appetite for taking physical risks, but a tendency to bond with other males of comparable age (Archer, 2019; Forbes and Dahl, 2010). One consequence is a tendency to band together, as in street gangs. These are particularly attractive to those from a lower socio-economic background, or from dysfunctional families. They offer companionship, security, and often financial gain, and have strict rules about membership, territoriality, loyalty, and status within the group. They are often highly hostile towards other gangs, and may be involved in criminal activities (Rowe et al., 2004). Young males from other strata of society have similar tendencies, but expressed in different ways (e.g. clubs, societies, corporate drinking, etc.).

The process of puberty includes rapid physical growth; sexually dimorphic alterations in facial structure, voice, and body; the activation of new motivations; altered sleep and circadian regulation; and a wide array of social, behavioural, and emotional changes, including heightened responses to threat and reward, social exclusion, and interactions with peers. It segues into adolescence. Adolescence is typically a time of individually variable

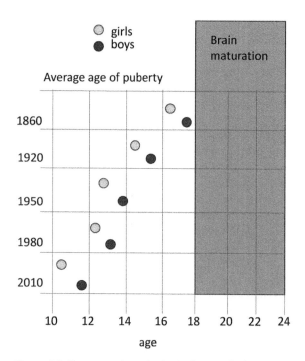

Figure 4.2 The progressive reduction in the age of puberty

psychological instability, mood disruptions, and increased risky behaviour (*Sturm und Drang*; Arnett, 1999). There is a progressive loosening of bonds with parents and family, and increased attachment to peers. This often translates into conflicts with parents (and other figures of authority), high emotional responsivity and volatility, increased tendency to rule- and law-breaking, and seeking situations of high physical or social risk (Becker, 2009). If these features were to persist during adulthood, they might well be classified as a mental disorder. Rates of crime, car accidents, drug abuse, and sexually transmitted diseases all peak in adolescence or early youth, more prominently in males than females. These features wane towards the end of adolescence (late teens, early 20s). One example, directly related to rising testosterone, is conflict over sexual issues. This involves both parents (permission etc.) and peers (the nature of interactions). Immaturity of the brain (particularly the frontal lobes) impacts individual decision-making, reflected in reduced social restraint and exacerbation of conflictual interpersonal relationships.

Sexuality and Gender

The emergence of sexuality can also pose other psychological difficulties. For example, individual realization of homosexuality can result in feelings of shame, guilt, or fear: emotions, or a state of persistent stress, that are highly influenced by the current mores of particular societies or groups within those societies. Those societies that take a more lenient view of homosexuality will reduce the likelihood of these emotional states evolving into more clinical syndromes of anxiety or depression. Fluid gender identity and dysphoria are common in very young children, and most (around 70%) will resolve. However, those that do not face both social and physical difficulties, as the individual's body transmutes at puberty into a form inconsistent with gender identity. This is the time when most transgender people seek medical advice (Costa et al., 2015).

The decision to transition socially and physically to the other gender is not always easy or simple (gender, like all other attributes, is not binary). One method of postponing the psychologically distressing effects of discordant pubertal development is to delay puberty until a more 'adult' decision can be reached (Mahfouda et al., 2017). This involves treatment with GnRH-like (agonist) compounds that prevent the expected surge in gonadotrophins. Only when they are withdrawn will puberty commence. This can be replaced by hormone treatment that aligns phenotype with gender identity. It is still controversial, though there is empirical evidence that it is safe and has psychologically beneficial results. Transgender adolescents who do not receive puberty-delaying treatment have higher rates of depression, anxiety, self-harm, and suicidal ideation (Puckett et al., 2019). Parental support can mitigate these detrimental states. Transgender children in the USA who transition socially have lower rates of anxiety and depression (which are no different from controls) than those who do not (Durwood et al., 2017).

XY babies with genetic 5α-reductase mutations (and hence deficiency in dihydrotestosterone (DHT) formation) may have female-type genitalia, and incorrect attribution of female gender at birth (Mendonca et al., 2016). There may be subsequent growth of male-type genitals (penis) at puberty. A proportion of these individuals (around 50%) are reassigned as males (Cohen-Kettenis, 2005). This raises interesting questions about the relative roles of early hormone exposure and upbringing on the formation of gender identity. As expected, males with this genetic variant have increased levels of anxiety, depression, and gender dysphoria. It should be noted that DHT seems more significant for development of the genitals than the brain, for which aromatization of testosterone to oestrogen is more important.

All transgender people, unless they choose to live simply as cross-dressers, have to deal with incongruities both in their overall body appearance (beards, breasts, etc.) and their genitalia. This involves treatment with appropriate steroids (testosterone in FtM, oestrogen and progestins in MtF), which requires medical supervision. It may also involve surgery to alter genital appearance and function and/or breast removal. The psychological outcome of these procedures, which commonly take place during adult life, depends not only on their efficacy, but also on the social and personal consequences of being transgender, which, as for homosexuality, has varied widely in different societies (Puckett et al., 2019). For a broader discussion of gender dysphoria in males, the reader is referred to Chapter 7.

Puberty and Depression

It seems reasonable to expect that the emotional and social turmoil of puberty and adolescence might increase the risk of mental disorder. About 75% of mental health problems are established by age 24 (WHO statistics). The onset of anxiety and depressive disorders peaks during adolescence and early adulthood, in males less prominently than females (Goodyer, 2003). Other diagnoses, such as bipolar disorder, do not show this gender difference (Van Meter et al., 2019). Then there are those disorders that occur before puberty, are mostly cognitive, but are more prevalent in males (e.g. autism, ADHD; see Chapters 2 and 3). Here we focus on affective disorders associated with the onset of puberty and adolescence. It is important to recognize that the likelihood of pathological events at puberty is strongly influenced by adversity in early childhood (e.g. abuse) or even during pregnancy (e.g. various kinds of maternal distress): these are discussed below.

Major depressive disorder (MDD) does occur in prepubertal children, but there are no apparent gender differences in rates. Its incidence increases sharply at puberty, more prominently in females, particularly those with a family history of MDD (Goodyer, 2003; Altemus et al., 2014). This suggests that some element of puberty is a risk factor, but that either this is greater for girls than boys, or that boys are protected to some degree from its impact (Harrington, 2003). Since the prevalence of MDD is around 1–5%, there must also be variable factors that represent risk or sensitize individuals to it. It is important to emphasize that depression is not a unitary disorder, though there is little agreement on the best ways to subdivide it (see also Chapter 12). Furthermore, there is overlap with anxiety and conduct disorders (Harrington, 2003). A major problem in defining mental disorders stems from lack of information on the pathological changes in the brain that underly depression, or their variety, and the absence of specific markers for MDD, which leaves undue reliance on symptoms or course as classifying features. There is recent evidence linking specific patterns of connections in the brain with current depression in adolescents (Mihalik et al., 2019). Risk factors are a concatenation of genetic, biological, environmental, and psychological events (Figure 4.3).

Most first episodes of MDD in pubertal or adolescent individuals follow a negative life event, usually involving a loss (such as loss of friends or pets, bereavement, bullying; Birmaher and Rozel, 2003; Figure 4.3). The converse is not true, so there are variations in the objective and subjective qualities of adverse life events, and/or individuals differ in their resilience to such events (van Harmelen et al., 2017). The perception of a negative life event is moderated both by the significance it has for the individual and by the resources they can call upon, whether psychological (e.g. family support) or concrete (e.g. financial). However, just as the impact of testosterone at puberty is moderated by previous exposure during embryonic life, so adverse events early in postnatal life (e.g. physical or psychological abuse, deprivation) can predispose a pathological, depressive response to subsequent adverse life events during puberty and adolescence (Kircanski et al., 2019).

The mechanisms underlying the sensitivity of the early brain to events in the environment remain uncertain. One contribution is the progressive development of perineuronal nets. These chondroitin sulphate proteoglycan structures surround the soma and dendrites of neurons and their appearance coincides with the end of developmental plasticity (Fawcett et al., 2019). It makes biological sense for a child's brain to be prepared for the environment in which they will live, but this can prove maladaptive. Epigenetic moderation of gene expression (for example by increased or decreased methylation or acetylation) results in long-lasting effects on behaviour and has been shown to occur in rodents following maternal deprivation (and other environmental events); one result is an exaggerated response to stress. Whether this occurs in the abused human brain is still not known, but it seems highly likely: certainly early neglect or abuse alters stress responses in later life (Garg et al., 2018; Meaney and Szyf, 2005).

More proximate psychological risk factors for MDD in young males include high levels of trait anxiety (sometimes called 'neuroticism') and a high rumination style: a tendency to focus on symptoms or features of adverse events. These psychological traits are likely to magnify the impact of adverse life events or other stressors (Wagner et al., 2015). Although they are sometimes analysed as independent variables, separating emotional and cognitive styles is not simple or precise; they interact. Furthermore, the neural mechanisms that may link these traits to events early in life are unknown.

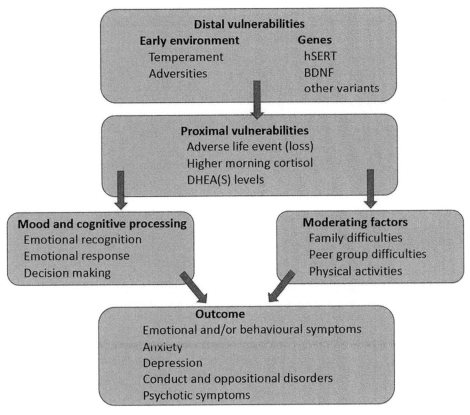

Figure 4.3 Risk and resilience factors in the onset of depression in adolescents

Endocrine Factors in the Risk for Depression

The impact of adverse life events on mood is also moderated by endocrine factors (Goodyer et al., 2003). High levels of cortisol can have damaging effects on the brain. Cushing's syndrome or the therapeutic administration of high doses of glucocorticoids can result both in affective disorder (depression) and cognitive malfunction (memory). The former tends to recover after treatment of Cushing's, the latter may not. Cortisol levels do not alter at puberty in males, nor does corticoid-binding globulin (CBG), so neither do free levels (which determine entry to the brain). However, basal cortisol levels differ between individuals (Halligan et al., 2004), and higher levels (but within the normal range) are a risk factor for subsequent MDD.

Several actions of cortisol on the brain might relate to this finding (see Box 4.3). Unlike its peripheral action, cortisol can be pro-inflammatory in the brain, activating microglia (Duque Ede and Munhoz, 2016). Elevated levels of pro-inflammatory cytokines

(e.g. IL6) are associated with increased risk for depression (Michopoulos et al., 2017) and can also be raised during an episode (Khandaker et al., 2018; Rainville and Hodes, 2019). Glucocorticoids also suppress the formation of new neurons in the hippocampus (Box 4.2), which continues in humans during adult life (Cameron and Gould, 1994) (Box 4.4). The formation of new neurons is stimulated by antidepressant drugs (e.g. selective serotonin reuptake inhibitors or SSRIs), and there are suggestions that reduced neurogenesis (which may be one result of increased inflammation) may underly the onset of MDD or its response to treatment. Testosterone has an activating effect on hippocampal neurogenesis, which might contribute to the reduced incidence of MDD in adolescent males compared to females (Duarte-Guterman et al., 2019). There are disputed reports of reduced hippocampal volumes in adults with MDD, but no evidence yet that treatment response or failure depends on changes in neurogenesis. Higher (e.g. stress-related) cortisol levels also exacerbate the actions of other toxic processes in the

---

Box 4.3 Cortisol and depression

Risk for depression

Higher morning cortisol (within normal range)

Excess cortisol (e.g. Cushing's) precipitates depression

Therapeutic corticoids increase incidence of depression

Genetic risk (small, disputed) linked to glucocorticoid receptor (GR) variants

During depression

Disturbed daily rhythm

Altered awakening effect (surge after waking)

Feedback resistance (dexamethasone test)

Neurobiology

Excess cortisol damages brain

Corticoids reduce hippocampal neurogenesis

Potentiate other toxic agents

Pro-inflammatory in the brain (microglia, cytokines)

Box 4.4 Hippocampal neurogenesis and depression

Formation of new neurons continues throughout adult life

Diminishes with age

Highly responsive to environmental events (e.g. stress)

Reduced by excess corticoids

Sensitive to serotonin

Drugs used as antidepressants stimulate neurogenesis

Intriguing parallels between factors regulating neurogenesis and those implicated in depression

No direct evidence yet of a central role in depression

Hippocampus implicated in episodic memory

---

brain ('neuroendangerment'; Sapolsky, 1996), though whether real-life adverse events raise cortisol – and if so, for how long – is not known. Male adolescents have lower levels of free cortisol than females (Netherton et al., 2004), and this might contribute to their reduced incidence of MDD, but elevated levels are a major risk for MDD in males as well as females (Owens et al., 2014). Unlike testosterone, cortisol receptors are widely distributed in the brain (Joels and de Kloet, 1994).

The actions of cortisol are, in turn, moderated by DHEA(S) (Box 4.3). DHEA levels increase rapidly during puberty (see above), only to fall progressively later in life. Both processes are individually variable. Lower levels of DHEA in adolescents, or a lower DHEA–cortisol molar ratio, predict increased risk of MDD (Goodyer et al., 2003), and this adds to the risk represented by an adverse life event. DHEA levels are also reported to be lowered during an episode of MDD, but this has not always been confirmed. Experimentally, giving DHEA to rats reduces the damaging effects of cortisol and other neurotoxins on the brain. The mechanisms of action of DHEA (S) are still not understood fully: unlike cortisol there is no identified intracellular receptor for DHEA, though it may interact with the sigma receptor (Moriguchi et al., 2013). Among its other actions, DHEA(S) acts as an anti-inflammatory agent, and can improve immune function. This may have direct relevance to a number of mental disorders related to puberty or adolescence.

Genes and Depression

MDD is moderately inheritable (*c.* 35%). Efforts to identify specific genes that might represent additional risks of mental illness during puberty and adolescence have not been very successful or consistent, though there are recent claims of improvement (Mullins and Lewis, 2017; Box 4.5). There are several reasons for this, including:

(1) MDD is not a homogenous disorder, so that including all cases will mix those with different aetiologies;

(2) Since it is likely that MDD has a polygenic foundation, very large numbers of subjects are required for genetic studies;

(3) Large-scale studies (e.g. genome-wide association studies (GWAS)) rarely take environmental factors into account, though it is likely that gene-environmental (G x E) interactions precipitate MDD;

(4) Interactions also occur between genes, and between genes and certain physiological measures (e.g. cortisol);

Heritability of depression about 30–50% (twin studies)

GWAS studies (SNPs only) either negative or show only small effects

Popular candidate genes (e.g. serotonin) generally show no association

But GWAS does not capture other variants (e.g. CNVs)

Recent identification of three phenotypes (1u7 loci)

Little consideration of environment

Candidate genes include: serotonin transporter (hSERT, 5HTT) and receptors (e.g. 5HT1A), BDNF, glucocorticoid receptor, immune-related (interleukins)

(5) GWAS are usually limited to single nucleotide polymorphisms (SNPs) and do not include other types of variation (e.g. copy number variations: CNVs). When there are positive results, they tend to show a contribution from multiple genes each with very small effects.

A highly cited paper – one of the earliest in the field – illustrates the significance of G x E interactions and the possible significance of copy number variants (CNVs; Caspi et al., 2003). Brain serotonin (the target of many anti-depressant therapies) is regulated by many processes, one being the reuptake of serotonin into presynaptic terminals. Reuptake depends on the presynaptic serotonin transporter (also called the 5HT transporter, 5HTT, SLC6A4), which has a copy number variation in the promotor region of its gene that alters its activity. This is a 44-base repeat sequence that occurs either 14 ('s') or 16 ('l') times (5HTTLPR). Late adolescent subjects experiencing increasing numbers of adverse life events had a corresponding increased incidence of depressive symptoms, but this was greatly accentuated in those possessing two 's' alleles of the 5HTT. However, two 's' alleles did not predict depression in the absence of such events. This result has not always been confirmed by others, though a large meta-analysis supported it (Karg et al., 2011; Uher and McGuffin, 2008). The point is that genetic variants alone cannot adequately explain variations in risk for mental illnesses, and appreciation of G x E interaction effects as well as developmental issues and those related to gender are crucial in this context.

The risk for MDD represented by higher morning cortisol is enhanced in those individuals with the 's' variant of the serotonin transporter (Goodyer et al., 2010). Cortisol interacts with other genetic variations. Glucocorticoids repress the formation and action of brain-derived neurotrophic factor (BDNF; Box 4.5). BDNF plays a major role in plasticity of the brain, stimulates hippocampal neurogenesis, and is thought to be involved in the onset of MDD (Zhang et al., 2016), though this depends largely on animal models of MDD, which are not very satisfactory. However, the risk for MDD in adolescents with higher morning cortisol is greater if they also possess a BDNF gene with a 'Val' variant at the Val/66/Met position (Goodyer et al., 2010). This mutation has effects on the expression and activity of BDNF.

A role for serotonin in the scale of risk for MDD fits well with its other known actions. This, however, does not imply that 'low' serotonin is the cause of depression, a view that was widely held in the 1980s but is no longer plausible (Cowen and Browning, 2015). Numerous studies have shown that variations in serotonin can alter the reactivity of the brain to incoming stimuli. The nature of the response is determined by the stimulus, but its likelihood by serotonin (among other factors). Sexual, appetitive, aggressive, and many other responses can be accentuated by lowering or blocking serotonin or its receptors, including a general tendency to react to stimuli (impulsivity), though impulsivity has many forms and a complex neural basis (Dalley and Roiser, 2012). There are essential differences between neural mechanisms that influence the level of risk for MDD from those that are responsible for its manifestation. The serotonin system encompasses a large array of post-synaptic receptors (at least 14) and much effort – mostly fruitless – has been expended trying to assign specific functions to given receptor types, given the span of action of serotonin on behaviour (Yohn et al., 2017). Serotonin receptors are active both post-synaptically and on the serotonin neurons themselves in the brain stem (sometimes with opposing actions). Considerable attention has been given to serotonin type 1A receptors in depression, but there is evidence for several others being involved (Yohn et al., 2017). Note, however, that – as already mentioned – much of this evidence is based on animal 'models' of MDD, which lack convincing validity in humans. Treatment with drugs that block the serotonin transporter (e.g. SSRIs) is likely to affect many of these receptors.

Anxiety Disorders

Anxiety disorders, which often overlap with MDD, are distinct in that anxiety (unlike depression) is a normal and necessary emotion in situations of danger, demand, threat, or uncertainty (see Chapter 9). It is when this emotional state becomes excessive, inappropriate, or disabling that it becomes a disorder. There are convincing animal models of anxiety (and fear) also unlike depression. There are several categories of anxiety disorder, including generalized, separation, claustrophobia, agoraphobia, and panic disorder. The life-changing alterations in social interactions that are precipitated by puberty are one reason why social phobia is a prominent dysfunction. The highest rates occur early in adolescence (i.e. immediately post-pubertal), sometimes remitting later. Co-morbidity between different categories of anxiety disorder is common as are other disorders such as those in eating (not considered further here, though more common in pubertal females; Ranta et al., 2017; Clarkson et al., 2019; see Chapter 8). Mean age of onset of other types of anxiety disorder may be earlier (e.g. separation) or later (e.g. panic or generalized disorders) and there are no major gender differences in rates (Lijster et al., 2017). Adolescent attitudes to others are highly influenced by relations with peers and friends, and whether they are accepted or rejected by their social groups (van Harmelen et al., 2017). It is unclear whether steroids such as testosterone have a direct effect on the liability for social phobia, or whether this is a secondary effect resulting from altered social interactions and the addition of sexual ones – both, of course, directly related to rising testosterone levels. This reservation applies to any other mental disorder that peaks at or just after puberty.

Bipolar Disorder

Bipolar disorder is highly heritable (*c.* 80%), but the gene(s) responsible have still not been identified. This casts a pall on attempts to define specific genetic factors in affective disorders with less prominent pedigrees (e.g. MDD). Although the risk for bipolar disorder is increased by early events (abuse, childhood anxiety, etc.; Duffy et al., 2015), unlike MDD the first manifestation is, in most cases, well after

puberty (Bauer et al., 2018; Goodyer and Wilkinson, 2019). Nevertheless, bipolar disorder can occur in childhood and adolescence, rates increasing with age, though there is no clear evidence that puberty itself plays a significant role. There has been considerable debate over diagnostic criteria, though recently there has been better agreement on prevalence in the USA and elsewhere (Van Meter et al., 2019). For a detailed discussion of bipolar disorder in males, see Chapter 14.

Puberty and the Brain

The information on how age- and puberty-related changes in the brain underly the behavioural events of puberty and adolescence is scanty. This is because it relies largely on neuroimaging of the brain (Foulkes and Blakemore, 2018). Whilst neuroimaging studies have been valuable, it is important to recognize their limitations. Magnetic resonance imaging (MRI) allows measures of the volumes of different brain areas. There are well-established developmental changes: for example, the cortical thinning that occurs during later adolescence and early adulthood (Herting et al., 2015), though this has been reinterpreted as increased myelination, rather than loss of grey matter (Natu et al., 2019). However, altered volume is a very indirect indicator of altered function. There does not need to be a change in volume following altered function, and interpretation of morphometric changes is highly uncertain. They may (or may not) be associated with altered volume. For example, the mechanism of neural maturity is not revealed by cortical thinning.

Functional MRI (fMRI) is an indirect measure of neural function, depending on overflow of oxygenated blood into the venules following local vasodilatation. It is not clear why this overflow occurs, or what exact relation it has to activity in the adjacent areas of the brain. While changes in either parameter at or after puberty can be recorded, their significance in functional terms remains blurred. Relating such changes as have been reported to mental health is even more problematic (Box 4.6).

The particular demands of post-pubertal adolescence on social interactions and decisions implies the importance of social cognition (Goddings et al., 2012). The 'social brain' involves many areas, but neuroimaging studies suggest that most of these are cortical. These include altered face processing (inferior occipital gyrus, fusiform gyrus); attributing qualities to the mental states of others and taking account of their views (dorsal frontal cortex, temporo-parietal junction, etc.); and social decision-making (dorso-lateral frontal cortex, temporo-parietal junction) (Kilford et al., 2016). Emotional responses to social interactions have been reflected in the ventro-lateral and orbito-frontal cortex. Accentuated responses have been found in the amygdala as well as the prefrontal cortex to aversive stimuli during adolescence (Silvers et al., 2017).

How much do these changes depend directly on rising levels of testosterone (Peper et al., 2011)? Androgen receptors are highly concentrated in limbic areas such as the hypothalamus and amygdala. These areas are not easily studied by (f)MRI. However, cortical thinning in boys (posterior occipital area) has been associated with individual differences in testosterone (Bramen et al., 2012). Experimental studies suggest that there are also androgen receptors in the cortical regions of young rats (Kritzer, 2004; Nunez et al., 2003), though it is uncertain whether this applies to boys (Bezdickova et al., 2007): the rat brain is deficient in those areas of the cortex most implicated in social interactions and cognition in humans. There is a high concentration of androgen receptors in the amygdala of both rats and humans. The role of the amygdala in emotionality is well established.

Conclusions

Puberty is a unique and dramatic event in a boy's life. It does not occur on the basis of a neutral brain, since both genetic and early endocrine and environmental events play powerful guiding roles on the response to the surge of testosterone at puberty. The upheaval in physical, psychological, and social function that this causes makes it a time that is ripe and ready for mental dysfunction of many kinds, or the accentuation of disorders or states already present. The consequences of such disorders can be severe: loss of friends, educational opportunities, increased family difficulties, low self-esteem, drug and/or alcohol abuse, reduced employment opportunities, risk of suicide, and recurrence of disorders during adulthood. Longer-term consequences include reduced financial assets, problems with relationships, an increased burden on family and community, and reduced socio-economic status. Recurrent adult depression is associated with increased risk for heart and Alzheimer's disease (Herbert and Lucassen, 2016). Puberty in males does not 'cause' mental dysfunction – though it may increase the risk for it – but it initiates sexual and social maturation. Though testosterone plays a major role, it is not the only significant event, and interactions between many other factors, both during puberty and preceding it, will determine whether or not puberty passes without accentuation or initiation of mental disorder.

References

Alexander, G. M. 2014. Postnatal testosterone concentrations and male social development. *Front Endocrinol (Lausanne)*, 5, 15.

Altemus, M., Sarvaiya, N., and Neill Epperson, C. 2014. Sex differences in anxiety and depression clinical perspectives. *Front Neuroendocrinol*, 35, 320–30.

Archer, J. 2019. The reality and evolutionary significance of human psychological sex differences. *Biol Rev Camb Philos Soc*, 94, 1381–1415.

Arnett, J. J. 1999. Adolescent storm and stress, reconsidered. *Am Psychol*, 54, 317–26.

Bauer, M., Andreassen, O. A., Geddes, J. R., Vedel Kessing, L., Lewitzka, U., Schulze, T. G., and Vieta, E. 2018. Areas of uncertainties and unmet needs in bipolar disorders:

clinical and research perspectives. *Lancet Psychiatry*, 5, 930–9.

Becker, J. B. 2009. Sexual differentiation of motivation: a novel mechanism? *Horm Behav*, 55, 646–54.

Berenbaum, S. A. and Beltz, A. M. 2011. Sexual differentiation of human behavior: effects of prenatal and pubertal organizational hormones. *Front Neuroendocrinol*, 32, 183–200.

Berenbaum, S. A., Beltz, A. M., and Corley, R. 2015. The importance of puberty for adolescent development: conceptualization and measurement. *Adv Child Dev Behav*, 48, 53–92.

Bezdickova, M., Molikova, R., Bebarova, L., and Kolar, Z. 2007. Distribution of nuclear receptors for steroid hormones in the human brain: a preliminary study. *Biomed Pap Med Fac Univ Palacky Olomouc Czech Repub*, 151, 69–71.

Birmaher, B. and Rozel, J. S. 2003. Unipolar depression – a lifespan perpsetive: 'the school age child'. In: Goodyer, I. M. (ed.) *Unipolar Depression: A Lifespan Perspective*. Oxford: Oxford University Press.

Bramen, J. E., Hranilovich, J. A., Dahl, R. E., Chen, J., Rosso, C., Forbes, E. E., Dinov, I. D., Worthman, C. M., and Sowell, E. R. 2012. Sex matters during adolescence: testosterone-related cortical thickness maturation differs between boys and girls. *PLoS One*, 7, e33850.

Cameron, H. A. and Gould, E. 1994. Adult neurogenesis is regulated by adrenal steroids in the dentate gyrus. *Neuroscience*, 61, 203–9.

Caspi, A., Sugden, K., Moffitt, T. E., Taylor, A., Craig, I. W., Harrington, H., Mcclay, J., Mill, J., Martin, J., Braithwaite, A., and Poulton, R. 2003. Influence of life stress on depression: moderation by a polymorphism in the 5-HTT gene. *Science*, 301, 386–9.

Clarkson, T., Eaton, N. R., Nelson, E. E., Fox, N. A., Leibenluft, E.,

Pine, D. S., Heckelman, A. C., Sequeira, S. L., and Jarcho, J. M. 2019. Early childhood social reticence and neural response to peers in preadolescence predict social anxiety symptoms in midadolescence. *Depress Anxiety*, 36, 676–89.

Cohen-Kettenis, P. T. 2005. Gender change in 46,XY persons with 5alpha-reductase-2 deficiency and 17beta-hydroxysteroid dehydrogenase-3 deficiency. *Arch Sex Behav*, 34, 399–410.

Cortes, M. E., Carrera, B., Rioseco, H., Pablo Del Rio, J., and Vigil, P. 2015. The role of kisspeptin in the onset of puberty and in the ovulatory mechanism: a mini-review. *J Pediatr Adolesc Gynecol*, 28, 286–91.

Costa, R., Dunsford, M., Skagerberg, E., Holt, V., Carmichael, P., and Colizzi, M. 2015. Psychological support, puberty suppression, and psychosocial functioning in adolescents with gender dysphoria. *J Sex Med*, 12, 2206–14.

Cowen, P. J. and Browning, M. 2015. What has serotonin to do with depression? *World Psychiatry*, 14, 158–60.

Dalley, J. W. and Roiser, J. P. 2012. Dopamine, serotonin and impulsivity. *Neuroscience*, 215, 42–58.

Duarte-Guterman, P., Lieblich, S., Wainwright, S. R., Chow, C., Chaiton, J., Watson, N. V., and Galea, L. A. M. 2019. Androgens enhance adult hippocampal neurogenesis in males but not females in an age-dependent manner. *Endocrinology*, 160(9), 2128–36.

Duffy, A., Jones, S., Goodday, S., and Bentall, R. 2015. Candidate risks indicators for bipolar disorder: early intervention opportunities in high-risk youth. *Int J Neuropsychopharmacol*, 19.

Duque Ede, A. and Munhoz, C. D. 2016. The pro-inflammatory effects of glucocorticoids in the brain. *Front Endocrinol (Lausanne)*, 7, 78.

Durwood, L., Mclaughlin, K. A., and Olson, K. R. 2017. Mental health and self-worth in socially transitioned transgender youth. *J Am Acad Child Adolesc Psychiatry*, 56, 116–23 e2.

Farooqi, N. A. I., Scotti, M., Yu, A., Lew, J., Monnier, P., Botteron, K. N., Campbell, B. C., Booij, L., Herba, C. M., Seguin, J. R., Castellanos-Ryan, N., Mccracken, J. T., and Nguyen, T. V. 2019. Sex-specific contribution of DHEA-cortisol ratio to prefrontal-hippocampal structural development, cognitive abilities and personality traits. *J Neuroendocrinol*, 31, e12682.

Fawcett, J. W., Oohashi, T., and Pizzorusso, T. The role of perineuronal nets and perinodal extracellular matrix in neuronal function. *Nat Rev Neurosci*. 2019 (8):451–465.

Forbes, E. E. and Dahl, R. E. 2010. Pubertal development and behavior: hormonal activation of social and motivational tendencies. *Brain Cogn*, 72, 66–72.

Foulkes, L. and Blakemore, S. J. 2018. Studying individual differences in human adolescent brain development. *Nat Neurosci*, 21, 315–23.

Garg, E., Chen, L., Nguyen, T. T. T., Pokhvisneva, I., Chen, L. M., Unternaehrer, E., Macisaac, J. L., Mcewen, L. M., Mah, S. M., Gaudreau, H., Levitan, R., Moss, E., Sokolowski, M. B., Kennedy, J. L., Steiner, M. S., Meaney, M. J., Holbrook, J. D., Silveira, P. P., Karnani, N., Kobor, M. S., O'Donnell, K. J., and Mavan Study, T. 2018. The early care environment and DNA methylome variation in childhood. *Dev Psychopathol*, 30, 891–903.

Goddings, A. L., Burnett Heyes, S., Bird, G., Viner, R. M., and Blakemore, S. J. 2012. The relationship between puberty and social emotion processing. *Dev Sci*, 15, 801–11.

Goodyer, I. M. 2003. *Unipolar Depression: A Lifespan Perspective.* Oxford: Oxford University Press.

Goodyer, I. M., Croudace, T., Dudbridge, F., Ban, M., and Herbert, J. 2010. Polymorphisms in BDNF (Val66Met) and 5-HTTLPR, morning cortisol and subsequent depression in at-risk adolescents. *Br J Psychiatry*, 197, 365–71.

Goodyer, I. M., Herbert, J., and Tamplin, A. 2003. Psychoendocrine antecedents of persistent first-episode major depression in adolescents: a community-based longitudinal enquiry. *Psychol Med*, 33, 601–10.

Goodyer, I. M. and Wilkinson, P. O. 2019. Practitioner review: therapeutics of unipolar major depressions in adolescents. *J Child Psychol Psychiatry*, 60, 232–43.

Gottlieb, B., Beitel, L. K., Nadarajah, A., Paliouras, M., and Trifiro, M. 2012. The androgen receptor gene mutations database: 2011 update. *Hum Mutat*.

Halligan, S. L., Herbert, J., Goodyer, I. M., and Murray, L. 2004. Exposure to postnatal depression predicts elevated cortisol in adolescent offspring. *Biol Psychiatry*, 55, 376–81.

Harrington, R. 2003. Adolescence. In: Goodyer, I. M. (ed.) *Unipolar Depression: A Lifespan Perspective.* Oxford: Oxford University Press.

Heim, C. and Binder, E. B. 2012. Current research trends in early life stress and depression: review of human studies on sensitive periods, gene–environment interactions, and epigenetics. *Exp Neurol*, 233, 102–11.

Herbert, J. 2017. *Testosterone: The Molecule Behind Power, Sex and the Will to Win.* Oxford: Oxford University Press.

Herbert, J. and Lucassen, P. J. 2016. Depression as a risk factor for Alzheimer's disease: genes, steroids, cytokines and neurogenesis – what do we need to know? *Front Neuroendocrinol*, 41, 153–71.

Herting, M. M., Gautam, P., Spielberg, J. M., Dahl, R. E., and Sowell, E. R. 2015. A longitudinal study: changes in cortical thickness and surface area during pubertal maturation. *PLoS One*, 10, e0119774.

Hines, M. 2006. *Brain Gender.* Oxford: Oxford University Press.

Hines, M. 2011. Gender development and the human brain. *Annu Rev Neurosci*, 34, 69–88.

Hines, M., Ahmed, S. F., and Hughes, I. A. 2003. Psychological outcomes and gender-related development in complete androgen insensitivity syndrome. *Arch Sex Behav*, 32, 93–101.

Hochberg, Z. and Belsky, J. 2013. Evo-devo of human adolescence: beyond disease models of early puberty. *BMC Med*, 11, 113.

Hodes, G. E. and Epperson, C. N. 2019. Sex differences in vulnerability and resilience to stress across the life span. *Biol Psychiatry*, 86(6), 421–32.

Joels, M. and De Kloet, E. R. 1994. Mineralocorticoid and glucocorticoid receptors in the brain. Implications for ion permeability and transmitter systems. *Prog Neurobiol*, 43, 1–36.

Karg, K., Burmeister, M., Shedden, K., and Sen, S. 2011. The serotonin transporter promoter variant (5-HTTLPR), stress, and depression meta-analysis revisited: evidence of genetic moderation. *Arch Gen Psychiatry*, 68, 444–54.

Khandaker, G. M., Stochl, J., Zammit, S., Goodyer, I., Lewis, G., and Jones, P. B. 2018. Childhood inflammatory markers and intelligence as predictors of subsequent persistent depressive symptoms: a longitudinal cohort study. *Psychol Med*, 48, 1514–22.

Kilford, E. J., Garrett, E., and Blakemore, S. J. 2016. The development of social cognition in adolescence: an integrated perspective. *Neurosci Biobehav Rev*, 70, 106–20.

Kircanski, K., Sisk, L. M., Ho, T. C., Humphreys, K. L., King, L. S.,

Colich, N. L., Ordaz, S. J., and Gotlib, I. H. 2019. Early life stress, cortisol, frontolimbic connectivity, and depressive symptoms during puberty. *Dev Psychopathol*, 31, 1011–22.

Kosti, K., Athanasiadis, L., and Goulis, D. G. 2019. Long-term consequences of androgen insensitivity syndrome. *Maturitas*, 127, 51–4.

Kritzer, M. 2004. The distribution of immunoreactivity for intracellular androgen receptors in the cerebral cortex of hormonally intact adult male and female rats: localization in pyramidal neurons making corticocortical connections. *Cereb Cortex*, 14, 268–80.

Lenroot, R. K. and Giedd, J. N. 2010. Sex differences in the adolescent brain. *Brain Cogn*, 72, 46–55.

Lijster, J. M., Dierckx, B., Utens, E. M., Verhulst, F. C., Zieldorff, C., Dieleman, G. C., and Legerstee, J. S. 2017. The age of onset of anxiety disorders. *Can J Psychiatry*, 62, 237–46.

Mahfouda, S., Moore, J. K., Siafarikas, A., Zepf, F. D., and Lin, A. 2017. Puberty suppression in transgender children and adolescents. *Lancet Diabetes Endocrinol*, 5, 816–26.

Matsuda, K. I., Mori, H., and Kawata, M. 2012. Epigenetic mechanisms are involved in sexual differentiation of the brain. *Rev Endocr Metab Disord*, 13, 163–71.

Meaney, M. J. and Szyf, M. 2005. Environmental programming of stress responses through DNA methylation: life at the interface between a dynamic environment and a fixed genome. *Dialogues Clin Neurosci*, 7, 103–23.

Melo, K. F., Mendonca, B. B., Billerbeck, A. E., Costa, E. M., Inacio, M., Silva, F. A., Leal, A. M., Latronico, A. C., and Arnhold, I. J. 2003. Clinical, hormonal, behavioral, and genetic characteristics of androgen insensitivity syndrome in a Brazilian cohort: five novel mutations in the androgen receptor gene. *J Clin Endocrinol Metab*, 88, 3241–50.

Mendonca, B. B., Batista, R. L., Domenice, S., Costa, E. M., Arnhold, I. J., Russell, D. W., and Wilson, J. D. 2016. Steroid 5alpha-reductase 2 deficiency. *J Steroid Biochem Mol Biol*, 163, 206–11.

Michopoulos, V., Powers, A., Gillespie, C. F., Ressler, K. J., and Jovanovic, T. 2017. Inflammation in fear- and anxiety-based disorders: PTSD, GAD, and beyond. *Neuropsychopharmacology*, 42, 254–70.

Mihalik, A., Ferreira, F. S., Rosa, M. J., Moutoussis, M., Ziegler, G., Monteiro, J. M., Portugal, L., Adams, R. A., Romero-Garcia, R., VErtes, P. E., Kitzbichler, M. G., Vasa, F., Vaghi, M. M., Bullmore, E. T., Fonagy, P., Goodyer, I. M., Jones, P. B., Consortium, N., Dolan, R., and Mourao-Miranda, J. 2019. Brain-behaviour modes of covariation in healthy and clinically depressed young people. *Sci Rep*, 9, 11536.

Moriguchi, S., Shinoda, Y., Yamamoto, Y., Sasaki, Y., Miyajima, K., Tagashira, H., and Fukunaga, K. 2013. Stimulation of the sigma-1 receptor by DHEA enhances synaptic efficacy and neurogenesis in the hippocampal dentate gyrus of olfactory bulbectomized mice. *PLoS One*, 8, e60863.

Mullins, N. and Lewis, C. M. 2017. Genetics of depression: progress at last. *Curr Psychiatry Rep*, 19, 43.

Natu V. S., Gomez J., Barnett M., Kirilina, E., Jaeger, C., Zhen, Z., Cox, S., Weiner, K. S., Weiskopf, N., and Grill-Spector, K. 8 October 2019. Apparent thinning of human visual cortex during childhood is associated with myelinisation. *Proc Natl Acad Sci USA*, 116(41), 20750–9, first published 23 September 2019.

Netherton, C., Goodyer, I., Tamplin, A., and Herbert, J. 2004. Salivary cortisol and

dehydroepiandrosterone in relation to puberty and gender. *Psychoneuroendocrinology*, 29, 125–40.

Nugent, B. M., Wright, C. L., Shetty, A. C., Hodes, G. E., Lenz, K. M., Mahurkar, A., Russo, S. J., Devine, S. E., and Mccarthy, M. M. 2015. Brain feminization requires active repression of masculinization via DNA methylation. *Nat Neurosci*, 18, 690–7.

Nunez, J. L., Huppenbauer, C. B., Mcabee, M. D., Juraska, J. M., and Doncarlos, L. L. 2003. Androgen receptor expression in the developing male and female rat visual and prefrontal cortex. *J Neurobiol*, 56, 293–302.

Ojeda, S. R. and Lomniczi, A. 2014. Puberty in 2013: unravelling the mystery of puberty. *Nat Rev Endocrinol*, 10, 67–9.

Owens, M., Herbert, J., Jones, P. B., Sahakian, B. J., Wilkinson, P. O., Dunn, V. J., Croudace, T. J., and Goodyer, I. M. 2014. Elevated morning cortisol is a stratified population-level biomarker for major depression in boys only with high depressive symptoms. *Proc Natl Acad Sci U S A*, 111, 3638–43.

Peper, J. S., Hulshoff Pol, H. E., Crone, E. A., and Van Honk, J. 2011. Sex steroids and brain structure in pubertal boys and girls: a mini-review of neuroimaging studies. *Neuroscience*, 191, 28–37.

Piekarski, D. J., Johnson, C. M., Boivin, J. R., Thomas, A. W., Lin, W. C., Delevich, K., E, M. G., and Wilbrecht, L. 2017. Does puberty mark a transition in sensitive periods for plasticity in the associative neocortex? *Brain Res*, 1654, 123–44.

Puckett, J. A., Matsuno, E., Dyar, C., MUstanski, B., and Newcomb, M. E. 2019. Mental health and resilience in transgender individuals: What type of support makes a difference? *J Fam Psychol*, 33(8), 954–64.

Rainville, J. R. and Hodes, G. E. 2019. Inflaming sex differences in mood

disorders. *Neuropsychopharmacology*, 44, 184–99.

Ranta, K., Vaananen, J., Frojd, S., Isomaa, R., Kaltiala-Heino, R., and Marttunen, M. 2017. Social phobia, depression and eating disorders during middle adolescence: longitudinal associations and treatment seeking. *Nord J Psychiatry*, 71, 605–13.

Rowe, R., Maughan, B., WorthmaN, C. M., Costello, E. J., and Angold, A. 2004. Testosterone, antisocial behavior, and social dominance in boys: pubertal development and biosocial interaction. *Biol Psychiatry*, 55, 546–52.

Sandberg, D. E. and Meyer-Bahlburg, H. F. 1994. Variability in middle childhood play behavior: effects of gender, age, and family background. *Arch Sex Behav*, 23, 645–63.

Sapolsky, R. M. 1996. Stress, glucocorticoids, and damage to the nervous system: the current state of confusion. *Stress*, 1, 1–19.

Silvers, J. A., Insel, C., Powers, A., Franz, P., Helion, C., Martin, R., Weber, J., Mischel, W., Casey, B. J., and Ochsner, K. N. 2017. The transition from childhood to adolescence is marked by a general decrease in amygdala reactivity and an affect-specific ventral-to-dorsal shift in medial prefrontal recruitment. *Dev Cogn Neurosci*, 25, 128–37.

Uenoyama, Y., Inoue, N., Nakamura, S., and Tsukamura, H. 2019. Central mechanism controlling pubertal onset in mammals: a triggering role of kisspeptin. *Front Endocrinol (Lausanne)*, 10, 312.

Uher, R. and Mcguffin, P. 2008. The moderation by the serotonin transporter gene of environmental adversity in the aetiology of mental illness: review and methodological analysis. *Mol Psychiatry*, 13, 131–46.

Van Harmelen, A. L., Kievit, R. A., Ioannidis, K., Neufeld, S., Jones, P. B., Bullmore, E., Dolan, R., Consortium, N., Fonagy, P., and

Goodyer, I. 2017. Adolescent friendships predict later resilient functioning across psychosocial domains in a healthy community cohort. *Psychol Med*, 47, 2312–22.

Van Meter, A., Moreira, A. L. R., and Youngstrom, E. 2019. Updated meta-analysis of epidemiologic studies of pediatric bipolar disorder. *J Clin Psychiatry*, 80.

Vermeersch, H., T'Sjoen, G., Kaufman, J. M., Vincke, J., and Van Houtte, M. 2010. Testosterone, androgen receptor gene CAG repeat length, mood and behaviour in adolescent males. *Eur J Endocrinol*, 163, 319–28.

Wagner, C. A., Alloy, L. B., and Abramson, L. Y. 2015. Trait rumination, depression, and executive functions in early adolescence. *J Youth Adolesc*, 44, 18–36.

Wierenga, L. M., Bos, M. G. N., Schreuders, E., VD Kamp, F., Peper, J. S., Tamnes, C. K., and Crone, E. A. 2018. Unraveling age, puberty and testosterone effects on subcortical brain development across adolescence. *Psychoneuroendocrinology*, 91, 105–14.

Yohn, C. N., Gergues, M. M., and Samuels, B. A. 2017. The role of 5-HT receptors in depression. *Mol Brain*, 10, 28.

Zhang, J., Yoa, W., and Hashimoto, K. 2016. Brain-derived neurotrophic factor (BDNF)-TrkB signaling in inflammation-related depression and potential therapeutic targets. *Current Neuropharmacology*, 14, 721–31.

5

Schizophrenia in Men

Erica Neill and David Castle

Schizophrenia is a severe psychiatric disorder that can have a devastating impact on the lives of those affected, their families, and their communities. Schizophrenia can affect both females and males but males tend to have both an earlier onset of symptoms and a worse longitudinal course of illness. This chapter explores the differences between males and females with schizophrenia, with a focus on how this difference impacts upon the lives of men. Areas discussed include prevalence and incidence rates, age at onset, and premorbid function. The role of sex hormones is discussed, followed by an examination of brain pathology and cognition. Symptom profile, response to antipsychotic medication, and psychosocial function post-diagnosis are also addressed. Finally, a typological model is proposed, with the thesis that males are differentially prone to an early-onset severe form of schizophrenia.

The Schizophrenia Construct

The causes of schizophrenia are poorly understood but evidence suggests both genetic and environmental factors play a role in its development. Genetic studies report a 40–50% concordance rate between identical twins (Tsuang, 2000) and meta-analytic data estimate heritability in liability to schizophrenia at 81%. The environmental factors associated with the development of schizophrenia are varied and include prenatal or early developmental injury, the impact of trauma, and drug use (with marijuana specifically implicated) along with an urban upbringing. The effects of immigration and membership of a minority group have also been implicated (Weiser et al., 2005) and more recently, older paternal age has been added to the list of potential contributing factors (van Os et al., 2010).

Both the International Classification of Diseases (ICD) and the Diagnostic Statistical Manual of Mental Disorders (DSM) define schizophrenia as a psychotic disorder associated with positive and

negative symptoms along with cognitive impairment. Positive symptoms encompass those associated with the addition/exaggeration or distortion of normal experiences. These include hearing voices or seeing visions in the absence of external stimuli. The presence of unusual thoughts, often paranoid or grandiose in nature, and disorganized speech leading to difficulties in communication are also common symptoms of schizophrenia.

Negative symptoms describe the loss of normal experience. Examples of negative symptoms include a reduction in the intensity of feelings and expressions of emotion. Thoughts and speed of thinking are also reduced, and there is a loss of energy, drive, and interest along with a decrease in the ability to feel pleasure.

Finally, cognitive dysfunction is recognized as a core symptom of schizophrenia. Impairments can be broad-ranging, impacting the speed of processing information, attention, and memory, as well as higher-level cognitive skills such as organization and problem solving. Social cognition, including interpreting social situations and understanding the feelings of others, can also be compromised.

The various combinations of these symptoms impact function and lead to a significant reduction in overall quality of life. While some 20% of people diagnosed with schizophrenia are reported to have a favourable outcome, many require medication and support for the length of their lives. Most, if employable, work at a lower level than their parents and a majority, particularly males, do not marry and have limited social contact outside of their family. In fact, it is widely accepted that males generally have a worse prognosis than females with a schizophrenia diagnosis.

Sex Differences in Incidence and Prevalence

First, it is important to understand the difference between incidence and prevalence rates as each has a different way of capturing, or missing, sex differences in the rates of schizophrenia. *Incidence* is the risk rate, describing the number of people who develop a disorder over a specified period in a given location. *Prevalence* is the burden rate, describing the number of people who are currently living with a particular disorder. In its simplest form, prevalence = incidence + course of illness. In relation to sex, incidence rates can be used to try to understand what the patterns of disease occurrence are and how sex might affect them. Prevalence describes the number of cases currently in the community and, as such, informs health care planning with sex-specific issues in mind.

In the case of schizophrenia, incidence and prevalence rate estimates differ somewhat around the world as a result of the various genetic and environmental factors involved in its development as well as help-seeking and service provision variations. The incidence rates reported are fairly uniform, ranging from 0.5 to 2.0 per 10,000 population (or between 0.05% to 0.2%) while there is greater variation in prevalence rates, with estimates between 1% and 12% (Räsänen et al., 2000).

Sex differences represent a significant complication in reporting schizophrenia risk, with some of this confusion stemming from the lack of consistency in research methodologies used between studies. First, the criteria used to diagnose schizophrenia vary and it has been shown that the broader the criteria used, the smaller the reported sex differences in incidence rates (Castle et al., 1995). Further, when affective psychoses, including schizoaffective disorder, are included, this can impact rates as more females receive affective diagnoses. Patterns of engagement with clinical services and the use of epidemiological versus clinical data can also complicate interpretation (Ochoa et al., 2012), and an early cut-off age for inclusion in research means that the later peak associated with females can be missed, falsely inflating the ratio of males to females diagnosed (Falkenburg and Tracy, 2014).

Despite these methodological problems, it has consistently been shown that incidence rates for schizophrenia are higher among males, with a male-to-female incidence ratio of around 1.42 (Falkenburg and Tracy, 2014). While this incidence rate is higher in males, there is information suggesting that this is only the case if one looks at the first half of the lifespan. After midlife, the numbers begin to even out, such that prevalence over the lifespan becomes close to equal (Häfner, 2003; Castle and Murray, 1993). Other factors that can distort incidence rates include a lower level of engagement with services and a higher suicide rate reported among males with schizophrenia (Hor and Taylor, 2010; Ösby et al., 2000; Ochoa et al., 2012).

It appears that while there is substantial variability in incidence and prevalence of schizophrenia around the world, there is convergence regarding a higher incidence rate among males (at least in the first half of life) and a prevalence rate that is similar between the sexes.

Age of Onset

There is evidence of differing patterns in the incidence of schizophrenia over the lifespan when examined separately by sex. Earlier studies suggest that males have an earlier age of onset by some 3–4 years (Häfner, 2003). A more recent large-scale meta-analysis including forty-six studies containing data for 29,218 males and 19,402 females found that males develop schizophrenia earlier but that this difference was smaller, with onset in males preceding that in females by just over a year (Eranti et al., 2012).

Research has explored whether this age of onset data varied over time – by examining incidence rates between 1955 and 1964 and comparing these to age of onset rates between 1982 and 1991 – and found that the sex difference remained stable over time (Takahashi et al., 2000). Further, the finding of earlier male onset has been replicated at multiple sites around the world, including England (Castle et al., 1998), Japan (Takahashi et al., 2000), Reunion Island (off the coast of Madagascar; Gorwood et al., 1995), the United States (Szymanski et al., 1995), and Germany (Häfner, 2003). Studies that have not confirmed this finding were in a South Indian population (Venkatesh et al., 2008) and an Ethiopian sample (Kebede et al., 2003). The first of these latter studies found no age difference (although trending towards male onset being earlier) and the second found a younger age of onset for females. This may reflect a difference between developing and developed countries. In saying that, however, the meta-analysis by Eranti et al. (2013) included a mix of developed and developing countries and meta-regression showed that country's developmental status did not affect the earlier onset among males. In terms of the possible influence of study design, both of those studies finding a sex difference and those that did not, included a mix of large and small samples (varying between as few as 25 females to as many as 300) and differing diagnostic categories (including ICD and DSM). Of the studies that did not find a younger onset in males, broader ICD diagnostic criteria were used. As mentioned, these broader inclusion criteria have been associated with a reduced differentiation in illness onset between the sexes (Eranti et al., 2013; Castle et al., 1995). Kebede et al. (2003) suggested that their finding of a younger onset in females in the Ethiopian sample may reflect a tendency for females in their study to report their age as lower than it actually was, which, they explain, is not uncommon in the Ethiopian culture. Other obvious possible confounding factors in these two studies include differences in help-seeking behaviours between the sexes and variation in service provisions in the countries included.

It is interesting to note that the age of onset difference exists in first-episode patients, indicating that the difference is not an artefact of averaging onset across the lifespan (females being more likely to develop schizophrenia later in life; Ochoa et al., 2012; Häfner et al., 1998).

Other research has examined age of onset in more depth, describing differing peaks in incidence over the lifespan. One such report found that males had two peaks for developing schizophrenia. The first was around 21 years and another at around 40. Females were found to have three peaks, one with a mean at around 22, another at 37, and a final peak at 62 years (Castle et al., 1998). More recently, we have run cluster analysis using the Australian SHIP data (Survey of High Impact Psychosis), which contains age of onset information for over 500 individuals with schizophrenia. We found, once again, evidence for two peaks for males (modal ages 20 and 40) and three peaks for females (modes 21, 26, and 42). While the Castle et al. (1998) study found a later onset peak of 62 among their female group, the SHIP later onset age was only 42. This may reflect the early cut-off age of 65 in the SHIP study while the Camberwell study data used by Castle et al. (1998) had no age limit for inclusion.

Overall, the data suggest that age of onset for schizophrenia is earlier for males, with support from both individual studies and meta-analytic review. In saying that, however, the picture is complicated by

---

Box 5.1

- Illness development trajectories differ between the sexes
- Males often develop schizophrenia earlier than females with a peak incidence in adolescence
- Males often have more negative symptoms and worse outcomes

---

the finding that age of onset does not hover around one specific age for males or females. In any analysis of age of onset, the influence of these peaks should be considered.

Premorbid Functioning

The often-reported finding of more obstetric complications in males compared to females who develop schizophrenia is inconsistent, with some finding more complications in females and some finding no difference between the sexes (Ochoa et al., 2012). However, when this relationship is explored among those with an early illness onset, the finding of an association between male sex and obstetric complications specifically is more robust (Dalman et al., 1999).

Delays in reaching developmental milestones have been reported for those who go on to develop schizophrenia. Differences in these delays analysed by sex find that males have more delayed development; however, these claims often stem from research that is confounded by normal developmental differences between the sexes. For example, females develop more quickly than males in certain domains (e.g. verbal), so depending at what age children are compared will impact the results. Further, females develop schizophrenia at a later age, so if the two sexes are compared at adolescence, more of the females who will develop schizophrenia will not be accounted for (Isohanni et al., 2001). As such, at this stage, it is difficult to say for certain whether delays in developmental milestones distinguish males from females with schizophrenia in terms of premorbid trajectory.

In terms of later development, males with schizophrenia tend to demonstrate worse premorbid function across a range of domains, including worse school, work, and interpersonal function (Leung and Chue, 2000); a finding confirmed by later studies (Allen et al., 2013). Males perform worse in both social and school function in early childhood, followed by a steep decline in social function in adolescence (in comparison to females), while both sexes demonstrated worse school performance compared to social function in late adolescence.

Overall, male sex is associated with obstetric complications in those cases of schizophrenia where age of onset is early. Differences between the sexes are not robust in relation to early developmental delays, but males demonstrate worse school, work, and interpersonal functioning starting from early childhood.

Hormones

Sex hormones are thought to have a role in the expression of schizophrenia. These include oestrogen, progesterone, testosterone, Dehydroepiandrosterone (DHEA), and its metabolite DHEA sulphate (DHEAS) (both of the latter adrenosteroid precursors to testosterone). Chapter 4 profiles details of the impact of the latter sex steroids on the male brain.

Given that females with schizophrenia tend to demonstrate a later age of onset, a milder course of illness, better response to antipsychotics, and better social function, it has been suggested that the female sex hormones (oestrogen and progesterone) may have a neuroprotective effect. This body of research has mixed findings (Abel et al., 2010), but a large review of the area was able to tease out some consistent results (da Silva and Ravindran, 2015). There is evidence that progesterone has anti-inflammatory effects and promotes neurogenesis and neuroplasticity. The evidence is stronger again for oestrogen, which also promotes neurogenesis and neuroplasticity and also enhances the expression of brain-derived neurotropic factor (BDNF) and reduces neuronal cell loss. Through its various actions, oestrogen is thought to provide some protection against dopamine depletion and glutamate toxicity, which are especially relevant to schizophrenia.

While there is research supporting some neuroprotective features of both the DHEA/S (including promoting neurogenesis and enhancing BDNF) and testosterone (e.g. neurogenesis and neurogeneration), neither provides the same level of protection as oestrogen. Further, both testosterone and DHEA/S are converted to oestrogen in the brain and it has been proposed that their neuroprotective actions occur after this conversion (da Silva and Ravindran, 2015).

Oestrogen, and to a lesser degree progesterone, are involved in the regulation of serotonin, noradrenaline, glutamate, dopamine, acetylcholine, and GABA in such a way that their actions are described as having atypical antipsychotic effects on the brain. While testosterone has been described as having some neuroprotective effects, its impact on glutamate and dopamine has been linked to increased negative symptoms and a more severe illness profile in males with schizophrenia.

The hypothesis that oestrogen has a protective function in schizophrenia has been used to explain the slightly later onset in females and the later in life peak which has been linked to the onset of menopause when oestrogen levels fall (Baldwin and Srivastava, 2015). Thus it has been proposed that oestrogen delays the onset of schizophrenia (Bergemann and Riecher-Rössler, 2005). Given the supposed neuroprotective effect of oestrogen, a small number of studies have explored the impact of oestrogen on males with schizophrenia and have produced mixed results (Kulkarni et al., 2011). Due to some inconsistency in the evidence, there have been updates to the oestrogen theory in recent times. Some authors have suggested that if oestrogen delays the onset of schizophrenia, then late onset schizophrenia should look more like early onset when it finally does appear. Research shows, however, that later onset schizophrenia in females is associated with greater positive and fewer negative symptoms (Baldwin and Srivastava, 2015). Authors have thus proposed that oestrogen's relationship with late onset symptoms may be more indirect. Instead of delaying the onset, it may be that it interacts with stress in females. Studies suggest that, due to differences in sexual dimorphism in the hypothalamus–pituitary–adrenal (HPA) axis, females may have a greater vulnerability to stress. This becomes enhanced after menopause and it has been posited that oestradiol is protective against this effect. As such, it may be that a greater vulnerability to stress post-menopause leads to a greater vulnerability to the development of psychosis (Baldwin and Srivastava, 2015).

A number of sex-specific hormones may provide some form of protection from psychosis. We are currently in the early stages of understanding how these hormones affect the development and course of schizophrenia and early attempts to remediate symptoms in males with these hormones have not provided clear improvements.

Box 5.2

- Female sex hormones may provide protection against the development of schizophrenia
- The impact of these hormones may explain why schizophrenia in women is more commonly associated with:
  - o A later illness onset
  - o A second risk period around menopause
  - o A milder form of the illness

Brain Differences

There is a large body of research investigating brain differences in schizophrenia by sex. See Chapters 1 and 4 for a broader discussion of male brain development and psychopathology. The results of this research are often conflicting depending on the techniques used (particularly in the early days of neuroimaging) and failures to include healthy control groups. A large meta-analysis of brain volume in schizophrenia, including 58 studies and 1588 participants (Wright et al., 2000), found that while sex differences did not exist across all areas of the brain, there was some evidence for larger ventricular volume among males than females. A more recent review (Mendrek and Mancini-Marïe, 2016) focusing specifically on sex differences in brain morphology found that males with schizophrenia manifest more significant brain abnormalities than females, including reductions in temporal and frontal regions. This study also confirmed earlier findings of a larger ventricle-to-brain ratio in males compared to females. It was also noted that amongst males with schizophrenia, normal sexual dimorphism is diminished or even reversed and, as negative symptoms increased, natural sex-related brain asymmetry was decreased (Mendrek and Mancini-Marïe, 2016).

Interestingly, the authors noted in their review of sex differences in cognition that cognitive performance was not clearly worse among males. Another meta-analysis found that intracranial volume and white matter tissue were both more reduced in males than females with schizophrenia (Haijma et al., 2013). These authors reflected that intracranial volume was mostly finalized by 5 years of age and complete by 14, supporting the theory that males have a more obvious neurodevelopmental subtype of schizophrenia.

Overall, it appears that males with schizophrenia do have more brain pathology than females. Interestingly, the link between this pathology and cognitive function is not direct.

Cognition

The relationship between sex and cognition in schizophrenia is complex. While there is a significant body of literature reporting greater cognitive dysfunction in males (Han et al., 2012; Vaskinn et al., 2011), there is other research finding no sex differences (particularly when psychotic symptoms are matched between groups; Ochoa et al., 2012) or even greater deficits among females. There is a very small body of evidence suggesting that females have worse cognition and a review of this research criticized the work for methodological shortcomings, including that the females included had an unusually early age of onset – or in another study, the male group demonstrated significantly more positive symptoms than the females (Mendrek and Mancini-Marïe, 2016). Further, length of illness, symptom profile, and antipsychotic use all complicate the exploration of the relationship between sex and cognitive function in schizophrenia (Mendrek and Mancini-Marïe, 2016). Despite these complexities, however, some relationships between sex and cognition hold true across a large number of studies. One relationship that has been repeatedly demonstrated is that between negative symptoms and worse performance on cognitive tests (Addington et al., 1991). As outlined below, male sex is more often associated with negative symptoms (Castle et al., 1994; Sham et al., 1996). Also, males with negative symptoms have been shown to perform more poorly on cognitive tasks than females; particularly once their illness has become chronic (Mendrek and Mancini-Marïe, 2016).

There is a small body of research examining sex differences in social cognition specifically. Studies suggest that males with schizophrenia perform worse than their female counterparts at interpreting facial expressions (Campellone and Kring, 2013; Scholten et al., 2005).

There is an interaction in schizophrenia between function and cognition for males and symptom severity and cognition for females with schizophrenia (Karilampi et al., 2011; Mendrek and Mancini-Marïe, 2016). This suggests that the role of cognition should be examined differently for each sex.

Symptom Profile

There is evidence that schizophrenia symptoms vary between the sexes. It has been shown that females are more likely to have prominent affective symptoms as a part of their illness and more auditory hallucinations (Falkenburg and Tracy, 2014) and persecutory delusions (Lindamer et al., 1999).

Males, on the other hand, have been described as exhibiting more negative and disorganized symptoms (Ochoa et al., 2012; Leung and Chue, 2000; Falkenburg and Tracy, 2014). A meta-analytic study found significant associations between male sex and a deficit profile of schizophrenia characterized by negative symptoms (pooled odds ratio=1.75, p= 0.000002; 95% C.I.1.39±2.21) (Roy et al., 2001). Further evidence for an association between male sex and negative symptoms has come from studies utilizing latent class analysis (a technique that allows grouping of individuals based on their related combination of symptoms). Results from two studies using this technique found that one group that emerged was characterized by both male predominance and the negative symptom of restricted affect, once again confirming the association between male sex and negative symptoms (Castle et al., 1994; Sham et al., 1996). This link between male sex and negative symptoms is important as it has implications for outcome. There is evidence that higher rates of negative symptoms are associated with more brain abnormalities (Sanfilipo et al., 2000), worse cognitive function (Lin et al., 2013), and worse long-term outcome (Strauss et al., 2013).

Response to Treatment

There are differences in the ways that males and females respond to pharmacological treatments for schizophrenia, such that males tend to need larger doses of antipsychotic drugs, sometimes as high as twice the dose in chronically ill samples (Seeman, 2004). Further, neuroleptic naïve males have a worse response to antipsychotic treatment than do neuroleptic naïve females, a difference that remains one year after treatment begins. Females have been found to respond more quickly, and this faster response is thought to contribute to their better adherence to medication early in the course of the illness (Smith, 2010). Males are more likely to struggle with extrapyramidal side effects, including dystonia, akathisia, and tardive dyskinesia (Smith, 2010).

In terms of taking prescribed antipsychotics, men more often have negative attitudes to these drugs and suffer more stigma due to being labelled with a mental illness (Smith, 2010). Further, while sexual dysfunction is reported amongst males and females, the rates are higher, at 54% for males versus 30% for females (Ghadirian et al., 1982).

Psychosocial Functioning

There is good evidence that females with schizophrenia have better social function and are better at managing their basic needs, such as food, daily activities, and accommodation. This may be related, in part, to age of onset. There is also some indication that females with schizophrenia are more resilient to stress than their male counterparts. Further, on objective measures of functionality (marriage and fertility) females also score more highly (Ochoa et al., 2012). A study comparing the sexes on measures of disability and global function found that males scored more poorly than females on all measures and this difference remained at follow-up two years later (Usall et al., 2002). Also, males tend to receive less family support and families demonstrate a lower tolerance for their symptomatic behaviour. It has been suggested that this more negative response to men's schizophrenia may stem in part from the higher aggression expressed by men when unwell and from some aspect of self-blame and guilt from parents given the often early onset of symptoms among males. These factors may contribute to higher relapse rates and worse illness outcomes for males (Falkenburg and Tracy, 2014). Other factors that can contribute to worse psychosocial function include higher rates of substance abuse and suicide among males with schizophrenia (discussed below).

Substance Abuse

Males with schizophrenia have higher levels of substance abuse across a range of drugs (Ochoa et al., 2012), including smoking, which can attenuate the benefits of some antipsychotic medications, including clozapine (Levin and Rezvani, 2007). There is also some suggestion that cannabis use is more closely linked to illness onset for males (Arendt et al., 2008). Further, substance abuse has also been linked to increased violence (Fazel et al., 2009). See Chapter 16 for a broader discussion of substance abuse in males.

Suicide

It also appears that a higher percentage of males than females with schizophrenia die by suicide. In their systematic review of suicide rate by sex, Hor and Taylor (2010) noted that this higher male suicide rate was particularly pronounced among young men with a higher education. The authors suggested that those with these characteristics should receive particular therapy in an attempt to reduce suicide amongst this group (see Chapter 15 for a broader discussion of male suicide).

Long-Term Outcomes

A German study investigated outcomes by sex for schizophrenia patients over an eight-year period and found that females had shorter hospital stays on average, a better response to treatment, and had longer gaps between hospitalizations (even after controlling for age and marital status) compared to males (Angermeyer et al., 1990). Males, on the other hand, spend longer in hospital and have more relapses (Ochoa et al., 2012) and are more likely than females to remain institutionalized for longer periods (Uggerby et al., 2011). A study of long-term outcome (over 14 years) in rural China found that males had worse long-term outcome in relation to suicidality, mortality generally, as well as higher rates of homelessness (Ran et al., 2018).

Conclusions

Before drawing conclusions from the review above, it must of course be acknowledged that schizophrenia is an umbrella term that likely describes a number of different neurological and psychiatric experiences that share an overlap in presentation. In saying that, however, there are consistent differences found between the sexes which make a discussion of such

---

Box 5.3

- Males with schizophrenia have worse psychosocial functioning
- This worse functioning is reflected in:
    o Worse social and occupational functioning
    o Less family support
    o More substance abuse
    o A higher suicide rate

---

differences valid. An understanding of these differences may improve prediction of illness trajectory, support a better understanding of the potentially different causes of schizophrenia, and inform a more nuanced approach to therapy for each of the sexes.

The evidence above paints a picture of a more *neurodevelopmental* pattern of schizophrenia in males. Specifically, the finding of a higher incidence in the earlier stages of life paired with premorbid developmental difficulties along with evidence of greater brain pathology supports this assertion. Further evidence comes from the profile of more negative symptoms in males, which are often linked to more brain abnormalities, worse cognition, and worse long-term outcomes. In addition, and likely arising due to the above features, male psychosocial trajectory post-diagnosis is worse. This includes worse social and occupational function along with more substance abuse, a higher suicide rate, and a higher mortality rate in general.

What is it that we can do to address the apparently worse form of schizophrenia seen in males? The following will focus on treatment options post-diagnosis. While the main method of treating schizophrenia is the use of antipsychotic medications, it is likely that adding other therapeutic options alongside medications will provide the most valuable support for males. Given their often long-standing social and educational difficulties, males may require different, and likely more intensive, psychosocial interventions for remediation of these issues. While overall cognition has not been shown to be clearly worse among males generally, there is evidence that higher levels of negative symptoms are related to worse cognitive performance. Given that negative symptoms are more prominent among males, it seems likely that those with this profile would benefit from the addition of cognitive remediation to their therapy. Further, there does appear to be some evidence that social cognition is specifically impaired in males with schizophrenia. There are now a number of cognitive remediation programs available that include remediation for social cognition along with the other more typically remediated areas of thinking.

Substance abuse rates are also higher among males and can lead to social and financial hardship along with negative interactions with antipsychotic medications. As such, psychological therapies with a focus on coping without the assistance of substances will likely be useful. Aggression is also reported as a bigger issue for males than females with schizophrenia and, as such, methods for dealing with such negative externalizing behaviours also need to be specifically addressed (Falkenburg and Tracy, 2014; Li et al., 2016). Given the research showing that the families of men are generally less supportive and tolerant of their illness, it would be useful to take steps to engage families in therapy around any potential guilt and self-blame for the illness and ways to better understand and manage illness behaviours.

> **Box 5.4**
>
> - Illness profiles differ between the sexes and these differences should be considered in therapy
> - Males may require more functional and cognitive rehabilitation to counter the more neurodevelopmental course of their illness
> - Further, more support aimed at preventing substance abuse and suicidality may improve outcomes for men

References

Abel, K. M., Drake, R., and Goldstein, J. M. 2010. Sex differences in schizophrenia. *International Review of Psychiatry*, 22, 417–28.

Addington, J., Addington, D., and Maticka-Tyndale, E. 1991. Cognitive functioning and positive and negative symptoms in schizophrenia. *Schizophrenia Research*, 5, 123–34.

Allen, D. N., Strauss, G. P., Barchard, K. A., Vertinski, M., Carpenter, W. T., and Buchanan, R. W. 2013. Differences in developmental changes in academic and social premorbid adjustment between males and females with schizophrenia. *Schizophrenia Research*, 146, 132–7.

Angermeyer, M. C., Kühn, L., and Goldstein, J. M. 1990. Gender and the course of schizophrenia: differences in treated outcomes. *Schizophrenia Bulletin*, 16, 293–307.

Arendt, M., Mortensen, P. B., Rosenberg, R., Pedersen, C. B., and Waltoft, B. L. 2008. Familial predisposition for psychiatric disorder: comparison of subjects treated for cannabis-induced psychosis and schizophrenia. *Archives of General Psychiatry*, 65, 1269–74.

Baldwin, C. H. and Srivastava, L. K. 2015. Can the neurodevelopmental theory account for sex differences in schizophrenia across the life span? *Journal of Psychiatry and Neuroscience*, 40, 75–7.

Bergemann, N. and Riecher-Rössler, A. 2005. *Estrogen Effects in Psychiatric Disorders*. Austria: Springer Science and Business Media.

Campellone, T. R. and Kring, A. M. 2013. Context and the perception of emotion in schizophrenia: sex differences and relationships with functioning. *Schizophrenia Research*, 149, 192–3.

Castle, D. J., Abel, K., Takei, N., and Murray, R. M. 1995. Gender differences in schizophrenia: hormonal effect or subtypes? *Schizophrenia Bulletin*, 21, 1–12.

Castle, D. J. and Murray, R. M. 1993. The epidemiology of late-onset schizophrenia. *Schizophrenia Bulletin*, 19, 691–700.

Castle, D. J., Sham, P., and Murray, R. 1998. Differences in distribution of ages of onset in males and females with schizophrenia. *Schizophrenia Research*, 33, 179–83.

Castle, D. J., Sham, P., Wessely, S., and Murray, R. 1994. The subtyping of schizophrenia in men and women: a latent class analysis. *Psychological Medicine*, 24, 41–51.

Da Silva, T. L. and Ravindran, A. V. 2015. Contribution of sex hormones to gender differences in schizophrenia: a review. *Asian Journal of Psychiatry*, 18, 2–14.

Dalman, C., Allebeck, P., Cullberg, J., Grunewald, C., and Köster, M. 1999. Obstetric complications and the risk of schizophrenia: a longitudinal study of a national birth cohort. *JAMA Psychiatry*, 56, 234–40.

Eranti, S. V., Maccabe, J. H., Bundy, H. and Murray, R. M. 2013. Gender difference in age at onset of schizophrenia: a meta-analysis. *Psychological Medicine*, 43(1), 155–67.

Falkenburg, J. and Tracy, D. K. 2014. Sex and schizophrenia: a review of gender differences. *Psychosis*, 6, 61–9.

Fazel, S., Gulati, G., Linsell, L., Geddes, J. R., and Grann, M. 2009. Schizophrenia and violence: systematic review and meta-analysis. *PLOS Medicine*, 6, e1000120.

Ghadirian, A. M., Chouinard, G., and Annable, L. 1982. Sexual dysfunction and plasma prolactin levels in neuroleptic-treated schizophrenic outpatients. *Journal of Nervous and Mental Disease*, 170, 463–7.

Gorwood, P., Leboyer, M., Jay, M., Payan, C., and Feingold, J. 1995. Gender and age at onset in schizophrenia: impact of family history. *Am J Psychiatry*, 152.

Häfner, H. 2003. Gender differences in schizophrenia. *Psychoneuroendocrinology*, 28, 17–54.

Häfner, H., An Der Heiden, W., Behrens, S., Gattaz, W. F., Hambrecht, M., Löffler, W., Maurer, K., Munk-Jørgensen, P., Nowotny, B., and Riecher-Rössler, A. 1998. Causes and consequences of the gender difference in age at onset of schizophrenia. *Schizophrenia bulletin*, 24, 99–113.

Haijma, S. V., Van Haren, N., Cahn, W., Koolschijn, P. C. M. P., Hulshoff Pol, H. E., and Kahn, R. S. 2013. Brain volumes in schizophrenia: a meta-analysis in over 18 000 subjects. *Schizophrenia Bulletin*, 39, 1129–38.

Han, M., Huang, X.-F., Chen, D. C., Xiu, M. H., Hui, L., Liu, H., Kosten, T. R., and Zhang, X. Y. 2012. Gender differences in cognitive function of patients with chronic schizophrenia. *Progress in Neuro-Psychopharmacology and Biological Psychiatry*, 39, 358–63.

Hor, K. and Taylor, M. 2010. Review: suicide and schizophrenia: a systematic review of rates and risk factors. *Journal of Psychopharmacology*, 24, 81–90.

Isohanni, M., Jones, P. B., Moilanen, K., Rantakallio, P., Veijola, J., Oja, H., Koiranen, M., Jokelainen, J., Croudace, T., and Järvelin, M. R. 2001. Early developmental milestones in adult schizophrenia and other psychoses. A 31-year follow-up of the Northern Finland 1966 Birth Cohort. *Schizophrenia Research*, 52, 1–19.

Karilampi, U., Helldin, L., and Archer, T. 2011. Cognition and global assessment of functioning in male and female outpatients with schizophrenia spectrum disorders. *The Journal of Nervous and Mental Disease*, 199, 445–8.

Kebede, D., Alem, A., Shibre, T., Negash, A., Fekadu, A., and Fekadu, D. 2003. Onset and clinical course of schizophrenia in Butajira-Ethiopia – a community-based study. *Soc Psychiatry Psychiatr Epidemiol*, 38(11), 325–31.

Kulkarni, J., De Castella, A., Headey, B., Marston, N., Sinclair, K., Lee, S., Gurvich, C., Fitzgerald, P. B., and Burger, H. 2011. Estrogens and men with schizophrenia: is there a case for adjunctive therapy? *Schizophrenia Research*, 125, 278–83.

Leung, A. and Chue, P. 2000. Sex differences in schizophrenia, a review of the literature. *Acta Psychiatrica Scandinavica*, 101, 3–38.

Levin, E. D. and Rezvani, A. H. 2007. Nicotinic interactions with antipsychotic drugs, models of schizophrenia and impacts on cognitive function. *Biochemical Pharmacology*, 74, 1182–91.

Li, R., Ma, X., Wang, G., Yang, J., and Wang, C. 2016. Why sex differences in schizophrenia? *Journal of Translational Neuroscience*, 1, 37–42.

Lin, C.-H., Huang, C.-L., Chang, Y.-C., Chen, P.-W., Lin, C.-Y., Tsai, G. E., and Lane, H.-Y. 2013. Clinical symptoms, mainly negative symptoms, mediate the influence of neurocognition and social cognition on functional outcome of schizophrenia. *Schizophrenia Research*, 146, 231–7.

Lindamer, L. A., Lohr, J. B., Harris, M. J., Mcadams, L. A., and Jeste, D. V. 1999. Gender-related clinical differences in older patients with schizophrenia. *The Journal of Clinical Psychiatry*, 60, 61–7; quiz 68–9.

Mendrek, A. and Mancini-Marïe, A. 2016. Sex/gender differences in the brain and cognition in schizophrenia. *Neuroscience and Biobehavioral Reviews*, 67, 57–78.

Ochoa, S., Usall, J., Cobo, J., Labad, X., and Kulkarni, J. 2012. Gender differences in schizophrenia and first-episode psychosis: a comprehensive literature review. *Schizophrenia Research and Treatment*, 1–9.

Ösby, U., Correia, N., Brandt, L., Ekbom, A., and Sparén, P. 2000. Mortality and causes of death in schizophrenia in Stockholm County, Sweden. *Schizophrenia Research*, 45, 21–8.

Ran, M.-S., Mao, W.-J., Chan, C. L.-W., Chen, E. Y.-H., and Conwell, Y. 2018. Gender differences in outcomes in people with schizophrenia in rural China: 14-year follow-up study. *British Journal of Psychiatry*, 206, 283–8.

Räsänen, S., Pakaslahti, A., Syvälahti, E., Jones, P., and Isohanni, M. 2000. Sex differences in schizophrenia: a review. *Nordic Journal of Psychiatry*, 54, 37–45.

Roy, M.-A., Maziade, M., Labbé, A., and Mérette, C. 2001. Male gender is associated with deficit schizophrenia: a meta-analysis. *Schizophrenia Research*, 47, 141–7.

Sanfilipo, M., Lafargue, T., Rusinek, H., Arena, L., Loneragan, C., Lautin, A., Feiner, D., Rotrosen, J., and Wolkin, A. 2000. Volumetric measure of the frontal and temporal lobe regions in schizophrenia: relationship to negative symptoms. *Archives of General Psychiatry*, 57, 471–80.

Scholten, M. R. M., Aleman, A., Montagne, B., and Kahn, R. S. 2005. Schizophrenia and processing of facial emotions: sex matters. *Schizophrenia Research*, 78, 61–7.

Seeman, M. V. 2004. Gender differences in the prescribing of antipsychotic drugs. *Focus*, 161, 1324–33.

Sham, P. C., Castle, D. J., Wessely, S., Farmer, A. E., and Murray, R. M. 1996. Further exploration of a latent class typology of schizophrenia. *Schizophrenia Research*, 20, 105–15.

Smith, S. 2010. Gender differences in antipsychotic prescribing. *International Review of Psychiatry*, 22, 472–84.

Strauss, G. P., Horan, W. P., Kirkpatrick, B., Fischer, B. A., Keller, W. R., Miski, P., Buchanan, R. W., Green, M. F., and Carpenter Jr, W. T. 2013. Deconstructing negative symptoms of schizophrenia: avolition–apathy and diminished expression clusters predict clinical presentation and functional outcome. *Journal of Psychiatric Research*, 47, 783–90.

Szymanski, S., Lieberman, J. A., Alvir, J. M., and Mayerhoff, D. 1995. Gender differences in onset of illness, treatment response, course, and biologic indexes in first-episode schizophrenic patients. *The American Journal of Psychiatry*, 152, 698.

Takahashi, S., Matsuura, M., Tanabe, E., Yara, K., Nonaka, K., Fukura, Y., Kikuchi, M., and Kojima, T. 2000. Age at onset of schizophrenia: gender differences and influence of temporal socioeconomic change. *Psychiatry and Clinical Neurosciences*, 54, 153–6.

Tsuang, M. 2000. Schizophrenia: genes and environment. *Biological Psychiatry*, 47(3), 210–20. doi:10 .1016/S0006-3223(99)00289-9

Uggerby, P., Nielsen, R. E., Correll, C. U., and Nielsen, J. 2011. Characteristics and predictors of long-term institutionalization in patients with schizophrenia. *Schizophrenia Research*, 131, 120–6.

Usall, J., Haro, J., Ochoa, S., Marquez, M., Araya, S., and Group, N. 2002. Influence of gender on social outcome in schizophrenia. *Acta Psychiatrica Scandinavica*, 106(5), 337–42.

Van Os, J., Kenis, G., and Rutten, B. P. F. 2010. The environment and schizophrenia. *Nature*, 468, 203.

Vaskinn, A., Sundet, K., Simonsen, C., Hellvin, T., Melle, I., and Andreassen, O. A. 2011. Sex differences in neuropsychological performance and social functioning in schizophrenia and bipolar disorder. *Neuropsychology*, 25, 499–510.

Venkatesh, B. K., Thirthalli, J., Naveen, M. N., Kishorekumar, K. V., Arunachala, U.,

Venkatasubramanian, G., Subbakrishna, D. K., and Gangadhar, B. N. 2008. Sex difference in age of onset of schizophrenia: findings from a community-based study in India. *World Psychiatry*, 7, 173–6.

Weiser, M., Davidson, M., and Noy, S. 2005. Comments on risk for schizophrenia. *Schizophrenia Research*, 79(1), 15–21.

Wright, I. C., Rabe-Hesketh, S., Woodruff, P. W., David, A. S., Murray, R. M., and Bullmore, E. T. 2000. Meta-analysis of regional brain volumes in schizophrenia. *American Journal of Psychiatry*, 157, 16–25.

Ethnicity and Male Mental Health

6

Matthew Kelly and Dinesh Bhugra

How mental health affects males is a topic of increasing interest within psychiatric research. This stems not only from public health campaigns looking at male suicide rates but also campaigns on so-called cultures of 'toxic masculinity'; a sociological concept suggested to be behind the creation of environments endorsing antisocial behaviour such as violence and sexual assault (see also Chapters 15 and 17). However, when first deciding to study epidemiology and modifying risk factors in the development of psychopathology in males, we must establish a way of measuring a socially constructed concept that varies hugely dependent on culture. In this chapter we explore the concept of gender identity and roles in society, its difference from biological sex, and how the concept of gender varies between cultures. By looking specifically at gender, we can then begin to investigate the stresses that can occur from psychosocial gender constructs and how these may contribute to male mental health problems and other risk behaviours. Of noticeable importance are the higher rates of psychiatric illness among male migrants along with other contributing factors such as sexual orientation in the development of mental illness. The clinical implications for identifying at-risk individuals and providing treatment in the area of male mental health, is discussed. A key aspect that must be remembered is that there are challenges in definition of gender and non-binary divisions (see also Chapter 8).

Concept of Gender across Cultures

When attempting to measure gender cultural differences we must first be clear as to what we define as an individual's 'gender'. When referring to gender we must make the distinction between the different elements of a person's gender identity. As articulated in Chapter 7, these characteristics include *sex* referring to the biological and physiological characteristics that define being male, female, or an intersex variation; and *gender*, which refers to the socially constructed roles, behaviours, activities, and attributes that a given society considers appropriate for men and women. Gender therefore can be seen as the range of characteristics pertaining to and differentiating between levels of masculinity and femininity. Gender identity is a combination of how someone chooses to identify their gender in line with their biological sex (Hankivsky, 2012).

How someone identifies their gender varies cross-culturally due to the socially constructed nature of gender traits. Traditionally, people who identify as men or women or use masculine or feminine gender pronouns are using a system of gender binary. The process of identifying as a certain gender is relevant to the particular culture in which they live. It is important to note that not all cultures have strictly defined gender roles and many cultures contain societally accepted gender roles outside of male and female, often termed 'third gender' (Towle and Morgan, 2002).

Examples of differing gender roles across cultures include the *hijra*, an institutionalized third gender role in India who are neither male nor female but contain elements of both, tending to be intersex or impotent males (Nanda, 1986). The *muxe* of Mexico are biologically male but with feminine characteristics. They perform gender in a different manner than men: that is, neither distinctly masculine nor feminine but a combination of the two (Stephen, 2002). The Dineh of the Southwestern USA, along with other North American Indigenous tribes, often don't have distinct gender roles and if they do they acknowledge four genders: feminine woman, masculine woman, feminine man, or masculine man. 'Third gendered' individuals are often referred to in North American Indigenous cultures as 'two spirit' people, differing from most Western, mainstream definitions of sexuality and gender identity being seen as a sacred and spiritual role within a society (Estrada, 2011).

Sociology and gender studies suggest that gender expression in the way of multiple gender roles was once the norm for many cultures, and it was colonialism that introduced a basic and universal social classification in terms of superiority and inferiority, one of which was gender binary. This was forced upon many colonized cultures replacing more traditional non-binary gender roles (Lugones, 2007). Today, according to more Western gender norms, those who exist outside of binary man and woman groups fall under the umbrella terms non-binary or genderqueer (Richards et al., 2016). As detailed in Chapter 7, individuals in a state of gender dysphoria who wish to reassign their biological sex in line with their perceived gender are referred to as 'transgender' (American Psychological Association, 2015).

How gender differences develop outside of biological sex – both within society and cross culturally – is a debate that opens up large discussions in the literature exploring nature and nurture explanations from a variety of fields from biology to clinical psychology, sociology, and gender studies. Theories focus largely on challenging the biology of gender and exploring the social construction of gender roles. Early social learning theory explanations, for example, argue that gender-stereotyped behaviours originate through cognitive processes that take place in a social context occurring purely through direct observation and/or the observation of rewards and punishments, a process known as vicarious reinforcement (Bandura, 1977). Social constructionist approaches and communication theory posit that humans rationalize experience by creating models of the social world, hence by sharing and constructing gender norms through language we create a joint assumption of a reality (Littlejohn and Foss, 2009).

Gender schema theory in particular proposes these ideas in a more empirical way, stating that an individual's gender identity is tied up in the socialized sex typing that an individual undergoes, heavily influenced by cultural transmission through parental upbringing, media, and peers (Bem, 1981). Four categories were suggested by Bem to describe where an individual's gender identity falls: sex-typed individuals who process and integrate information in line with their gender; cross-sex-typed individuals who process and integrate information in line with the opposite gender; androgynous individuals who process and integrate traits and information from both genders; and undifferentiated individuals who do not show efficient processing of sex-typed information. The level of masculine and feminine traits can be measured by the Bem Sex Role Inventory (BSRI) (Bem, 1974) and gives us an interesting starting point for measuring the gender differences that occur both in the presentation of mental distress across the general population and within ethnic groups.

Stresses Related to Masculinity

When considering the masculine gender role and its relation to mental distress, researchers and practitioners are increasingly aware of the need for theory, research, and intervention in men's mental health. Work in this area is slowly moving to viewing gender – and more specifically masculinity – as a concept that expands beyond the genetic sex differences between men and women (Addis and Cochane, 2005). Examples using the Bem Sex Role Inventory and Beck's Depression Inventory have identified significant links between masculinity and, to a lesser extent, femininity, as predictors of depression (Stoppard and Paisley, 1987). This effect has attempted to be explained by Gender Role Strain Theory, namely the concept that the gender role we become socialized to conform to can result in psychological stressors due to internalizing extreme gender norms (Pleck, 1995).

'Hegemonic masculinity' is a type of gender strain that refers to practices that signify the dominant and most societally endorsed forms of masculinity: what would be seen as socio-typical heterosexual, white Western norms, including traits such as competitiveness, strength, and self-reliance (Connell and Messerschmidt, 2005). However controversial and attracting criticism, 'toxic masculinity' is a concept that is increasingly attracting attention in popular culture as the exposure of gender issues intensifies due to coverage in the media. The term toxic masculinity refers to 'aspects of hegemonic masculinity that are socially destructive, associated with misogyny, homophobia, greed and violence which become integrated along with traits that are culturally accepted and valued' (Kupers, 2005, p. 716). How such a concept is measured empirically becomes more problematic.

The Masculine Gender-Role Stress Questionnaire (MGRS) was developed to measure masculine stress empirically. It consists of 66 items relating to masculine-related stressful scenarios, each rated on a 7-point scale of level of stress. It has provided evidence through both correlational data and multiple regression to validate and measure gender-related stress in men. Early use of the tool found (as expected) that males experienced more masculine-role stress than women, but interestingly increased masculine-role stress also predicted a significant increase in anger, anxiety, and even poorer health behaviours such as engaging in risky behaviour or lack of help seeking (Eisler, Skidmore, and Ward, 1988). Investigation into the five cluster-specific factors that make up the MGRS have found interesting results in clinical samples, for example looking at gender role stress among violent men court-mandated to attend domestic violence intervention programs. MGRS total scores were associated with intimate partner violence, but gender role stress regarding failure to perform in work and sexual performance were the only factors associated with psychological intimidation. Gender role stress regarding appearing physically fit and not appearing feminine was the only factor associated with sexual coercion, and gender role stress regarding intellectual inferiority was the only factor associated with injury to partners (Moore et al., 2008).

Continuing psychological research has attempted to develop multiple questionnaires to demonstrate psychological distress correlated to masculine gender role. The Subjective Masculinity Stress Scale (SMSS) was developed to assesses the stress associated with men's subjective experiences of what it means to be male. SMSS scores were significantly and positively related to psychological distress and demonstrated how stress resulting from subjective expectations of masculinity leads to wider distress (Wong et al., 2013). More recent meta-analyses exploring the relationships between conformity to masculine norms and mental health-related outcomes found conformity to masculine norms to be associated with mental health issues as well as poor psychological help seeking. Moderation effects such as correlated negative social functioning and conformity to the specific masculine norms of self-reliance and power over women served as predictors of negative mental health outcomes. Conversely, conformity to more positive masculine norms such as work ethic did not have any specific associated mental health-related outcome (Wong et al., 2017).

Psychiatric Disorders in Men, Especially Migrants

When it comes to the epidemiology of psychiatric disorders, males are at an increased risk of suicide, quite often choosing violent and successful methods to end their life (Hawton, 2000, and also see Chapter 11). The reasons for this remain unclear, but stress originating from the masculine gender role could well be a causative factor. Reviews into male suicide rates now explicitly state the need to explore prevention policy and practice by taking into account men's views of what it is to 'be a man' in today's society. In addition, they raise the explicit links between alcohol and substance misuse reduction and suicide prevention in men, noting the links between masculinity and responding to stress by risk taking (Wyllie et al., 2012).

Rates of psychiatric disorders in male migrants warrant particular attention. Ödegaard (1932) performed one of the first studies showing that hospital admission rates for schizophrenia were much higher among Norwegians who had migrated to the United States than Norwegian natives. This increase was explained on the basis of migration. The association between migration and mental health difficulties has been shown in multiple studies, with meta-analyses repeatedly showing a personal or family history of migration is an important risk factor for schizophrenia. In a review and meta-analysis, the relative risk for developing schizophrenia among first-generation migrants was shown to be higher than for the general population (RR=2.7); and second-generation migrants were at a larger risk still (RR=4.5). Even greater relative risks were seen for migrants from developing countries and from areas where the majority of the population is black (RR=4.8) (Cantor-Graae and Selten, 2005).

Studies using a number of different methods have shown elevated rates of schizophrenia between African-Caribbeans and whites in the UK varying from 2.5 to 8.4 times. Using a diathesis stress model, it could appear that elevated rates of schizophrenia may well be a result of postmigration delay in progression (Bhugra, 2004). However, the associations between racism and mental health among Black individuals cannot be underestimated. In a study of of Black Americans, a positive association was found between perceived racism and psychological distress, including anxiety, depression, and other psychiatric symptoms (Pieterse et al., 2012).

Interestingly, prevalence rates of common mental disorders among migrants are not as clear-cut as those in the case of schizophrenia. Nazroo (1997) found lower rates of depression in migrants compared with the white groups, while anxiety varied greatly between ethnic groups and differed also by gender. However, when using migration as a variable, ethnic minority individuals who were either born in Britain or migrated below the age of 11 were found much more likely to report anxiety. Difficulty with collecting these data include language barriers, as lack of English fluency and different cultural help-seeking behaviours may impact the prevalence of patients reporting such issues to health services. Asian men, for example, are generally more likely to consult a GP than their white counterparts, despite having fewer health issues and less emotional distress (Murray and Williams, 1986).

Reasons for the inconsistency in findings for mental health prevalence lie in part in the process of migration being a highly variable and heterogeneous process: an individual may move to study, seek better employment and a future, or to avoid persecution. Acculturation is mentioned regularly within the migration literature to refer to the phenomenon of 'when groups of individuals from different cultures come into continuous first-hand contact with subsequent changes in original cultural patterns'. These can be elements such as language or religion or more abstract concepts of cognitive style, behavioural patterns, attitudes, self-esteem, and identity issues, including gender role. Issues associated with acculturation appear to result in higher rates of severe psychological stress, with a tendency to then manifest psychiatric symptoms (Bhugra, 2004).

More recent analyses of the literature on prevalence and risk factors for common mental health problems related to migration have found that while communication difficulties due to language barriers and cultural differences influence the presentation of symptoms, coping, and the shaping of diagnosis/ treatment of mental health problems, the process of acculturation is also important. It is, however, noted that above all it is the migration trajectory that can be divided into three components: premigration, migration, and postmigration resettlement, with each phase carrying associated specific risks. As would be expected, specific mental health problems are influenced by the migration experience and the adversity experienced before, during, and after resettlement (Kirmayer et al., 2011).

The role of gender identity in the process of acculturation should not be underestimated. More recent studies have begun to expand gender role stress to migrants who have experienced significant cultural shock in male identity, referred to as 'minority masculinity stress theory'. This term was first applied to US-born Asian American men and how they experience Western concepts of 'masculinity'. Open-ended questionnaires were employed to explore two experiences of masculinity-related stress: trying to live up to the masculine ideal of toughness, body image, restrictive emotionality, and heterosexuality; and work-related behaviours, being the achiever and provider. Results found that Asian American men's role identities contradicted hegemonic masculinity concepts, resulting in reflected appraisals that predispose them toward stress (Lu and Wong, 2013). Attempts to integrate hegemonic masculinity, racial stereotypes, different societal gender norms, and mental health to examine the impact in male migrants should be explored in a variety of ethnicities to investigate the role of gender identity in the acculturation process and as potentially modifying effects in increased psychopathology in migrants, particularly second-generation immigrants.

Sexuality and the Role of Sex across Cultures

Studying the role of sex across cultures can become difficult due to the large differences between more religiously conservative countries and more liberally open Western societies. Social anthropologists studying the role of sex often look to the sexual behaviour of other mammals, in particular other great apes. A notable example is the Bonobo, which along with the common chimpanzee are the closest genetic relative to humans. Male and female bonobos engage in sexual behaviour with both the opposite sex and the same sex, not just for procreation but also in what is believed to be for sociosexual purposes using sex to resolve conflict and form social bonds for societal cohesion (De Waal, 1995).

One of the main proposed reasons for the existence of gender role differences is socially communicating sexual desire. For example, research suggests masculine people are not only generally perceived to be more interested in sex than feminine people but also more actively express sexual desire as opposed to those with feminine qualities, who are usually more passive or submissive (Baumeister et al., 2001). Interestingly, when looking at institutional third gender roles across the world, despite their often sacred role in the society, they often begin fulfilling a sexual purpose. For example, the Hijra in India quite often serve as prostitutes to married men (Nanda, 1986). As a result, gender identity is often and sometimes wrongly associated with sexual orientation. An example is the current legal and medical use of gender reassignment in Iran, as a sanctioned option for 'heteronormalizing' people with same-sex desires and practices so their sexual behaviour falls in line with their gender (Najmabadi, 2011).

Sexual orientation and conflict with gender appear to be largely modifying factors with gender in the presence of psychological distress. Despite growing public support across many countries, mental health problems remain higher in LGBT communities then the general population (Russell and Fish, 2016). This is particularly true when looking at the mental health of gay or bisexual men – often referred to clinically as MSM (men who have sex with men). Using samples from four large American cities (Chicago, Los Angeles, New York, and San Francisco), recreational drug use (52%) and alcohol use (85%) were found highly prevalent among urban MSM, with levels of frequent drug use (19%) and heavy–frequent alcohol use (8%) also being common (Stall et al., 2001). Lived experienced of discrimination may be one reason for this, but explanations also encompass internalization of homophobia and the effects of 'minority stress'. The reader is referred to Chapter 7 of this book for a more detailed discussion of gender dysphoria in men.

While looking at non-affirming religious settings, higher internalized homophobia and worse psychological well-being supports the idea that a non-affirming religious environment is associated with higher internalized homophobia. For example, Latino LGBT people had higher internalized homophobia compared to White and Black heterosexuals as mediated by their greater exposure to religion (Barnes and Meyer, 2012). Minority stress, traditional masculine gender roles, and perceived violation of social norms have been advanced as contributors to gay male risk behaviour, including the use of alcohol, tobacco, illicit drugs, and risky sexual practices (Hatzenbuehler et al., 2008).

Studies using correlations and regressions in response to multiple questionnaire outcomes from MSM have found links to social norms and masculinity variables in particular, being significantly related to health-risk behaviours (Hamilton and Mahalik, 2009). Minority stress factors have also been associated with body image dissatisfaction and masculine body ideal distress in MSM using similar methods (Kimmel and Mahalik, 2005). Further studies examining the impact of minority stress theory upon risk behaviours among gay and bisexual (MSM) men lend support to these findings, demonstrating minority stress associations with participant sexual risk behaviours, illicit drug use, and partner type (Dentato et al., 2013). It appears – as with heterosexual males – that gender role-related stress can result in mental ill health that is expressed as risk behaviours. While in typical male samples this usually presents as anger, for MSM behaviour tends to be more inwardly violent, indulging recklessness. These similarities and differences in the presentation of symptoms can be useful in the treatment of mental health in applied clinical practice.

Clinical Approaches

Men's mental health has not been a topic of specific major research or clinical interest until recent years. Epidemiologic studies suggest that the majority of mood and anxiety disorders are found in women (see also Chapters 9 and 12). Why this difference occurs has sparked many debates but one line of thought is that men are more likely to 'mask' emotional distress with substance abuse and violence, two problems for which prevalence is far higher in males. Men also typically underutilize health services relative to women, for the majority of mental and physical health problems for which help-seeking has been studied (Addis and Mahalik, 2003). In addition, it is males engaging in more risk-taking unhealthy behaviours throughout their lives compared to women which is thought to be one of the factors involved in increased mortality rates, with men on average dying seven years younger than women (Courtenay, 2000). Drawing on the areas of male mental health vulnerabilities discussed in this chapter, it is suggested that encompassing a range of social sciences to consider several theoretical paradigms of masculinity is critical for progress in both research and clinical practice when treating male mental ill health (Addis and Cochane, 2005).

In order to address male mental health issues fully, it is suggested that research recognize that gender is about much more than sex differences between men and women. Thus, it is important to understand – from the highly personal to the wider cultural context – how gender impacts society and vice versa. As discussed in this chapter, high scores on measures of gender-role conflict have been repeatedly associated with a range of negative mental health outcomes, including increased symptoms of depression, anxiety, anger, and substance abuse. It follows that improving male mental health would have profound effects on society and those closely affected by the current expression of male mental health problems, including female partners and children (Addis and Cochane, 2005). An example is the use of masculine gender-role stress measures in the predication and prevention of male intimate partner violence towards women (see also Chapter 17). Current research assessing a large sample of college men found that adult attachment insecurity (i.e., attachment anxiety and attachment avoidance) and gender-related stress were associated with tendencies to experience stress from violations of rigidly internalized traditional male role norms, which, in turn, were associated with 'acceptance' of intimate partner violence (McDermott and Lopez, 2013).

Clinical approaches to improving male mental health should encompass gender-related responses to distress. Adherence to particular masculine norms such as emotional stoicism (hiding of symptoms) and indulging in risk behaviours only further exacerbates problems and distress. Interventions should focus on providing males with new ways of responding to emotions that are less influenced by negative 'hegemonic' aspects of traditional masculinity. In addition, aspects of narrative therapy's notably gradual retelling of critical events in the past to reconstruct the masculinity experience of distress in ways that challenge typical male norms and maladaptive coping shows promise clinically. It is important to note, however, that masculinity gender identity begins to develop in early childhood socialization and continues to take shape through middle childhood and adolescence (Bem, 1981). As such, preventative mental health psycho-education at school level is suggested to be effective in particular for male acceptability of emotional expression and help-seeking behaviour (Addis and Cochane, 2005). It is important also to address cultures where male gender stress can

be intensified by the interplay between environment and individual male characteristics. This can be cross-cultural and subcultural with an extreme clinical example being the toxic masculinity that occurs within the institutional dynamics of male prisons, fostering hostile environments where emotional stoicism results in resistance to psychotherapy (see also Chapter 16). Suggested successful interventions focus on male resistances to build relationships through having open discussions about confidentiality, being realistic about treatment aims and focusing on providing practical support and advocacy (Kupers, 2005).

For clinical interventions in male migrants it is noted that risk factors for migrant mental health problems can differ between men and women. In males, language proficiency often has a great influence on employment, which also appears to have subsequent impacts on mental health (Takeuchi et al., 2007), potentially due to stress from gender role expectation to be the provider for the family. However, language barriers also prevent the disclosure of mental health issues in immigrant patients presenting to primary care, with depression or anxiety manifesting as physical complaints or the use of culture-specific bodily idioms to express distress (Kirmayer, 2001). Professional interpreters can improve communication and increase disclosure of psychological symptoms among migrants, with use of specific medical translators being associated with better clinical outcomes then standard translators in randomize control trials (Leng et al., 2010). Along with early identification, prevention can also be achieved by looking at evidence showing migrants living in communities with a high proportion of immigrants from the same background having better well-being. Interventions that are specific to various ethnic backgrounds can provide a sense of belonging and support for a particular ethnocultural identity and assist the process of acculturation (Kirmayer et al., 2011).

Conclusions

In conclusion, the area of specific male mental health research has received far more focus in recent years. The role of gender-related stresses that arise from the masculine gender role appear to have implications for the overrepresentation of violence, suicidal behaviour, and general risk taking in males. This propensity seems to be further intensified when gender role is in conflict with culture, for example in the mental health of migrants or men with sexual orientation issues. Future research should explore the risks that arise from masculine gender role adherence, not just male biological sex; and focus on how the measurement of gender role stress could be used to predict, measure, and treat psychological ill health in males.

References

Addis, M. E. and Cohane, G. H. 2005. Social scientific paradigms of masculinity and their implications for research and practice in men's mental health. *Journal of Clinical Psychology*, 61(6), 633–47.

Addis, M. E. and Mahalik, J. 2003. Men, masculinity and the context of help-seeking. *American Psychologist*, 58, 5–14.

American Psychological Association. 2015. Guidelines for psychological practice with transgender and gender nonconforming people. *American Psychologist*, 70 (9), 832–64.

Bandura, A. 1977. *Social Learning Theory*. Englewood Cliffs, NJ: Prentice Hall.

Barnes, D. M. and Meyer, I. H. 2012. Religious affiliation, internalized homophobia, and mental health in lesbians, gay men, and bisexuals. *American Journal of Orthopsychiatry*, 82(4), 505.

Baumeister, R. F., Catanese, K. R., and Vohs, K. D. 2001. Is there a gender difference in strength of sex drive? Theoretical views, conceptual distinctions, and a review of relevant evidence. *Personality and Social Psychology Review*, 5(3), 242–73.

Bem, S. L. 1974. The measurement of psychological androgyny. *Journal of Consulting and Clinical Psychology*, 42(2), 155.

Bem, S. L. 1981. Gender schema theory: a cognitive account of sex typing. *Psychological Review*, 88(4), 354.

Bhugra, D. 2004. Migration and mental health. *Acta Psychiatrica Scandinavica*, 109, 243–58.

Cantor-Graae, E. and Selten, J. P. 2005. Schizophrenia and migration: a meta-analysis and review. *American Journal of Psychiatry*, 162(1), 12–24.

Connell, R. W. and Messerschmidt, J. W. 2005. Hegemonic masculinity: rethinking the concept. *Gender and Society*, 19(6), 829–59.

Courtenay, W. H. 2000. Constructions of masculinity and their influence on men's well-being: a theory of gender and health. *Social Science and Medicine*, 50(10), 1385–1401.

Dentato, M. P., Halkitis, P. N., and Orwat, J. 2013. Minority stress theory: an examination of factors surrounding sexual risk behavior among gay and bisexual men who use club drugs. *Journal of Gay and Lesbian Social Services*, 25(4), 509–25.

De Waal, F. B. 1995. Bonobo sex and society. *Scientific American*, 272(3), 82–8.

Eisler, R. M., Skidmore, J. R., and Ward, C. H. 1988. Masculine gender-role stress: predictor of anger, anxiety, and health-risk behaviors. *Journal of Personality Assessment*, 52(1), 133–41.

Estrada, G. 2011. Two spirits, Nadleeh, and LGBTQ2 Navajo gaze. *American Indian Culture and Research Journal*, 35(4), 167–90.

Hamilton, C. J. and Mahalik, J. R. 2009. Minority stress, masculinity, and social norms predicting gay men's health risk behaviors. *Journal of Counseling Psychology*, 56(1), 132.

Hankivsky, O. 2012. Women's health, men's health, and gender and health: implications of intersectionality. *Social Science and Medicine*, 74(11), 1712–20.

Hatzenbuehler, M. L., Nolen-Hoeksema, S., and Erickson, S. J. 2008. Minority stress predictors of HIV risk behavior, substance use, and depressive symptoms: results from a prospective study of bereaved gay men. *Health Psychology*, 27(4), 455.

Hawton, K. 2000. Sex and suicide: gender differences in suicidal behaviour. *British Journal of Psychiatry*, 177(6), 484–5.

Kimmel, S. B. and Mahalik, J. R. 2005. Body image concerns of gay men: the roles of minority stress and conformity to masculine norms. *Journal of Consulting and Clinical Psychology*, 73(6), 1185.

Kirmayer, L. J. 2001. Cultural variations in the clinical presentation of depression and anxiety: implications for diagnosis and treatment. *Journal of Clinical Psychiatry*, 62, 22–30.

Kirmayer, L. J., Narasiah, L., Munoz, M., Rashid, M., Ryder, A. G., Guzder, J. and Canadian Collaboration for Immigrant and Refugee Health CCIRH. 2011. Common mental health problems in immigrants and refugees: general approach in primary care. *Canadian Medical Association Journal*, cmaj-090292.

Kupers, T. A. 2005. Toxic masculinity as a barrier to mental health treatment in prison. *Journal of Clinical Psychology*, 61(6), 713–24.

Leng, J. C., Changrani, J., Tseng, C. H., and Gany, F. 2010. Detection of depression with different interpreting methods among Chinese and Latino primary care patients: a randomized controlled trial. *Journal of Immigrant and Minority Health*, 12(2), 234–41.

Littlejohn, S. W. and Foss, K. A. 2009. *Encyclopedia of Communication Theory* (Vol. 1). Los Angeles, CA: Sage, pp. 892–5.

Lu, A. and Wong, Y. J. 2013. Stressful experiences of masculinity among

US-born and immigrant Asian American men. *Gender and Society*, 27(3), 345–71.

Lugones, M. 2007. Heterosexualism and the colonial/modern gender system. *Hypatia*, 22(1), 186–219.

McDermott, R. C. and Lopez, F. G. 2013. College men's intimate partner violence attitudes: contributions of adult attachment and gender role stress. *Journal of Counseling Psychology*, 60(1), 127.

Moore, T. M., Stuart, G. L., McNulty, J. K., Addis, M. E., Cordova, J. V., and Temple, J. R. 2008. Domains of masculine gender role stress and intimate partner violence in a clinical sample of violent men. *Psychology of Men and Masculinity*, 9(2), 82.

Murray, J. and Williams, P. 1986. Self-reported illness and general practice consultations in Asian born and British born residents of West London. *Social Psychiatry*, 21, 136–45.

Najmabadi, A. 2011. Verdicts of science, rulings of faith: transgender/sexuality in contemporary Iran. *Social Research: An International Quarterly*, 78(2), 533–56.

Nanda, S. 1986. The Hijras of India: cultural and individual dimensions of an institutionalized third gender role. *Journal of Homosexuality*, 11 (3–4), 35–54.

Nazroo, J. Y. 1997. Ethnicity and mental health: findings from a national community survey. Policy Studies Institute, London, 115pp., http://hdl.handle.net/10068/432676

Odegaard, O. 1932. Emigration and insanity. *Acta Psychiatrica Neurologica*, 4(Suppl.), 1–206.

Pieterse, A. L., Todd, N. R., Neville, H. A., and Carter, R. T. 2012. Perceived racism and mental health among Black American adults: a meta-analytic review. *Journal of Counseling Psychology*, 59(1), 1.

Pleck, J. H. 1995. The gender role strain paradigm: an update. In: R. F. Levant and W. S. Pollack (eds), *A New Psychology of Men*. New York: Basic Books, pp. 11–32.

Richards, C., Bouman, W. P., Seal, L., Barker, M. J., Nieder, T. O., and T'Sjoen, G. 2016. Non-binary or genderqueer genders. *International Review of Psychiatry*, 28(1), 95–102.

Russell, S. T. and Fish, J. N. 2016. Mental health in lesbian, gay, bisexual, and transgender (LGBT) youth. *Annual Review of Clinical Psychology*, 12, 465–87.

Stall, R., Paul, J. P., Greenwood, G., Pollack, L. M., Bein, E., Crosby, G. M., . . . and Catania, J. A. 2001. Alcohol use, drug use and alcohol-related problems among men who have sex with men: the Urban Men's Health Study. *Addiction*, 96(11), 1589–1601.

Stephen, L. 2002. Sexualities and genders in Zapotec Oaxaca. *Latin American Perspectives*, 29(2), 41–59.

Stoppard, J. M. and Paisley, K. J. 1987. Masculinity, femininity, life stress, and depression. *Sex Roles*, 16(9–10), 489–96.

Takeuchi, D. T., Zane, N., Hong, S., Chae, D. H., Gong, F., Gee, G. C., . . . and Alegría, M. 2007. Immigration-related factors and mental disorders among Asian Americans. *American Journal of Public Health*, 97(1), 84–90.

Towle, E. B. and Morgan, L. M. 2002. Romancing the transgender native: rethinking the use of the 'third gender' concept. *GLQ: Journal of Lesbian and Gay Studies*, 8(4), 469–97.

Wong, Y. J., Shea, M., Hickman, S. J., LaFollette, J. R., Cruz, N., and Boghokian, T. 2013. The Subjective Masculinity Stress Scale: Scale development and psychometric properties. *Psychology of Men and Masculinity*, 14(2), 148.

Wong, Y. J., Ho, M. H. R., Wang, S. Y., and Miller, I. S. 2017. Meta-analyses of the relationship between conformity to masculine norms and mental health-related outcomes. *Journal of Counseling Psychology*, 64(1), 80.

Wyllie, C., Platt, S., Brownlie, J., Chandler, A., Connolly, S., Evans, R., Kennelly, B., et al. 2012. *Men, Suicide and Society. Why Disadvantaged Men in Mid-Life Die by Suicide*. Surrey: Samaritans.

Chapter

7

Gender Dysphoria in Men

Jaco Erasmus

For the purpose of this chapter, it is important that we first review what is understood by the term 'men'. Historically and conventionally, the terms 'man' and 'male' have referred to sex but this has often been conflated with gender, resulting in 'sex' and 'gender' being used interchangeably. In recent times, our understanding of the differences between sex and gender has evolved. *Sex* refers to the biological characteristics (chromosomes, genitalia, hormones) that categorize people into male or female. *Gender*, however, is understood as a social construct that reflects a range of feelings, beliefs, and behaviours that a person may experience and exhibit, along a male–female spectrum. Other chapters in this book focus solely on the mental health of individuals whose sex was assigned male at birth (usually due to the appearance of their external genitalia) and who identify with the male gender. Some individuals, however, do not identify with the sex that was assigned to them at birth. In discussing gender dysphoria in men, this chapter, therefore, departs from the conventional definition of men to also include individuals who were not assigned male at birth but do identify as male. There is increasing awareness of the importance of inclusivity (Kaplan et al., 2018), and that a discussion about the mental health care needs of men must also include the needs of men who were not assigned male at birth.

Trans, gender diverse, and non-binary (TGDNB) is an umbrella term that relates to individuals whose gender identity does not match the sex assigned to them at birth. Many of these individuals will experience gender dysphoria, where the incongruence between their gender identity and the sex assigned to them at birth is associated with distress. As TGDNB people continue to become more visible in our society, our understanding and acceptance of gender diversity is also increasing. This may explain why specialist gender clinics across the world have seen a rapid increase in recent times in the number of people experiencing gender dysphoria (Fielding and Bass, 2018). This increase in awareness and desire to seek professional assistance has overwhelmed current resources and has highlighted the need to broaden education initiatives to include general mental health professionals who are likely to encounter TGDNB individuals in their everyday practice (Byne et al., 2018). This chapter reviews the terminology, prevalence, diagnosis, management, mental health concerns, and outcomes for TGDNB individuals who experience gender dysphoria. The reader is also referred to Chapter 6 for a consideration of ethnocultural aspects of gender.

Terminology

Definitions of terms that relate to gender diversity continue to evolve. Language and how it gets used is important and so it is essential to be aware of the contemporary use of terms to be respectful of, and avoid causing harm to, TGDNB individuals. It is also important to acknowledge that not all individuals will identify with every term due to a number of factors, including cultural and generational differences. It is therefore always

---

Box 7.1   General issues relating to gender dysphoria in men

- Not all men identify with the sex that was assigned to them at birth and for some this causes significant distress
- Around 0.4% of the population identify as trans, gender diverse, or non-binary (TGDNB)
- Gender dysphoria can present in many ways with no classic history
- Emerging evidence supports the biological basis for gender identity development
- Treatment is individualized and aims to affirm a person's gender identity
- Gender minority stress underpins many of the mental health difficulties that TGDNB people experience

helpful to check which terms the individual prefers. Although not an exhaustive list, the following summarizes commonly used terms and their definitions:

Sex: Biological characteristics (chromosomes, hormones, genitalia) that categorize people into male or female.

Sex assigned at birth: The sex initially recorded on a person's birth certificate and usually determined by examination of the external genitalia.

Gender: A social construct that reflects a range of feelings, beliefs, and behaviours along a male–female spectrum.

Gender identity: A person's intrinsic sense of their gender.

Gender expression: Outward appearance and behaviours that in a given culture are designated along a male–female spectrum.

Gender non-conformity: Expression, interests, or behaviours that do not align with the sociocultural expectations of the sex assigned at birth.

Gender dysphoria: Distress associated with an incongruence between a person's gender identity and their sex assigned at birth.

Non-binary: A gender identity that does not fit into a binary male or female understanding of gender.

TGDNB: An umbrella term used to describe those individuals whose gender identity does not match the sex assigned to them at birth, and includes those individuals who are non-binary.

Transgender/Trans: Alternative umbrella terms to describe those individuals whose gender identity does not match the sex assigned to them at birth.

Cisgender: A person whose gender identity is congruent with the sex assigned to them at birth.

Transsexual: A term preferred by some TGDNB individuals who have undergone genital gender affirmation surgery and who have a binary understanding of their gender identity.

Transman: A person assigned female at birth who identifies as male.

Transwoman: A person assigned male at birth who identifies as female.

FTM: A dated term describing the direction of gender transition from female to male.

MTF: A dated term describing the direction of gender transition from male to female.

Miscellaneous terms and expressions (generally considered offensive, and to be avoided): tranny, ladyboy, he-she, shemale, 'real' man, 'real' woman, 'real' name, male role, female role.

Prevalence

Considerable variation in the prevalence rate of gender dysphoria has been reported in studies, due to differences in methodology and diagnostic classifications. One of the difficulties in determining the prevalence accurately has been the challenge in clearly defining the population. Some studies have focused on the transsexual population, defined as only those who had undergone sex reassignment surgery, and estimated the prevalence to be 1 in 12,900 birth-assigned males and 1 in 33,800 birth-assigned females (De Cuypere et al., 2007). Other studies have estimated prevalence based on changes to name or sex in national registers (Dhejne et al., 2014) or attendance at a specialist gender clinic (Becerra-Fernández et al., 2017). In a meta-analysis of eleven studies, the prevalence of transsexualism in birth-assigned males was calculated to be 6.8 per 100,000 or 1 in every 14,705 individuals; and the prevalence of transsexualism in birth-assigned females was calculated to be 2.6 per 100,000 or 1 in every 38,461 individuals (Arcelus et al., 2015). The prevalence of transsexualism in birth-assigned males is often reported as higher than in birth-assigned females, with a ratio of 2.6:1 in this meta-analysis (Arcelus et al., 2015). Although the reason for this is unclear, it has often been surmised that society is less tolerant of gender non-conformity in birth-assigned males, which may increase motivation to undergo sex reassignment. This ratio does, however, appear to be narrowing (Garrett et al., 2000).

Large-scale population-based studies have aimed to estimate the prevalence of those people who self-identify as TGDNB within the broader community. A meta-regression of twelve surveys in the United States estimated a prevalence of 0.39% (Meerwijk and Sevelius, 2017) or 390 per 100,000. The study highlights the significant heterogeneity that may be due to the large number of ways in which questions are asked to determine gender identity. Other population-based studies outside of the USA have reported prevalence rates between 0.5% and 0.9% of the adult population (Winter et al., 2016). An increase in prevalence per year has also been reported and is likely to be a result of increasing awareness of the concept of gender variance and greater willingness to identify as TGDNB in surveys (MacCarthy et al., 2015).

The reason for the substantial difference in prevalence rates between population-based surveys and other cohorts has not been fully investigated. While some TGDNB individuals may not wish to undergo medical or social transition, it is likely that other factors, such as cost and fear of discrimination, present barriers to people seeking medically assisted gender transition. It is plausible, nonetheless, that the number of people seeking medical interventions will continue to rise in the years to come, and this has significant implications for the planning of health service delivery.

Diagnosis and Presentation

People who experience gender dysphoria present in various ways and there is no 'classic' history. While some may develop an awareness of their gender identity during their childhood, for others this may occur during their teenage years or even in late adulthood. Gender dysphoria may have a rapid onset resulting in a sense of urgency in seeking treatment, or an insidious onset resulting in a lag of years before seeking treatment. Some people who experience dysphoria may indeed never seek medical interventions. The onset may be triggered by the development of sex characteristics during puberty, first sexual experiences, exposure to information about TGDNB identities, or exposure to the TGDNB community. Gender identity cannot be assumed from how a person presents or from their behaviour or interests. Some cisgender men, for example, can be nurturing and emotional, or choose to have long hair, wear makeup, and enjoy reading fashion magazines, or engage in acts or pursuits that are stereotypically considered feminine. Gender identity is, instead, self-determined.

A diagnosis related to gender identity was first included in the Diagnostic and Statistical Manual of Mental Disorders in 1983 (American Psychiatric Association, 1983). Efforts to destigmatize the diagnosis in the most recent edition have included changing the name from Gender Identity Disorder to Gender Dysphoria and emphasizing that the core pathology is distress and not the incongruence between gender identity and sex assigned at birth per se (American Psychiatric Association, 2013). Despite these changes, the ongoing inclusion of the diagnosis in a manual for mental disorders remains controversial. For a DSM-5 diagnosis to be made, two or more indicators of the incongruence between gender identity and sex assigned at birth are required, over a six-month period, together with distress or functional impairment. Examples of these indicators include: 'a strong desire to be rid of one's primary and/or secondary sex characteristics', 'a strong desire to acquire the sex characteristics of another gender', 'a strong desire to be treated as another gender' and 'a strong conviction that one has the typical feelings and reactions of another gender' (American Psychiatric Association, 2013).

In a historic decision, the World Health Organization, in updating its International Classification of Diseases (ICD-11), has retained a diagnosis related to gender identity but has moved the diagnosis from the chapter on Mental and Behavioural Disorders to the chapter on Conditions Related to Sexual Health (Reed et al., 2016). The condition has also been renamed 'Gender Incongruence'. It is hoped that this attempt to de-psychopathologize gender diversity will lead to an increase in societal acceptance with a subsequent reduction in prejudice and discrimination.

It is important to consider alternative explanations for why an individual may be experiencing gender dysphoria, although these are rarely encountered. Some people with schizophrenia may hear command hallucinations telling them to pursue gender transition or may have developed an understanding of their gender identity as part of a delusional belief. Patients with dissociative identity disorder may present with gender dysphoria if their alters have different genders. At times, instability and confusion about one's gender identity may form part of a more global disturbance in identity, as seen in borderline personality disorder. A preoccupation with a perceived or actual minor flaw in sex characteristics may be better explained by body dysmorphic disorder (see Chapter 8), particularly if the individual does not have concerns about their gender identity. Where the desire to wear female clothing is primarily a means to achieve or enhance sexual arousal, a transvestic fetish may be a likely explanation. Obsessive preoccupations are common in patients with an autism spectrum disorder (see Chapter 2); such obsessions may be gender non-conforming and can be misconstrued as a reflection of their gender identity. Other factors to consider include internalized homophobia, which leads to believing that gender transition is preferable to same-sex relationships; confusing sexuality with gender identity, where gender identity is wrongly inferred from one's sexual orientation; and intolerance of gender non-conformity, where gender transition is deemed more culturally acceptable than living as an effeminate male.

Aetiology

The exact mechanisms guiding gender identity development are ill-understood and are likely to be complex and multifactorial. Psychological and sociocultural factors appear to have a stronger influence over gender expression, whereas there has been an increase in the scientific evidence supporting the biological basis of gender identity. The US Endocrine Society has recently summarized the following four key areas of evidence in a Position Statement (Endocrine Society, 2017):

(1) Attempts to change the gender identity of intersex patients so that their gender identity matches their genitals or chromosomes, are often unsuccessful and distressing (Saraswat et al., 2015);

(2) Concordance rates are higher in monozygotic twins than dizygotic twins (39% versus 0%) (Heylens et al., 2012);

(3) Rates of male gender identity are higher in individuals with XX chromosomes who were exposed to high levels of androgens in utero, whilst rates of female gender identity are higher in individuals with XY chromosomes who have androgen insensitivity syndrome (Dessens et al., 2005);

(4) Structural and functional brain studies have found differences between TGDNB individuals and controls (Saraswat et al. 2015).

Improving our understanding of the aetiology of gender diversity is important as there is evidence that holding the belief that gender diversity has a biological origin is associated with greater tolerance by our society (Landen and Innala, 2000). This may, therefore, result in less harassment and discrimination. It is important, however, for us to be cautious not to inadvertently pathologize gender diversity by excessively focusing on trying to understand how TDGNB identities have developed, but instead to focus on how diversity in gender identity formation can be welcomed and embraced by society.

Management

Research has shown that TGDNB individuals mostly have negative experiences when accessing health care, irrespective of whether that care was provided for gender dysphoria or not (Riggs et al., 2014). Some such individuals are categorically denied service while others encounter clinicians who do not have adequate knowledge or skills. Waiting times are often long due to the limited number of specialists in the field and the costs of accessing services can be substantial as these services are often available only in the private health care sector. Discrimination and harassment within health care settings are also not uncommon, with more than one in four patients being victim to verbal harassment according to one large survey (Grant et al., 2010). Not only are these added stresses detrimental to the mental health of those seeking health care, but there is evidence that discrimination by health care providers results in TGDNB individuals avoiding health care, including preventative health care, when it is needed (Grant et al., 2010). Discrimination in health care settings may also explain why some TGDNB people choose to access unmonitored hormone therapy online, which is not prescribed by a clinician (de Haan et al., 2015).

Many clinicians will have therapeutic encounters with TGDNB individuals that are not related to their gender dysphoria. It is crucial therefore for all clinicians to develop an inclusive practice that is sensitive to the needs of TGDNB individuals. This includes accurately recording the individual's preferred name, salutation, pronouns, and gender in their medical records and in all correspondence. It is important for all staff to be aware of the significance of these and to use these in all interactions with clients. It is also important for staff to be flexible depending on the needs of the person at a particular time. A transwoman, for example, who has not socially transitioned in the workplace, attends an appointment during her lunch break presenting as a male. Although administrative records may reflect that she uses female pronouns and prefers a female name, on this occasion she may prefer to use a different name and pronouns. Privacy, too, is of paramount importance and extra effort needs to be adopted to avoid accidental disclosure of a person's gender history. Bathrooms can also be a source of great anxiety. Single-sex bathrooms may need to be redesigned to be inclusive of all genders. Where this is not possible, a policy that allows TGDNB people to use the bathroom that matches their gender identity should be developed. Waiting rooms should reflect an attitude of respecting diversity and intolerance of discrimination and harassment. Educational materials provided to clients should appropriately reflect the diversity of their needs. Finally, it is important to have a clear process whereby TGDNB individuals can provide feedback on the cultural awareness of the clinic and staff.

The guiding principle in medical treatment aimed at alleviating gender dysphoria, as pioneered by Dr Harry Benjamin, is to assist TGDNB individuals in affirming their gender (Benjamin, 1966). This may be achieved socially by changes to outer appearance, such as clothing and hairstyle, legal change of name and identity documents, and through medical interventions that help align physical appearance and voice with gender identity. Feminization may be achieved through oestrogen and antiandrogen hormone therapy, voice therapy, hair removal therapies, and/or various surgeries including facial feminization, tracheal shave, and vaginoplasty. Masculinization may be achieved through testosterone hormone therapy and/ or surgeries including chest reconstruction and phalloplasty. Treatment is always tailored to the individual's goals. Not everyone requests hormone replacement, surgery and voice therapy. Some people, for example, undergo chest reconstruction surgery without commencing masculinizing hormones. Others commence feminizing hormones and undergo voice feminization therapy but never undergo genital surgery, while others may never seek any medical intervention.

A number of guidelines have been published to assist clinicians in providing safe and effective care for TGDNB individuals. The World Professional Association for Transgender Health (WPATH) has developed Standards of Care based on best available research evidence and expert professional consensus. In the most recent version, a comprehensive assessment by a suitably experienced mental health clinician is recommended to assess whether the person fulfils certain criteria to commence hormone therapy or undergo surgery (Coleman et al., 2012). These are shown in Boxes 7.2 and 7.3.

In recent years, a number of clinicians and gender clinics have viewed the current requirements for hormone therapy as unnecessary hurdles that delay

---

Box 7.2 Hormone therapy and/or chest surgery

- Persistent, well-documented gender dysphoria;
- Age of majority;
- If significant medical or mental health concerns are present, they must be well controlled; and
- Capacity to make an informed decision and to consent to treatment.

Box 7.3 Genital surgery: the following additional criteria are included

- Twelve continuous months of hormone therapy; and
- Twelve continuous months of living according to their gender identity, if the person is undergoing phalloplasty, metoidioplasty, or vaginoplasty.

---

access to care, and have subsequently adopted an informed consent model of care in which provision of hormone therapy is at the discretion of the primary care provider. A comprehensive mental health assessment is only undertaken if requested by the individual or deemed necessary by the primary care clinician due to existing severe mental health problems. Although no head-to-head comparisons have been conducted between these two models of care, clinics using an informed consent model of care are held in high regard by patients and there do not appear to be significant legal risks (Deutsch, 2012).

Specific tasks for the mental health professional in providing ongoing care for TGDNB clients include the following:

(1) Providing a safe and validating environment in which the individual can explore and develop an understanding of their gender identity.

(2) Ensuring that a person's gender identity development has not been unduly influenced by a mental illness.

(3) Providing information about medical interventions aimed at reducing gender dysphoria.

(4) Ensuring that the individual has been provided with adequate information about the possible effects and risks of the medical intervention from a biopsychosocial perspective.

(5) Assessing the person's capacity to give informed consent to treatment.

(6) Identifying and providing optimal management of coexisting mental health problems.

(7) Facilitating 'coming out' to significant others.

(8) Recognizing and addressing the impact of minority stress and building resilience by developing emotion regulation skills, improving self-esteem, and forming strong peer and family support networks.

Mental Health

The Gender Minority Stress Model was adapted from the Minority Stress Model for sexual minorities (Hendricks and Testa, 2012) and is based on the premise that TGDNB individuals are subject to a unique form of stigma and prejudice, and that the stress associated with this results in adverse health outcomes. 'Transphobia' refers to the prejudicial attitudes, beliefs, and behaviours directed at TGDNB individuals. This usually comes from an external source in the form of harassment or discrimination but may also manifest as internalized transphobia where the prejudice is internally directed at the self. This has been strongly associated with mental health difficulties, particularly in young adults (Nuttbrock et al., 2010).

Many studies have reported elevated rates of psychiatric disorders amongst TGDNB individuals. In a review of thirty-eight studies, Dhejne et al. (2016) reported that although the prevalence of psychiatric disorders amongst those attending specialist gender clinics was high, it was not possible, due to the lack of controlled studies, to conclude with confidence that the rates were higher in this population than in the cisgender population or the TGDNB population who do not seek medical care. In a community survey of over 27,000 TGDNB people in the USA, where one-third had never received gender-related health care, 39% of respondents reported experiencing serious psychological distress in the previous month (James et al., 2016). Only one study has reported prevalence rates of mental illness prior to commencing treatment for gender dysphoria, and found rates of 38% for current Axis I disorders and 70% for lifetime Axis I disorders (Heylens et al., 2014). These higher rates were mostly attributable to depression and anxiety disorders. Interestingly, the prevalence rate of affective disorders was equal between birth-assigned males and birth-assigned females. The prevalence rate for Axis II disorders was 15%, with Cluster C personality disorders being the most common (Heylens et al., 2014). The higher prevalence of autism spectrum disorder amongst TGDNB individuals has also been

gaining attention and further research is needed into cultural competence when working with neurodiverse individuals who are also TGDNB (Pasterski et al., 2014).

In addition to standard psychiatric care, it is important to address factors associated with the development and maintenance of psychopathology. Resilience can be improved by building self-esteem through strategies to increase acceptance and a sense of pride in gender identity (Mizock, 2017). Facilitating family support and peer support may increase help-seeking behaviour. Improving interpersonal skills, problem-solving skills, and mood regulation skills may all mitigate the stresses associated with gender transition (Witcomb et al., 2018). Clinicians should be mindful of potential situations where a person can be exposed to transphobic harassment, not only within the broader community but also within health care settings such as psychiatric inpatient units. Finally, clinicians play a key role in advocating on behalf of TGDNB clients to ensure access to gender-affirming health care given the positive impact this has on mental well-being (Dhejne et al., 2016).

Outcomes

Over fifty studies have found that gender transition improves the overall well-being of those people who have experienced gender dysphoria. The quality of these studies, however, has generally been low with lack of control groups, lack of randomization, and reliance on self-report measures. Furthermore, it has been very difficult to tease out the benefits of each individual component of gender-affirmative care. In the largest meta-analysis to date, Murad et al. (2010) identified 28 studies that enrolled a total of 1833 participants. Only three studies had a control group and eight were longitudinal. Significant improvement in psychological functioning was reported by 78% of participants, with 80% reporting significant improvement in gender dysphoria and quality of life.

In a systematic review of the impact of hormone therapy alone on psychological functioning, White and Reisner (2016) found only three prospective studies. Notwithstanding methodological flaws, the review shows low-quality evidence for a positive effect on mental health and quality of life, 3–12 months after initiation of hormone therapy.

Patients consistently report high levels of satisfaction with surgical interventions (Van De Grift et al.,

2018). Surgical complication rates tend to vary depending on the nature of the procedure. Although high patient satisfaction has been reported in those undergoing phalloplasty, a review of nineteen studies reported that complication rates were high (39.4%; Remington et al., 2018). Complication rates for chest reconstructive surgery in transmen, on the other hand tend, to be lower (11.8%) with high levels of satisfaction (Wolter et al., 2015). Major surgical complications in transwomen who undergo vaginoplasty are rare (Sigurjonsson et al., 2015) and quality of life improves within the first year after surgery (Lindqvist et al., 2017). Although some studies have reported worsening of quality of life, especially in birth-assigned males (Murad et al., 2010), this appears to occur in patients with significant psychiatric morbidity, poor social support, later onset of gender dysphoria, and poor surgical outcomes. Major regret (defined as the desire to detransition) is rare. In a file review of 6793 people who attended the Amsterdam gender clinic between 1972 and 2015 (Wiepjes et al., 2018), regret was only experienced in 0.6% of transwomen and 0.3% of trans men who had undergone gonadectomy.

Of significant concern has been the high prevalence of lifetime suicide attempts amongst TGDNB individuals. In a large survey of over 6000 participants, 41% of respondents reported attempting suicide at some point in their life (Grant et al., 2010).

Discrimination and victimization are factors that have been shown to contribute to the risk of suicide attempts (Haas, Rodgers, and Herman, 2014). Completing medical transition, however, is associated with a reduction in suicide attempts (Bauer et al., 2015). Despite this reduction in suicide attempts after medical transition, the rate remains higher than the general population (Murad et al., 2010).

Conclusions

This chapter highlights the importance of not making assumptions. Some men were not assigned male at birth and some people who were assigned male at birth do not identify as male. There are also many ways to be a male and this cannot be inferred based on clothing choice, hairstyles, interests, sexual orientation, or genitals. Gender identity is a core element of identity and, as with many others aspects of identity, is self-determined. Having your gender identity invalidated, either overtly or in subtle covert ways, can lead to profound mental health difficulties. Our current generation is witnessing a turning point in how society views gender diversity. By approaching gender diversity with compassion through affirmative care we can begin to heal the wounds that have been inflicted over many years on the trans, gender diverse, and non-binary community.

References

American Psychiatric Association. 1983. *Diagnostic and Statistical Manual of Mental Disorders.* 3rd ed. Washington, DC: American Psychiatric Association.

American Psychiatric Association. 2013. *Diagnostic and Statistical Manual of Mental Disorders.* 5th ed. Washington, DC: American Psychiatric Association.

Arcelus, J., Bouman, W. P., Van Den Noortgate, W., Claes, L., Witcomb, G., and Fernandez-Aranda, F. 2015. Systematic review and meta-analysis of prevalence studies in transsexualism. *European Psychiatry*, 30(6), 807–15.

Bauer, G. R., Scheim, A. I., Pyne, J., Travers, R., and Hammond, R. 2015. Intervenable factors associated with suicide risk in transgender persons: a respondent driven sampling study in Ontario, Canada. *BMC Public Health*, 15(1), 525.

Becerra-Fernández, A., Rodríguez-Molina, J. M., Asenjo-Araque, N., Lucio-Pérez, M. J., Cuchí-Alfaro, M., García-Camba, E., Pérez-López, G., Menacho-Román, M., Berrocal-Sertucha, M. C., Ly-Pen, D., and Aguilar-Vilas, M. V. 2017. Prevalence, incidence, and sex ratio of transsexualism in the autonomous region of Madrid (Spain) according to healthcare demand. *Archives of Sexual Behavior*, 46(5), 1307–12.

Benjamin, H., Lal, G. B., Green, R., and Masters, R. E. 1966. *The Transsexual Phenomenon.* New York: Ace Publishing Company.

Byne, W., Karasic, D. H., Coleman, E., Eyler, A. E., Kidd, J. D., Meyer-Bahlburg, H. F., Pleak, R. R., and Pula, J. 2018. Gender dysphoria in adults: an overview and primer for psychiatrists. *Transgender Health*, 3 (1), 57–73.

Coleman, E., Bockting, W., Botzer, M., Cohen-Kettenis, P., DeCuypere, G., Feldman, J., Fraser, L., Green, J., Knudson, G., Meyer, W. J., and Monstrey, S. 2012. Standards of care for the health of transsexual, transgender, and gender-nonconforming people, version 7. *International Journal of Transgenderism*, 13(4), 165–232.

De Cuypere, G., Van Hemelrijck, M., Michel, A., Carael, B., Heylens, G., Rubens, R., Hoebeke, P., and Monstrey, S. 2007. Prevalence and demography of transsexualism in

Belgium. *European Psychiatry*, 22 (3), 137–41.

Dessens, A. B., Slijper, F. M., and Drop, S. L. 2005. Gender dysphoria and gender change in chromosomal females with congenital adrenal hyperplasia. *Archives of Sexual Behavior*, 34(4), 389–397.

Deutsch, M. B. 2012. Use of the informed consent model in the provision of cross-sex hormone therapy: a survey of the practices of selected clinics. *International Journal of Transgenderism*, 13(3), 140–6.

Dhejne, C., Öberg, K., Arver, S., and Landén, M. 2014. An analysis of all applications for sex reassignment surgery in Sweden, 1960–2010: prevalence, incidence, and regrets. *Archives of Sexual Behavior*, 43(8), 1535–45.

Dhejne, C., Van Vlerken, R., Heylens, G., and Arcelus, J. 2016. Mental health and gender dysphoria: a review of the literature. *International Review of Psychiatry*, 28(1), 44–57.

Endocrine Society. 2017. An Endocrine Society position statement. Available at: www.endocrine.org/-/media/endosociety/files/advocacy-and-outreach/position-statements/2017/position_statement_transgender_health.pdf?la=en (accessed 15 July 2018).

Fielding, J. and Bass, C. 2018. Individuals seeking gender reassignment: marked increase in demand for services. *BJPsych Bulletin*, 1–5.

Garrels, L., Kockott, G., Michael, N., Preuss, W., Renter, K., Schmidt, G., Sigusch, V., and Windgassen, K. 2000. Sex ratio of transsexuals in Germany: the development over three decades. *Acta Psychiatrica Scandinavica*, 102(6), 445–8.

Grant, J. M., Mottet, L. A., Tanis, J., Herman, J. L., Harrison, J., and Keisling, M. 2010. *National Transgender Discrimination Survey Report on Health and Health Care*. Washington, DC: National

Center for Transgender Equality and the National Gay and Lesbian Task Force.

Grift, T. C. van de, Elaut, E., Cerwenka, S. C., Cohen-Kettenis, P. T., and Kreukels, B. P. 2018. Surgical satisfaction, quality of life, and their association after gender-affirming surgery: a follow-up study. *Journal of Sex and Marital Therapy*, 44(2), 138–48.

Haan, G. de, Santos, G. M., Arayasirikul, S., and Raymond, H. F. 2015. Non-prescribed hormone use and barriers to care for transgender women in San Francisco. *LGBT Health*, 2(4), 313–23.

Haas, A. P., Rodgers, P. L., and Herman, J. L. 2014. Suicide attempts among transgender and gender non-conforming adults. *work*, 50, 59.

Hendricks, M. L. and Testa, R. J. 2012. A conceptual framework for clinical work with transgender and gender nonconforming clients: An adaptation of the Minority Stress Model. *Professional Psychology: Research and Practice*, 43(5), 460.

Heylens, G., De Cuypere, G., Zucker, K. J., Schelfaut, C., Elaut, E., Vanden Bossche, H., De Baere, E., and T'sjoen, G. 2012. Gender identity disorder in twins: a review of the case report literature. *The Journal of Sexual Medicine*, 9(3), 751–7.

Heylens, G., Elaut, E., Kreukels, B. P., Paap, M. C., Cerwenka, S., Richter-Appelt, H., Cohen-Kettenis, P. T., Haraldsen, I. R., and De Cuypere, G. 2014. Psychiatric characteristics in transsexual individuals: multicentre study in four European countries. *The British Journal of Psychiatry*, 204(2), 151–6.

James, S. E., Herman, J. L., Rankin, S., Keisling, M., Mottet, L., and Anafi, M. 2016. *The Report of the 2015 U.S. Transgender Survey*. Washington, DC: National Center for Transgender Equality.

Kaplan, R. L., El Khoury, C., and Lize, N. 2018. Discussions about the

health of women should include transgender women. *The Lancet Public Health*, 3(6), e269.

Landén, M. and Innala, S. 2000. Attitudes toward transsexualism in a Swedish national survey. *Archives of Sexual Behavior*, 29(4), 375–88.

Lindqvist, E. K., Sigurjonsson, H., Möllermark, C., Rinder, J., Farnebo, F., and Lundgren, T. K. 2017. Quality of life improves early after gender reassignment surgery in transgender women. *European Journal of Plastic Surgery*, 40(3), 223–6.

MacCarthy, S., Reisner, S. L., Nunn, A., Perez-Brumer, A., and Operario, D. 2015. The time is now: attention increases to transgender health in the United States but scientific knowledge gaps remain. *LGBT Health*, 2(4), 287–91.

Meerwijk, E. L. and Sevelius, J. M. 2017. Transgender population size in the United States: a meta-regression of population-based probability samples. *American Journal of Public Health*, 107(2), e1–e8.

Mizock, L. 2017. Transgender and gender diverse clients with mental disorders: treatment issues and challenges. *Psychiatric Clinics*, 40(1), 29–39.

Murad, M. H., Elamin, M. B., Garcia, M. Z., Mullan, R. J., Murad, A., Erwin, P. J., and Montori, V. M. 2010. Hormonal therapy and sex reassignment: a systematic review and meta-analysis of quality of life and psychosocial outcomes. *Clinical Endocrinology*, 72(2), 214–31.

Nuttbrock, L., Hwahng, S., Bockting, W., Rosenblum, A., Mason, M., Macri, M., and Becker, J. 2010. Psychiatric impact of gender-related abuse across the life course of male-to-female transgender persons. *Journal of Sex Research*, 47 (1), 12–23.

Pasterski, V., Gilligan, L., and Curtis, R. 2014. Traits of autism spectrum disorders in adults with gender dysphoria. *Archives of Sexual Behavior*, 43(2), 387–93.

Reed, G. M., Drescher, J., Krueger, R. B., Atalla, E., Cochran, S. D., First, M. B., Cohen-Kettenis, P. T., Arango-de Montis, I., Parish, S. J., Cottler, S., and Briken, P. 2016. Disorders related to sexuality and gender identity in the ICD-11: revising the ICD-10 classification based on current scientific evidence, best clinical practices, and human rights considerations. *World Psychiatry*, 15(3), 205–21.

Remington, A. C., Morrison, S. D., Massie, J. P., Crowe, C. S., Shakir, A., Wilson, S. C., Vyas, K. S., Lee, G. K., and Friedrich, J. B. 2018. Outcomes after phalloplasty: do transgender patients and multiple urethral procedures carry a higher rate of complication? *Plastic and Reconstructive Surgery*, 141(2), 220e–229e.

Riggs, D. W., Coleman, K., and Due, C. 2014. Healthcare experiences of gender diverse Australians: a mixed-methods, self-report survey. *BMC Public Health*, 14(1), 230.

Saraswat, A., Weinand, J., and Safer, J. 2015. Evidence supporting the biologic nature of gender identity. *Endocrine Practice*, 21(2), 199–204.

Sigurjonsson, H., Rinder, J., Möllermark, C., Farnebo, F., and Lundgren, T. K. 2015. Male to female gender reassignment surgery: surgical outcomes of consecutive patients during 14 years. *JPRAS Open*, 6, 69–73.

White Hughto, J. M. and Reisner, S. L. 2016. A systematic review of the effects of hormone therapy on psychological functioning and quality of life in transgender individuals. *Transgender Health*, 1 (1), 21–31.

Wiepjes, C. M., Nota, N. M., de Blok, C. J., Klaver, M., de Vries, A. L., Wensing-Kruger, S. A., de Jongh, R. T., Bouman, M. B., Steensma, T. D., Cohen-Kettenis, P., and Gooren, L. J. 2018. The Amsterdam cohort of gender dysphoria study (1972–2015): trends in prevalence, treatment, and regrets. *The Journal of Sexual Medicine*, 15(4), 582–90.

Winter, S., Diamond, M., Green, J., Karasic, D., Reed, T., Whittle, S., and Wylie, K. 2016. Transgender people: health at the margins of society. *The Lancet*, 388(10042), 390–400.

Witcomb, G. L., Bouman, W. P., Claes, L., Brewin, N., Crawford, J. R., and Arcelus, J. 2018. Levels of depression in transgender people and its predictors: results of a large matched control study with transgender people accessing clinical services. *Journal of Affective Disorders*, 235, 308–15.

Wolter, A., Diedrichson, J., Scholz, T., Arens-Landwehr, A., and Liebau, J. 2015. Sexual reassignment surgery in female-to-male transsexuals: an algorithm for subcutaneous mastectomy. *Journal of Plastic, Reconstructive and Aesthetic Surgery*, 68(2), 184–91.

Chapter

8

Body Image Disorders in Men

Scott Griffiths, Stuart B. Murray, and David Castle

This chapter provides an overview of body image disorders as they pertain to men. Body image encapsulates thoughts, beliefs, and feelings about one's physical appearance. For some men, these thoughts, beliefs, and feelings are neutral, or even positive. This is ideal, insofar as one's body ought to be a functional and useful asset that allows an individual to live life on their own terms. Yet for others, these thoughts, beliefs, and feelings are decidedly negative.

Whilst body image disorders – notably the eating disorders – are often thought of as the preserve of women, many men experience dissatisfaction with their physical appearance. Prevalence estimates vary, but it is clear that substantial numbers of men dislike their body in at least some respects. One general population study of Australian adults found that 60% of males reported at least some dissatisfaction with their body (Griffiths et al., 2016). A more difficult question is whether body dissatisfaction in men is becoming more common. One meta-analysis suggests that men's body dissatisfaction has remained stable since the early 1990s (Karazsia et al., 2017). Nevertheless, in recent decades there has been a demonstrated intensification of the social and cultural pressures on men to 'improve' their bodies (Pope et al., 2000, 1999; Leit et al. 2001; Boepple and Thompson, 2016; Murray et al., 2016). For some men, these environmental pressures, combined with genetic predispositions and personal life events, may cause a level of body dissatisfaction that is severe enough to warrant clinical intervention.

Body Image Disorders

Body image disorders are intrinsically related to, but not synonymous with, body dissatisfaction. As aforementioned, most men experience some dissatisfaction with their appearance. The key element that distinguishes a body image concern from a body image disorder is that the latter causes psychological distress

and significantly impedes normal, everyday functioning. For example, a man who sees his reflection in a bathroom mirror and laments his receding hairline, but who then promptly forgets this shortly after leaving the bathroom, has experiencing body dissatisfaction but is not experiencing a body image disorder. By contrast, a man who sees his receding hairline in the mirror, becomes profoundly upset by this, and who subsequently finds it difficult to engage in social conversation with his friends due to being unable to stop thinking about his hairline and others' judgements of his hairline, may very well be experiencing a body image disorder.

Hereafter, we use the term 'body image disorder' as an umbrella term to refer to a number of specific psychological disorders for which body image is a key psychological component. Body image disorders covered in this chapter include anorexia nervosa, bulimia nervosa, binge-eating disorder, body dysmorphic disorder, muscle dysmorphia, and anabolic-androgenic steroid dependence. Some of these disorders are subsumed by broader categories. Throughout the chapter, we distinguish these categories and highlight important areas of overlap.

Anorexia Nervosa

Anorexia nervosa (AN) is historically the oldest body image disorder recognized in contemporary psychiatric classification systems, having first been described by physicians Charles Lasègue and William Gull in the late eighteenth century (Russell and Treasure, 1989). Until the mid-nineteenth century, AN was widely viewed as a disorder of sexual and emotional immaturity. Few, if any, references to body image were made in early accounts of the disorder (Russell and Treasure, 1989). In subsequent decades, body image has risen in prominence to become a defining feature of AN, such that contemporary diagnostic criteria now explicitly and centrally implicate body image disturbance (APA, 2013). AN is distinct from other body image disorders in that it focuses on aspects of physical appearance that are modifiable through diet and exercise; namely, body weight and body shape.

To receive a diagnosis of AN (see Box 8.1), an individual must persistently restrict their energy intake such that it results in a significantly low body weight. Moreover, individuals must report an intense fear of gaining weight or becoming fat, be disturbed in the way they experience their body weight or shape (e.g., perceiving oneself as obese despite being very slender), and/or overvalue their body shape and weight (e.g., 'nobody will ever love me if I get fat'). The previous edition of the DSM, the DSM-IV (APA, 2000), was criticized for including amenorrhea (the absence of menstruation) as a diagnostic criterion. The presence of amenorrhea as a criterion reinforced the perception that AN is a 'female disorder' and may have resulted in men with AN being precluded from receiving a corresponding diagnosis (Wooldridge and Lytle, 2012). Fortunately, in the DSM 5, this criterion has been removed.

In absolute terms, anorexia is relatively rare. Studies of the general population suggest that between 0.1% and 0.3% of men will develop AN during their lifetime (Allen et al., 2013; Hudson et al., 2007; Kjelsås et al., 2004; Smink et al., 2013; Woodside et al., 2001). Prevalence estimates for AN differ between men and women. Studies of the general population suggest that males account for 25% to 33% of AN diagnoses (Hudson et al., 2007; Madden et al., 2009). By contrast, studies of clinical populations suggest that males constitute just 5% to 10% of such diagnoses (Sweeting et al., 2015). This discrepancy between general population and clinical population studies may be because the various intersecting stigmas attached to men who experience body dissatisfaction, eating disorders, and psychological issues more generally, arguably

disincentivize and discourage males from seeking help for AN (Griffiths et al., 2015b, 2015; Robinson et al., 2012; Räisänen and Hunt, 2014). Another contributing factor may be poor mental health literacy regarding eating disorders. It may be that both men and the health professionals who diagnose men have relatively poor and/or inaccurate knowledge about men and AN (Mond, 2014).

The manifestation of AN differs between men and women. In a study of nearly 120 males and 350 females with diagnoses of AN confirmed by clinical interviews, males were found to score systematically lower on two of the most widely used self-report eating disorder symptom measures: the Eating Disorders Examination – Questionnaire (EDE–Q; Fairburn and Beglin, 1994) and the Eating Disorders Inventory – 3 (EDI-3; Garner, 2004). While it is possible that AN in men is less severe than in women, a more plausible explanation is that there are substantive gender differences in the manifestation of the disorder. The EDE-Q, EDI-3 and other eating disorder measures were developed largely in samples of women with AN. Consequently, these measures may have inherited an insensitivity to men with the disorder (Griffiths et al., 2013). Gender differences identified to date include that men with AN are less concerned with body weight than women, but equally concerned with body shape (Murray et al., 2017). This discrepancy is consistent with men's tendency to desire a lean and muscular body rather than a thin and emaciated body (Murray et al., 2017). Moreover, males are less likely to desire a 'flat stomach' so much as a 'six-pack' of overt abdominal muscles (Murray et al., 2017). Compulsive exercise may also feature more prominently in men with AN in terms of its embeddedness, rigidity, and resistance to treatment. Compulsive exercise in men with AN may also function differentially, with evidence suggesting that men are more likely than women to rely on exercise to regulate their emotions, both positive and negative (Murray et al., 2013).

Bulimia Nervosa

Bulimia nervosa (BN) was the second eating disorder to be identified after AN (Russell, 1979) and was recognized in the third edition of the *Diagnostic and Statistical Manual of Mental Disorders*, DSM-III (APA, 1987). BN is distinct from AN in that is characterized by recurrent episodes of binge eating with

> **Box 8.1** Core features of anorexia nervosa (APA, 2013)
>
> Restriction of energy intake leading to significantly low weight
>
> Intense fear of gaining weight or becoming fat
>
> Disturbance in view of one's body in terms of weight and shape
>
> Two subtypes: restricting and binge-purge

subsequent compensatory behaviours designed to offset the impact of the binge episodes. In this context, a binge-eating episode occurs when an individual eats a large amount of food whilst simultaneously experiencing a loss of control over their eating (e.g., feeling unable to stop themselves from eating). Common compensatory behaviours include self-induced vomiting, the use of laxatives or diuretics, and exercise. As with AN, a diagnosis of BN has an explicit body image component. Specifically, an individual must experience their body weight or shape as central to their self-evaluation. Box 8.2 summarizes the diagnostic criteria for BN

Similar to AN, prevalence estimates for BN differ between men and women; although, in general, the evidence base pertaining to gender differences in BN is smaller than for AN. General population studies suggest that men account for 33% of BN diagnoses (Hudson et al., 2007; Hay et al., 2015). In absolute terms, BN is more common than AN: between 0.1% and 1.6% of men will develop BN during their lifetime (Allen et al., 2013; Hudson et al., 2007; Kjelsås et al., 2004; Woodside et al., 2001).

Men and women with BN may differ with respect to binge-eating episodes and compensatory behaviours. First, there may be differences in perceptions of what constitutes a 'large amount' of food (Forney et al., 2015), with men typically eating more than women and also being more likely to report eating an objectively large amount of food (Lewinsohn et al., 2002; Moore et al., 2009). Second, there may be differences in the types of food eaten by men and women during binge-eating episodes. Men appear more likely to crave high-fat and high-protein foods, such as meats, while women tend towards high-sugar food, such as desserts (Wansink et al., 2003). Third, men

may be less likely than women to engage in purging-related compensatory behaviours, inducing self-induced vomiting and using laxatives or diuretics; rather, men may be more likely to restrict their diet and exercise (Moore et al., 2009; Lavender et al., 2010). As with AN, these differences may cause substantive discrepancies on widely used self-report measures of eating disorder symptoms: men with BN score considerably lower than their female counterparts on both the EDE-Q and EDI-3 (Smith et al., 2017).

Binge-Eating Disorder

Binge-Eating Disorder (BED) has only recently been granted full diagnostic status by the American Psychiatric Association (APA, 2013) and thus is much less researched than AN or BN. The drive to include BED as a discrete diagnostic entity was driven by the appreciation that many people who would under DSM-IV rules have been considered to have a non-specific eating disorder actually manifested a relatively discrete disorder characterized by episodic binge eating but with few of the compensatory behaviour characteristics of BN (Box 8.3). People with BED are usually overweight rather than underweight and often carry much shame about their disorder.

In a large study spanning fourteen mostly high- or upper/middle-income countries, Kessler et al. (2013) reported a median lifetime prevalence rate of BED of 1.4% (interquartile range 0.8–1.9%). Mean age at onset was in the early 20s and the disorder tended to persist. A BED diagnosis was associated with high rates of psychiatric and general health morbidities,

---

Box 8.2 Core features of bulimia nervosa (APA, 2013)

Recurrent episodes of binge eating, characterized by:

- Eating a large amount of food (more than most people would consume over that time period) in a limited time period
- A sense of loss of control during the binge period
- Recurrent compensatory behaviours (e.g., self-induced vomiting, misuse of diuretics, and/or laxatives, excessive exercise)
- Self-evaluation impacted to a large extent by weight/shape concerns

---

Box 8.3 Core features of binge-eating disorder (APA, 2013)

Recurrent episodes of binge eating, characterized by:

- Eating a large amount of food (more than most people would consume over that time period) in a limited time period
- A sense of loss of control during the binge period

Three of the following:

- Eating more rapidly than usual
- Eating till feeling uncomfortably full
- Eating when not hungry
- Eating alone through embarrassment of amount eaten
- Feelings of disgust with self

including arthritis (odds ratio (OR) 1.7), diabetes (OR 2.9), hypertension (OR 2.2), and stroke (OR 1.6). Role impairment subsequent upon BED was reported by nearly half of respondents.

Of the eating disorders, BED is most likely to afflict males, with a M:F ratio of 1:1.75 (Hudson et al., 2007). We are aware of no studies that have specifically addressed BED in men, or have systematically compared men with BED with women with BED. However, it does not seem that there are any substantial differences in the illness parameters between the sexes. Understanding how BED afflicts males in particular is an area for future research.

Body Dysmorphic Disorder

Body dysmorphic disorder (BDD) was formally recognized as a diagnostic entity in DSM-III in 1987 (APA 1987). It is distinct from AN and BN in that the predominating body image psychopathology cannot (by definition) be focused on body weight or body fat. Indeed, the DSM-5 criteria for BDD (Box 8.4) are explicit in stating that the diagnosis can be sustained only if an individual's body image concerns cannot instead be explained by an eating disorder. The range of body image concerns reported by people with BDD is more varied than those with eating disorders. To receive a diagnosis of BDD, an individual must obsesses over one or more apparent flaws in their physical appearance that others would regard as small, slight, unnoticeable, or non-existent. In addition, an individual must perform recurrent behaviours, such as mirror-checking, excessive grooming, comparing their appearance to that of others, or undertaking cosmetic surgeries (these examples are not exhaustive). Finally, individuals with BDD may differ in the level of insight they have into their body image disturbance. For instance, an individual may have good insight,

meaning they are able to recognize that their beliefs about their physical appearance are definitely, or at least probably, false (e.g., 'I know I don't have the biggest nose in the world, but that's the way I feel about it most of the time'). By contrast, an individual with limited insight may endorse delusional beliefs that are wholly divorced from reality (e.g., 'I have the biggest nose in the world; nobody has ever had a nose as big as mine').

Men and women with BDD differ with respect to the foci of their body image concerns. Men are more likely than women to obsess over their genitals, their thinning/receding hairlines (and balding more generally), and their body size and build (Phillips et al., 2006). Men are less likely to obsess over their skin, stomach, breasts/chest, buttocks, thighs, legs, hips, toes, and excessive hair on the body or face (Phillips et al., 2006). In descending order, the body areas most frequently obsessed over by men with body dysmorphic disorder are the skin (70%), hair (64%), nose (38%), body size and build (37%), teeth (22%), and the face in general (22%) (Phillips et al., 2006). There is also evidence to suggest that relative to women, men with BDD experience greater impairment in their functioning, including being less likely to be working due to their symptoms, and being more likely to be receiving disability payments than their female counterparts (Phillips et al., 2006).

Muscle Dysmorphia

Muscle dysmorphia is a relatively newly recognized body image disorder insofar as it was first formally described by a Harvard academic, Professor Harrison Pope, in 1993 (Pope et al., 1993). Whilst conducting a study of bodybuilders, Pope noticed a conspicuous pattern of psychological dysfunction in some of his participants. He described nine large and muscular men who were adamant that they appeared scrawny and weak to others, including partners, friends, and family members. The men were obsessed about their perceived lack of muscle. They refused to be seen shirtless in public spaces and wore heavy body-camouflaging clothing even in the middle of summer. All nine injected anabolic steroids. Seeing the parallels with anorexia nervosa, Pope tentatively named the condition 'reverse anorexia' (Pope et al., 1993). Four years later, Pope formally named the disorder muscle dysmorphia and positioned it as a subtype of body dysmorphic disorder (Pope et al., 1997).

> **Box 8.4 Criteria for body dysmorphic disorder**
>
> Similar to AN and BN, BDD appears more common in women than men, albeit by a smaller margin. General population studies suggest that men may account for approximately 45% of BDD diagnoses, whilst studies of student populations suggest men account for approximately 38% of such diagnoses (Veale et al., 2016). The absolute prevalence of body dysmorphic disorder may be similar to that for bulimia nervosa: between 1.3% and 2.1% of men will experience BDD during their lifetime (Veale et al., 2016).

The nosology of muscle dysmorphia is embroiled in debate. The disorder is currently recognized as one of two specifiers for BDD in the DSM-5. By contrast, muscle dysmorphia will not be recognized in the upcoming International Statistical Classification of Diseases and Related Health Problems – 11th revision (ICD-11; World Health Organization, 2018). In making this decision, the ICD-11 Working Group on the Classification of Obsessive-Compulsive and Related Disorders determined that there was insufficient empirical evidence to support the clinical utility of including muscle dysmorphia as a specifier of body dysmorphic disorder (Veale and Matsunaga, 2014). Furthermore, researchers unaffiliated with the above-mentioned psychiatric classification systems vary in their opinions on the nosology of muscle dysmorphia. Some experts believe that the available empirical evidence is inadequate to support the inclusion of muscle dysmorphia in the above-mentioned psychiatric diagnostic systems (Santos Filho et al., 2015). Others opine that provisional incorporation of muscle dysmorphia into these systems is necessary to incentivize the very research that may inform the nosology of the disorder (Griffiths et al., 2016).

Unfortunately, muscle dysmorphia has yet to receive the high-quality general population studies that are required to inform reliable prevalence estimates. However, studies conducted to date suggest that the disorder is more common among men than women, with men accounting for 80% to 100% of diagnoses of muscle dysmorphia in published clinical studies (Cafri et al., 2008; Olivardia et al., 2000; Murray et al., 2012; Pope et al., 1993, 2005; Hitzeroth et al. 2001; Choi et al. 2002). Relatedly, it is estimated that approximately 25% of men with body dysmorphic disorder have muscle dysmorphia; for women, this proportion is probably less than 10% (Simmons and Phillips, 2017).

The clinical presentation of muscle dysmorphia (Box 8.5) is characterized by preoccupation with thoughts about one's muscularity (4 to 6 hours per day on average), frequent mirror checking (9 to 13 times per day on average), and frequent body weighing (4 to 5 times per week on average) (Cafri et al., 2008; Olivardia et al., 2000). Nearly 90% of men with muscle dysmorphia actively avoid exposing their bodies in public spaces (Olivardia et al., 2000). Insight in muscle dysmorphia ranges from good to zero (the latter indicating delusional beliefs), with an average level-of-insight of fair through poor (Olivardia et al.,

> **Box 8.5 Presenting features of muscle dysmorphia**
>
> Men with muscle dysmorphia engage in many of the same types of disordered eating practices that characterize AN (e.g., rule-driven and rigid rules around what can and cannot be eaten; Murray et al., 2013; Mosley, 2009). In muscle dysmorphia, these disordered eating practices are oriented toward muscularity rather than thinness. Men with muscle dysmorphia report stronger adherence to traditional male gender roles than weightlifting controls without muscle dysmorphia (Murray et al., 2013). This finding accords with the 'gender roles hypothesis': namely, that adherence to traditional male and female gender roles may predispose individuals to the development of thinness- and muscularity-oriented body image disorders, respectively (Griffiths et al., 2015; Mishkind et al., 1986; Lakkis et al., 1999; Meyer et al., 2001). Finally, men with muscle dysmorphia often report ego-syntonic beliefs, such as the beliefs that their (pathological) behaviours are admirable, laudable, or life-affirming (Griffiths et al., 2015a). Disconfirmation of these beliefs can be especially difficult (Griffiths and Murray, 2018).

2000; Cafri et al., 2008). Men with muscle dysmorphia often use anabolic steroids to help them build muscle. Estimates of anabolic steroid use range from 40% to 50% (Olivardia et al., 2000; Cafri et al., 2008; Hitzeroth et al., 2001), though these may be underestimates given the legal ramifications and social stigma associated with anabolic steroid use (Griffiths et al., 2016). In most cases, symptoms of muscle dysmorphia develop before the decision is made to use anabolic steroids (Olivardia et al., 2000). Muscle dysmorphia can cause extreme functional impairment and substantial degradation in quality of life (Pope et al., 2005; Cafri et al., 2008).

Anabolic-Androgenic Steroid Dependence

Anabolic steroids are highly effective at building muscle in men (Bhasin et al., 1996; Bhasin, 2001). This makes anabolic steroids an attractive option for men who are unhappy with their level of muscularity (Griffiths et al., 2016). When a man decides to stop using anabolic steroids, muscle loss of some degree (often a large degree) is inevitable, and he is confronted by the preoccupations and anxieties that fuelled his decision to start using anabolic steroids in the first place (Griffiths et al., 2017). In the context of body image disorders, anabolic-androgenic steroid dependence is concerned with the psychological phenomena surrounding these decisions to start and stop using anabolic steroids.

Anabolic-androgenic steroid dependence predates muscle dysmorphia in that scattered case-reports describing individuals with symptoms of steroid dependence were published during the 1980s and 1990s (Brower et al., 1989; Hays et al., 1990; Tennant et al., 1988). In recent years, however, there has been a surge of public and scientific interest in steroid dependence. Two factors have driven this interest. First, the advent and public popularization of muscle dysmorphia (Pope et al., 2000) has drawn attention to anabolic steroids because 40% to 50% of men with muscle dysmorphia use anabolic steroids (Olivardia et al., 2000; Cafri et al., 2008; Hitzeroth et al., 2001). Second, rates of anabolic steroid use are rising in Australia, the United Kingdom, and elsewhere (McVeigh and Begley, 2016; Memedovic et al., 2017; Iversen et al., 2013). Steroid dependence was formally recognized in 2009 when Kanayama and colleagues (2009a, b) published provisional diagnostic criteria based on the DSM-IV-TR (APA, 2000) criteria for substance use. Two of these criteria are notably relevant: tolerance and withdrawal. In the context of anabolic steroids, tolerance is exemplified by an individual using more potent doses of anabolic steroids to offset the dissatisfaction experienced with the muscle acquired at lower doses. Withdrawal is exemplified by the fatigue, anxiety, insomnia, depression, and other adverse psychological phenomena that frequently occur after stopping anabolic steroids. Users of anabolic steroids have created various terms for this period of psychological instability (e.g., the 'post-cycle blues') and may use a variety of substances to try to normalize their endocrine functioning and ameliorate their malaise (Griffiths et al., 2017).

Three mechanisms of steroid dependence have been proposed to date (Kanayama et al., 2010). The most relevant of these (and arguably the most common) is the body image mechanism. For men preoccupied with their muscles, the improvement in psychological well-being caused by starting anabolic steroids acts as a positive reinforcer that facilitates continued use of these agents. Subsequently, the deterioration in psychological well-being caused by stopping anabolic steroids acts as a negative reinforcement mechanism that maintains psychological dependence. Studies of this mechanism are limited. One study of 74 male steroid users found that symptoms of steroid dependence were strongly linked with body image anxieties (Griffiths et al., 2018). By contrast, a study of 102 male steroid users found no association of body image psychopathology with steroid dependence (Kanayama et al., 2018). Additional research on steroid dependence in the context of body image disorders is urgently needed.

Treatment for Men with Body Image Disorders

Evidence of effective treatments for men with AN and BN is lacking. The landscape of treatment studies for these disorders is dominated almost entirely by randomized controlled trials populated by women. Indeed, it is common for randomized controlled studies of treatments for AN and BN to exclude men because they often comprise only a minority of the sample (Murray et al., 2017) and because men score differently on symptom measures compared to women (Smith et al., 2017), complicating data analyses.

Nevertheless, we can draw upon the available literature to inform treatment approaches for men with AN and BN. A meta-analysis of psychological treatments for AN suggests that cognitive behavioural therapy and family-based therapy improve weight-related outcomes at end-of-treatment, but not at follow-up (Murray et al., 2018). The psychological symptoms of anorexia nervosa have proven especially resistant: neither cognitive behavioural therapy nor family-based therapy improved psychological outcomes at end-of-treatment or follow-up (Murray et al., 2018). These findings have proven highly controversial in the field. Whilst we believe it is still reasonable to adopt either of these therapies for AN, it is clear that additional work is urgently needed to innovate or otherwise improve treatments for this condition. For BN, a recent meta-analysis of psychological treatments suggests that both individual cognitive behavioural therapy and guided cognitive-behavioural self-help improve psychological outcomes at end-of-therapy; the data were insufficient for an analysis of psychological outcomes at follow-up (Slade et al., 2018).

Treatments for BED include cognitive behavioural and dietary strategies but it often recurs and excess weight is often not lost. A number of pharmacological treatments have been explored, with perhaps the most encouraging results for the binge cycles as well as reduction in weight being seen with the anticonvulsant topiramate and the stimulant lisdexamphetamine (Reas and Grilo, 2014). We are aware of no specific treatment implications pertinent to males.

The evidence base for effective treatments for BDD is smaller than for AN and BN. Men are better represented in randomized control trials of treatments for BDD than the eating disorders; on average, men accounted for 30% of the participants in these trials (Phillipou et al., 2016). A systematic review of treatment trials for body dysmorphic disorder suggests that cognitive behavioural therapy and metacognitive therapy may improve psychological outcomes (Phillipou et al., 2016); however, the data were insufficient for meta-analysis. Serotonergic antidepressants also have an established place in treatment of BDD but no studies have investigated males specifically in this regard (Phillipou et al., 2016). There is a clear need for more trials of treatments for BDD as well as an exploration of novel psychological and biological approaches.

Evidence of effective treatments for muscle dysmorphia and anabolic-androgenic steroid dependence is generally unavailable. There exist no published randomized controlled trials of treatments for either of these disorders; a fact that reflects the nascency of these disorders and the expense and time required to develop or adapt psychological treatments, let alone evaluate those treatments. There are, however, scattered published case-reports of the successful adaptation of treatments for eating disorders to the muscle dysmorphia context (Murray and Griffiths, 2014; Murray et al., 2017). Because muscle dysmorphia shares many parallels with AN and BN in particular, and because muscle dysmorphia is a specifier for

BDD, it is sensible to recommend the adaptation of treatments that are effective for these disorders.

Conclusions

Body dissatisfaction is common among men. Body image disorders, by comparison, are rarer. Six body image disorders are well delineated (albeit, to various degrees) in the psychological and psychiatric literatures: anorexia nervosa, bulimia nervosa, binge-eating disorder, body dysmorphic disorder, muscle dysmorphia, and anabolic-androgenic steroid dependence. AN and BN belong to the broader category of eating disorders and men account for a minority of these cases. By contrast, men account for nearly half of BDD diagnoses. Muscle dysmorphia is a diagnostic specifier for BDD and men account for the vast majority of diagnoses. Muscle dysmorphia may account for one-quarter of BDD diagnoses in men. Anabolic-androgenic steroid dependence is a syndrome of dependence on anabolic steroids and body image disturbance is purported to be a key mechanism that drives this dependence. Around half of men with muscle dysmorphia use anabolic steroids.

Body image is a key component of each of the above-mentioned disorders. Men with AN and BN are typically concerned with thinness, while men with muscle dysmorphia and anabolic-androgenic steroid dependence are typically concerned with muscularity. By contrast, men with BDD report a broad range of body image concerns, but tend to focus on the skin, hair, nose, teeth, face in general, and genitals. Evidence of effective treatments for men with body image disorders is sparse and limited. Nevertheless, the core body image phenomenology of these disorders suggests that it is sensible to adapt therapies that are effective for any one of these disorders, at least until more and better evidence becomes available.

References

Allen, K. L. et al. 2013. DSM–IV–TR and DSM-5 eating disorders in adolescents: prevalence, stability, and psychosocial correlates in a population-based sample of male and female adolescents. *Journal of Abnormal Psychology*, 122, 720–32.

APA. 1980. *Diagnostic and Statistical Manual of Mental Disorders*. 3rd ed.

Washington, DC: American Psychiatric Association.

APA. 1987. *Diagnostic and Statistical Manual of Mental Disorders*. 4th ed. Washington, DC: American Psychiatric Association.

APA. 2000. *Diagnostic and Statistical Manual of Mental Disorders*. 4th ed., revised. Washington, DC: American Psychiatric Association.

APA. 2013. *Diagnostic and Statistical Manual of Mental Disorders*. 5th ed. Washington, DC: American Psychiatric Association.

Bhasin, S. 2001. Testosterone dose–response relationships in healthy young men. *American Journal of Physiology – Endocrinology and Metabolism*, 281, 1172–81.

Bhasin, S. et al. 1996. The effects of supraphysiologic doses of testosterone on muscle size and strength in normal men. *New England Journal of Medicine*, 335, 1–7.

Boepple, L. and Thompson, J. K. 2016. A content analytic comparison of fitspiration and thinspiration websites. *International Journal of Eating Disorders*, 49, 98–101.

Brower, K. J. et al. 1989. Anabolic-androgenic steroid dependence. *The Journal of Clinical Psychiatry*, 50, 31–3.

Cafri, G., Olivardia, R., and Thompson, J. K. 2008. Symptom characteristics and psychiatric comorbidity among males with muscle dysmorphia. *Comprehensive Psychiatry*, 49, 374–9.

Choi, P. Y. L., Pope Jr., H. G., and Olivardia, R. 2002. Muscle dysmorphia: a new syndrome in weightlifters. *British Journal of Sports Medicine*, 36, 375–6.

Fairburn, C. and Beglin, S. 1994. Assessment of eating disorders: interview or self-report questionnaire? *International Journal of Eating Disorders*, 16, 363–70.

Forney, K. J. et al. 2015. Determining empirical thresholds for 'definitely large' amounts of food for defining binge-eating episodes. *Eating Disorders: The Journal of Treatment & Prevention*, 23, 15–30.

Garner, D. M. 2004. *Eating Disorder Inventory – 3 Professional Manual*. Lutz, FL: Psychological Assessment Resources.

Griffiths, S. and Murray, S. B. 2018. Muscle dysmorphia: clinical presentation and treatment strategies. In: L. K. Anderson, S. B. Murray, and W. H. Kaye (eds.) *Clinical Handbook of Complex and Atypical Eating Disorders* (pp. 235–52). Oxford: Oxford University Press.

Griffiths, S. et al. 2017. Post-cycle therapy for performance and image enhancing drug users: a qualitative investigation. *Performance Enhancement & Health*, 5, 103–7.

Griffiths, S. et al. 2018. Physical appearance concerns are uniquely associated with the severity of steroid dependence and depression in anabolic-androgenic steroid users. *Drug and Alcohol Review*, 24, 383.

Griffiths, S., Hay, P., et al. 2016. Sex differences in the relationships between body dissatisfaction, quality of life and psychological distress. *Australian and New Zealand Journal of Public Health*, 40, 518–22.

Griffiths, S., Mond, J. M., Li, Z., et al. 2015. Self-stigma of seeking treatment and being male predict an increased likelihood of having an undiagnosed eating disorder. *International Journal of Eating Disorders*, 48, 775–8.

Griffiths, S., Mond, J. M., Murray, S. B., and Touyz, S. 2015a. Positive beliefs about anorexia nervosa and muscle dysmorphia are associated with eating disorder symptomatology. *Australian and New Zealand Journal of Psychiatry*, 49, 812–20.

Griffiths, S., Mond, J. M., Murray, S. B., and Touyz, S. 2015b. The prevalence and adverse associations of stigmatization in people with eating disorders. *International Journal of Eating Disorders*, 48, 767–74.

Griffiths, S., Murray, S. B., and Mond, J. M. 2016. The stigma of anabolic steroid use. *Journal of Drug Issues*, 46(4), 446–56.

Griffiths, S., Murray, S. B., and Touyz, S. 2013. Disordered eating and the muscular ideal. *Journal of Eating Disorders*, 1:15.

Griffiths, S., Murray, S. B., Mitchison, D., et al. 2016. Anabolic steroids: lots of muscle in the short-term, potentially devastating health consequences in the long-term. *Drug and Alcohol Review*, 35, 375–6.

Griffiths, S., Murray, S. B., and Touyz, S. 2015. Extending the masculinity hypothesis: an investigation of gender role conformity, body dissatisfaction, and disordered eating in young heterosexual men. *Psychology of Men & Masculinity*, 16, 108–14.

Hay, P., Girosi, F., and Mond, J. 2015. Prevalence and sociodemographic correlates of DSM-5 eating disorders in the Australian population. *Journal of Eating Disorders*, 3, article no. 19.

Hays, L. R., Littleton, S., and Stillner, V. 1990. Anabolic steroid dependence. *American Journal of Psychiatry*, 147, 122.

Hitzeroth, V. et al. 2001. Muscle dysmorphia: a South African sample. *Psychiatry and Clinical Neurosciences*, 55, 521–3.

Hudson, J. I. et al. 2007. The prevalence and correlates of eating disorders in the National Comorbidity Survey replication. *Biological Psychiatry*, 61, 348–58.

Iversen, J. et al. 2013. Are people who inject performance and image-enhancing drugs an increasing population of Needle and Syringe Program attendees? *Drug and Alcohol Review*, 32, 205–7.

Kanayama, G. et al. 2010. Treatment of anabolic–androgenic steroid dependence: emerging evidence and its implications. *Drug and Alcohol Dependence*, 109, 6–13.

Kanayama, G., Brower, K., Wood, R., Hudson, J. I., and Pope, H. G. 2009a. Issues for DSM-V: clarifying the diagnostic criteria for anabolic-androgenic steroid dependence. *American Journal of Psychiatry*, 166, 642–4.

Kanayama, G., Brower, K. J., Wood, R. I., Hudson, J. I., and Pope, H. G., Jr. 2009b. Anabolic-androgenic steroid dependence: an emerging disorder. *Addiction*, 104, 1966–78.

Kanayama, G., Pope, H. G., and Hudson, J. I. 2018. Associations of anabolic-androgenic steroid use with other behavioral disorders: an analysis using directed acyclic graphs. *Psychological Medicine*, 57, 1–8.

Karazsia, B. T., Murnen, S. K., and Tylka, T. L. 2017. Is body dissatisfaction changing across time? A cross-temporal meta-analysis. *Psychological Bulletin*, 143(3), 293–320.

Kessler, R. C., Berglund, P. A., Chiu, W. T., et al. 2013. The prevalence and correlates of binge eating disorder in the World Health Organization World Mental Health Surveys. *Biological Psychiatry*, 73, 904–14.

Kjelsås, E., Bjørnstrøm, C., and Götestam, K. G. 2004. Prevalence of eating disorders in female and male adolescents (14–15 years). *Eating Behaviors*, 5, 3–25.

Lakkis, J., Ricciardelli, L. A., and Williams, R. J. 1999. Role of sexual orientation and gender-related traits in disordered eating. *Sex Roles*, 41, 1–16.

Lavender, J. M., De Young, K. P., and Anderson, D. A. 2010. Eating Disorder Examination Questionnaire (EDE-Q): norms for undergraduate men. *Eating Behaviors*, 11, 119–21.

Leit, R., Pope, H. G., and Gray, J. 2001. Cultural expectations of muscularity in men: the evolution of Playgirl centerfolds. *International Journal of Eating Disorders*, 29, 90–3.

Lewinsohn, P. M. et al. 2002. Gender differences in eating disorder symptoms in young adults. *International Journal of Eating Disorders*, 32, 426–40.

Madden, S. et al. 2009. Burden of eating disorders in 5–13-year-old children in Australia. *Medical Journal of Australia*, 190, 410–14.

McVeigh, J. and Begley, E. 2016. Anabolic steroids in the UK: an increasing issue for public health. *Drugs: Education, Prevention, and Policy*, 24, 278–85.

Memedovic, S. et al. 2017. *Australian Needle and Syringe Program National Data Report 2012–2016*. Sydney: Kirby Institute, University of New South Wales.

Meyer, C., Blissett, J., and Oldfield, C. 2001. Sexual orientation and eating psychopathology: the role of masculinity and femininity. *International Journal of Eating Disorders*, 29, 314–18.

Mishkind, M. E. et al. 1986. The embodiment of masculinity: cultural, psychological, and behavioral dimensions. *American Behavioral Scientist*, 29, 545–62.

Mond, J. M. 2014. Eating disorders 'mental health literacy': an introduction. *Journal of Mental Health*, 23, 51–4. https://pubmed.ncbi.nlm.nih.gov/32041463/

Moore, R. H. S. et al. 2009. Gender difference in the prevalence of eating disorder symptoms. *International Journal of Eating Disorders*, 42, 471–4.

Mosley, P. E. 2009. Bigorexia: bodybuilding and muscle dysmorphia. *European Eating Disorders Review*, 17, 191–8.

Murray, S. B. and Griffiths, S. 2014. Adolescent muscle dysmorphia and family-based treatment: a case report. *Clinical Child Psychology and Psychiatry*, 20, 324–30.

Murray, S. B. et al. 2012. A comparison of eating, exercise, shape, and weight related symptomatology in males with muscle dysmorphia and anorexia nervosa. *Body Image*, 9, 193–200.

Murray, S. B. et al. 2018. Treatment outcomes for anorexia nervosa: a systematic review and meta-analysis of randomized controlled trials. *Psychological Medicine*, 194, 1–10.

Murray, S. B., Griffiths, S., and Mond, J. M. 2016. Evolving eating disorder psychopathology: conceptualising muscularity-oriented disordered eating. *British Journal of Psychiatry*, 208, 414–15.

Murray, S. B., Griffiths, S., et al. 2013. A comparison of compulsive exercise in male and female presentations of anorexia nervosa: what is the difference? *Advances in Eating Disorders: Theory, Research and Practice*, 2, 65–70.

Murray, S. B., Griffiths, S., et al. 2017. The transition from thinness-oriented to muscularity-oriented disordered eating in adolescent males: a clinical observation. *Journal of Adolescent Health*, 60, 353–5.

Murray, S. B., Griffiths, S., Hazery, L., et al. 2016. Go big or go home: a thematic content analysis of pro-muscularity websites. *Body Image*, 16, 17–20.

Murray, S. B., Nagata, J. M., et al. 2017. The enigma of male eating disorders: a critical review and synthesis. *Clinical Psychology Review*, 57, 1–11.

Murray, S. B., Rieger, E., et al. 2013. Masculinity and femininity in the divergence of male body image concerns. *The Journal of Eating Disorders*, 1, 1–8.

Olivardia, R., Pope, H. G., and Hudson, J. 2000. Muscle dysmorphia in male weightlifters: a case-control study. *American Journal of Psychiatry*, 157, 1291–6.

Phillipou, A. et al. 2016. Randomised controlled trials of psychological & pharmacological treatments for body dysmorphic disorder: a systematic review. *Psychiatry Research*, 245, 179–85.

Phillips, K. A., Menard, W., and Fay, C. 2006. Gender similarities and differences in 200 individuals with body dysmorphic disorder. *Comprehensive Psychiatry*, 47, 77–87.

Pope, C. G. et al. 2005. Clinical features of muscle dysmorphia among males with body dysmorphic disorder. *Body Image*, 2, 395–400.

Pope, H. G. et al. 1999. Evolving ideals of male body image as seen through action toys. *International Journal of Eating Disorders*, 26, 65–72.

Pope, H. G. et al. 1997. Muscle dysmorphia: an underrecognized form of body dysmorphic disorder. *Psychosomatics*, 38, 548–57.

Pope, H. G., Jr, Katz, D. L., and Hudson, J. I. 1993. Anorexia nervosa and 'reverse anorexia' among 108 male bodybuilders. *Comprehensive Psychiatry*, 34, 406–9.

Pope, H. G., Phillips, K., and Olivardia, R. 2000. *The Adonis Complex: The Secret Crisis of Male Body Dissatisfaction*. New York: Free Press.

Räisänen, U. and Hunt, K. 2014. The role of gendered constructions of eating disorders in delayed help-seeking in men: a qualitative interview study. *BMJ Open*, 4, e004342.

Reas, D. L. and Grilo, C. M. 2014. Current and emerging drug treatments for binge eating disorder. *Expert Opinion Emerging Drugs*, 19, 1–44.

Robinson, K. J., Mountford, V. A., and Sperlinger, D. J. 2012. Being men with eating disorders: perspectives of male eating disorder service-users. *Journal of Health Psychology*, 18(2), 176–86.

Russell, G. 1979. Bulimia nervosa: an ominous variant of anorexia nervosa. *Psychological Medicine*, 9, 429–48.

Russell, G. F. M. and Treasure, J. 1989. The modern history of anorexia nervosa: an interpretation of why the illness has changed. *Annals of the New York Academy of Sciences*, 575, 13–30.

Santos Filho, dos, C. A. et al. 2015. Systematic review of the diagnostic category muscle dysmorphia.

Australian and New Zealand Journal of Psychiatry, 50, 322–33.

Simmons, R. A. and Phillips, K. A. 2017. Core clinical features of body dysmorphic disorder: appearance preoccupations, negative emotions, core beliefs, and repetitive and avoidance behaviors. In: K. A. Phillips (ed.) *Body Dysmorphic Disorder: Advances in Research and Clinical Practice*. Oxford: Oxford University Press.

Slade, E. et al. 2018. Treatments for bulimia nervosa: a network meta-analysis. *Psychological Medicine*, 10, 1–8.

Smink, F. R. E., van Hoeken, D., and Hoek, H. W. 2013. Epidemiology, course, and outcome of eating disorders. *Current Opinion in Psychiatry*, 26, 543–8.

Smith, K. E. et al. 2017. Male clinical norms and sex differences on the Eating Disorder Inventory (EDI) and Eating Disorder Examination Questionnaire (EDE-Q). *International Journal of Eating Disorders*, 13, 305.

Sweeting, H. et al. 2015. Prevalence of eating disorders in males: a review of rates reported in academic research and UK mass media. *International Journal of Mens Health*, 14.

Tennant, F., Black, D. L., and Voy, R. O. 1988. Anabolic steroid

dependence with opioid-type features. *New England Journal of Medicine*, 319, 578.

Veale, D. and Matsunaga, H. 2014. Body dysmorphic disorder and olfactory reference disorder: proposals for ICD-11. *Revista Brasileira de Psiquiatria*, 36, 14–20.

Veale, D. et al. 2016. Body dysmorphic disorder in different settings: a systematic review and estimated weighted prevalence. *Body Image*, 18, 168–86.

Wansink, B., Cheney, M., and Chan, N. 2003. Exploring comfort food preferences across age and gender. *Physiology & Behavior*, 79, 739–47.

Woodside, D. B. et al. 2001. Comparisons of men with full or partial eating disorders, men without eating disorders, and women with eating disorders in the community. *American Journal of Psychiatry*, 158, 570–4.

Wooldridge, T. and Lytle, P. P. 2012. An overview of anorexia nervosa in males. *Eating Disorders: The Journal of Treatment & Prevention*, 20, 368–78.

World Health Organization. 2018. *International Statistical Classification of Diseases and Related Health Problems – 11th revision*. Geneva, Switzerland: World Health Organization.

Chapter

9

Anxiety Disorders and OCD in Men

Rupert Goodman, Christine Lochner, and Dan J. Stein

Fear and anxiety are common and often transient human responses to stressors, danger, or traumatic events. However, when fear and anxiety persist over time, and result in functional impairment, an anxiety disorder may be present. In both the *Diagnostic and Statistical Manual of Mental Disorders*, fifth edition (DSM-5) (APA, 2013) and the ICD-11 (World Health Organization, 2018) the category of 'anxiety disorders' includes a range of conditions that share characteristics of excessive fear or anxiety with consequent distress and impairment. These include generalized anxiety disorder, panic disorder, agoraphobia, and social anxiety disorder (social phobia), among others. This chapter focuses on these conditions with particular reference to how they affect adult men. In addition, obsessive-compulsive disorder (OCD), an anxiety-related disorder placed in a separate DSM-5 and ICD-11 category called 'Obsessive-Compulsive and Related Disorders', is also included here due to its historical positioning as an anxiety disorder in earlier editions of the DSM and ICD. Posttraumatic stress disorder (PTSD) has also been reclassified in DSM-5 and ICD-11 from an anxiety disorder to a new diagnostic category known as 'Trauma and Stressor-Related Disorders', and is discussed in Chapter 10.

Anxiety disorders are the most prevalent group of psychiatric disorders. A systematic review of eighty-seven studies across forty-four countries in 2013 estimated the current (three-month) global prevalence of anxiety disorders (including OCD) to be 7.3% (4.8–10.9%) when adjusted for methodological differences (Baxter et al., 2013). The prevalence of anxiety disorders is consistently found to be significantly lower in men than women. For example, a large community study from the United States (N = 20,013) estimated male:female prevalence ratios of DSM-IV anxiety disorders to be 1:1.7 for lifetime prevalence and 1:1.79 for 12-month prevalence (Mclean et al., 2011). Similarly, in the World Mental Health Survey (WMHS) collaboration, lifetime

prevalence of anxiety disorders was lower in males than females (Seedat et al., 2009). Box 9.1 presents some key gender differences amongst these disorders.

Both anxiety disorders and OCD are associated with substantial co-morbidity, particularly with other anxiety and mood disorders, although overall co-morbidity is also consistently lower in men. Patterns of co-morbidity also differ between men and women. For example, men with a lifetime diagnosis of an anxiety disorder are significantly more likely be diagnosed with co-morbid attention deficit hyperactivity disorder (ADHD) (see Chapter 3), intermittent explosive disorder (IED), and substance use disorders (see Chapter 18), whereas women are more likely to have another lifetime anxiety disorder, bulimia nervosa, or major depressive disorder (Mclean et al., 2011). No significant difference has been found between men and women in age of onset or chronicity of anxiety disorders as a whole (Mclean et al., 2011). However, some studies (detailed later in this chapter) have found gender differences in the clinical course of certain anxiety and anxiety-related disorders.

The following sections of this chapter cover the epidemiology, clinical characteristics, and course of some of the more prevalent anxiety disorders and OCD in adult men, along with a discussion of some of the theories explaining differences between the genders.

Box 9.1 Gender differences in anxiety disorders

- Prevalence of anxiety disorders is lower in men than women in the community, and there may also be gender differences in treatment-seeking.
- There are different patterns of symptoms and co-morbidity in males and females with anxiety disorders.
- Gender does not appear to be a consistent moderator of treatment outcome in the anxiety disorders.

Generalized Anxiety Disorder

DSM-5 defines generalized anxiety disorder (GAD) as persistent and excessive anxiety or worry that is hard to control, in relation to a number of different events or activities, resulting in a number of physical and cognitive symptoms such as restlessness, fatigability, and impaired concentration. GAD is characterized by significant distress and impairment of functioning, including difficulties at work or in social relationships (APA, 2013). In the WMHS, cross-national 12-month and lifetime prevalence of DSM-5 GAD was estimated to be 1.8% and 3.7% (N = 147,261), with estimates varying widely across countries (Ruscio et al., 2017). In the USA alone, the National Comorbidity Study Replication (NCS-R), a large, nationally representative community survey of mental disorders (N = 9282), estimated the lifetime prevalence of DSM-IV GAD to be 6.2%, with significantly lower prevalence among men: 4.6% for men compared to 7.7% for women (Kessler et al., 2012). This gender difference was also observed globally (Ruscio et al., 2017) with the divergence in prevalence emerging in mid-adolescence (Beesdo et al., 2009).

Men and women have also reported different clinical presentations of GAD. In the 2001–2002 National Epidemiologic Survey on Alcohol and Related Conditions (NESARC), a large US community survey (N = 43,093), men with GAD were more likely to report using substances, alcohol, or medication to relieve symptoms, as well as being more likely to report social friction with relatives and friends due to excessive or uncontrollable worry. In contrast, women more frequently reported somatic discomfort such as cardiovascular and gastrointestinal symptoms, along with fatigue, irritability, and muscle tension (Vesga-López et al., 2008).

GAD is highly co-morbid with other mental disorders, in particular mood disorders. For example, it is estimated that approximately 90% of individuals with GAD have another mental disorder either concurrently or at some time in their life (Beesdo-Baum and Hilbert, 2015). There are also commonly reported differences between men and women with GAD in terms of co-morbidity. In NESARC, for example, men with lifetime or 12-month GAD were more likely than women to have any alcohol or substance use disorder or antisocial personality disorder, and were less likely than women to have co-morbid mood and anxiety disorders (Vesga-López et al., 2008).

The clinical course of GAD is generally chronic, and does not appear to differ significantly between men and women in terms of number and duration of episodes. GAD typically begins in adulthood, with a mean age of onset of 32 (Vesga-López et al., 2008). However, it is notable that some clinical studies have found the age of onset to be later in men than in women (Simon et al., 2006; Yonkers et al., 2003). Although males with GAD seek treatment less frequently (Vesga-López et al., 2008), gender is not a significant predictor of psychotherapy or pharmacotherapy outcome (Beesdo-Baum and Hilbert, 2015).

Panic Disorder

Panic disorder is characterized by recurrent, often unexpected panic attacks, typified by a surge of fear or discomfort and a range of physical and cognitive symptoms, such as dizziness, shortness of breath, or fear of losing control. To meet diagnostic criteria for panic disorder, at least one panic attack must be followed by one month or more of continual fear of having additional attacks or a change of behaviour in an effort to avoid future attacks, to the extent that normal functioning is impaired (APA, 2013). In earlier editions of the DSM, panic disorder was defined as being either with or without agoraphobia; however, DSM-5 now categorizes agoraphobia as a discrete diagnosis.

In the WMHS, cross-national lifetime prevalence of DSM-5 panic disorder was estimated to be 1.7% (de Jonge et al., 2016). Using the earlier DSM-IV criteria, the NCS-R estimated lifetime and 12-month prevalence of panic disorder (with or without agoraphobia) in the USA to be 4.7% and 2.8%, respectively (Kessler et al., 2006). In the earlier National Comorbidity Survey (NCS), lifetime prevalence estimates for panic disorder were approximately 2.5 times lower in men than women (Kessler et al., 1994), with the gender difference found to increase with age: among respondents aged 15 to 24, lifetime prevalence was 1.3% for men and 2.5% for women, whilst for those aged 35 to 44, it was 0.6% for men and 2.1% for women (Eaton et al., 1994).

The clinical characteristics of panic disorder have also been found to differ between men and women. Men of all ages report lower rates of anxiety sensitivity (the fear of anxiety-related behaviours or sensations) than women in both non-clinical (Deacon et al., 2003) and clinical samples with a diagnosis of panic disorder (Schmidt and Koselka, 2000). In addition, men are more likely than women to report a fear of the social consequences of panic attacks, but less likely to report respiration-related symptoms, such as difficulty breathing or feeling faint (Sheikh et al., 2002).

Psychiatric co-morbidities are very common among those with panic disorder. In particular, panic disorder is often accompanied by agoraphobia, explaining the historical linkage of these two disorders in the DSM. Agoraphobia may co-occur frequently with panic disorder as a means of avoiding places or situations where panic attacks might occur. Overall, co-morbidity does not differ significantly between the genders, but findings in this area have been mixed. For example, one study of middle-aged and older adults in the USA has suggested that men with panic disorder have a lower risk of exhibiting a pattern of binge drinking (Chou et al., 2011), while another US study found that men with panic disorder are more likely to report a past history of alcohol or substance dependence/abuse (Clayton et al., 2006).

While panic disorder is generally a chronic and relapsing condition, it has been suggested that men may have a lower risk of relapse than women. A five-year longitudinal study (N = 412) of men and women diagnosed with panic disorder (with and without agoraphobia) found that after remission, men were twice less likely than women to have a recurrence of panic symptoms (Yonkers et al., 1998). Reflecting its chronic and relapsing nature, panic disorder has one of the highest rates of help-seeking among common mental disorders: 45% of NESARC respondents with panic disorder had sought help within the past year, compared to 19.3% for anxiety disorders overall (MacKenzie et al., 2012). This study also showed that men and women are equally likely to seek treatment for panic disorder. There is no evidence to suggest that gender moderates response to either pharmacotherapy or psychotherapy for this condition (Grant and Odlaug, 2015).

Agoraphobia

Agoraphobia is the fear of multiple situations or places where escape might be difficult or help might not be available in the event of developing panic-like or embarrassing symptoms. These situations or places are either avoided, endured with intense anxiety, or require the presence of a companion (APA, 2013).

The re-categorizing of agoraphobia as an independent disorder in DSM-5 reflects research demonstrating that the fear associated with agoraphobia may not necessarily be a fear of developing panic-like symptoms, but may also include excessive fear or anxiety that occurs in, or in anticipation of, multiple situations where escape might be difficult or help might not be available, such as using public transportation or being in crowds. As with other anxiety disorders, this fear causes significant impairment in everyday functioning.

Agoraphobia is one of the least prevalent anxiety disorders, with the WMHS estimating lifetime and 12-month prevalence of DSM-5 agoraphobia at 1.5% and 1.0%, respectively (Roest et al., 2019). The WMHS also highlighted a significant gender difference, with men significantly less likely to have a lifetime diagnosis of agoraphobia. Similarly, a 2010 review of European studies estimated that men were approximately three times less likely than women to have a diagnosis of agoraphobia in the previous 12 months (Wittchen et al., 2011). In addition, quality of life for men with agoraphobia seems to be less affected than it is for women. This is exemplified by the finding that men with agoraphobia are significantly less likely to avoid being in unfamiliar places alone and are less reliant on a companion (Starcevic et al., 1998).

As reflected in its historical categorization, agoraphobia most commonly occurs with panic disorder. The NCS-R also found that agoraphobia with panic disorder is significantly co-morbid with all other anxiety and mood disorders (Kessler et al., 2006). Alcohol dependence is also a common co-morbidity. Men with agoraphobia and panic disorder are significantly more likely than women to experience alcoholism (Starcevic et al., 1998; Yonkers et al., 1998). However, it is important to interpret these studies in light of the overall higher rate of hazardous alcohol abuse among men (Kessler et al., 1994). Importantly, some have argued that agoraphobia may be under-reported by men due to its incongruence with traditional masculine norms of strength and bravery (Barlow, 2002). Men may rather present with alcoholism than acknowledge agoraphobic symptoms. Whether or not this is true, both men and women with agoraphobia report drinking alcohol as a coping strategy for managing agoraphobic inhibition (Cox et al., 1993; Turgeon et al., 1998).

The majority of research into the clinical course of agoraphobia involves individuals with both panic disorder and agoraphobia. However, studies such as the longitudinal study of Yonkers and colleagues (1998) show that the course for men with both disorders is less chronic than for women, evidenced by less re-occurrence of symptoms and relapse after remission. Again, there is no evidence of any gender differences in treatment response.

Social Anxiety Disorder (Social Phobia)

Social anxiety disorder (SAD) is characterized by persistent fear or anxiety about social situations, such as having a conversation or performing in front of others, due to the fear of negative evaluation by others. As such, the feared situation is either avoided or endured with intense difficulty (APA, 2013). SAD can be highly debilitating, with fear, anxiety, or avoidance causing significant distress or impairment in daily functioning, whether at work or in social relationships. SAD is also known as social phobia, although DSM-5 recognizes SAD as its principal name in order to reflect the broad nature of fears and impairment that characterize the disorder. Another change from DSM-IV to DSM-5 is the removal of the requirement that an individual recognizes that their anxiety is excessive or unreasonable. This has been replaced with the requirement that the anxiety must be out of proportion to the actual threat of the situation and taking into account the sociocultural context.

SAD is one of the most common psychiatric disorders with estimated cross-national 12-month and lifetime prevalence rates of 2.4% and 4.0% (Stein et al., 2017). The WHMS also estimated prevalence rates to be significantly lower among men than women. In the USA, a recent study using data from the NCS-R found that the prevalence of lifetime and 12-month SAD was 10.9% and 5.8%, respectively, for men, compared to 13.5% and 8% for women (Asher and Aderka, 2018). Similar results have been observed in a European study involving 18,980 participants aged 15 or over from the UK, Germany, Italy, Spain, and Portugal, with the prevalence of SAD being higher in women, with an odds ratio of 1.6 (Ohayon and Schatzberg, 2010).

Men and women with SAD tend to report different types of social fears. For example, men with lifetime SAD are significantly more likely to report a fear of dating, whereas women are significantly more likely to report a fear of speaking up in groups or in work situations (Xu et al., 2012). Men also tend to report a lower number of social fears, less severe SAD symptoms, and less suicidal ideation compared to women (Asher et al., 2017).

SAD is often accompanied by other anxiety disorders as well as depression and substance use in both men and women (Fehm et al., 2005). Whether there are co-morbidity trends that are specific to men is less clear. In some studies of SAD, however, men are more likely to have co-morbid externalizing disorders, particularly alcohol use disorder, gambling disorder, conduct disorder, or antisocial personality disorder, whereas women are more likely to have co-morbid internalizing disorders, such as mood and anxiety disorders. This is consistent with gender differences in prevalence of these various conditions. However, inconsistencies in findings regarding gender differences in co-morbidity rates exist; for example, one study found that men with SAD are more likely to have a lifetime major depressive episode (Asher et al., 2017).

There is no significant difference between men and women in the age of onset (typically the mid-teens: Compton et al. 2000), or chronicity of SAD (Asher et al., 2017). Interestingly, whilst the prevalence of SAD tends to decline with age, the gender difference in prevalence rates also appears to narrow. A large study of older adults in Canada (N = 12,792) found no significant difference in prevalence rates between men and women over the age of 54 (Cairney et al., 2007).

Although it is more common for women to have a diagnosis of SAD, men are more likely to seek treatment for this condition (Asher et al., 2017). This is particularly interesting given that women seek treatment more than men for anxiety disorders in general (Shear et al., 2000) and for OCD (Goodwin et al., 2002). In terms of treatment response, gender has not been found to be a significant moderator of response to medication or psychotherapy (Stein et al., 2004).

Obsessive-Compulsive Disorder

As noted earlier, obsessive-compulsive disorder (OCD) is no longer categorized as an anxiety disorder in DSM-5 and ICD-11 and is now included under 'Obsessive-Compulsive and Related Disorders'. This category places OCD alongside disorders such as body dysmorphic disorder (see Chapter 8) and trichotillomania due to evidence demonstrating commonalities between these conditions, such as obsessive thoughts and/or repetitive behaviours. However, OCD has been labelled as an anxiety-related disorder, given that anxiety is commonly present and that CBT for anxiety disorders and OCD shares many features. Earlier editions of the DSM classified OCD as an anxiety disorder to reflect this similarity of symptoms and the co-morbidity between OCD and other anxiety disorders. The ICD-11 follows DSM-5, with a new grouping of Obsessive-Compulsive and Related Disorders (OCRD). The proposed OCRD category is located in the ICD-11 immediately following the Anxiety and Fear-Related Disorders given their phenomenological and psychobiological similarities. Not all researchers agree with this move, arguing that OCRDs should not be separate from the Anxiety and Fear-Related Disorders (Storch et al., 2008).

OCD is characterized by obsessions (recurrent, persistent and intrusive thoughts, images, or urges that can cause anxiety or distress) and compulsions (repetitive behaviours, such as hand washing or checking) or mental acts (such as counting or repeating words). To meet diagnostic criteria an individual must have obsessions, compulsions, or both, and will either attempt to ignore or suppress their obsessions or try to neutralize them with compulsions/mental acts according to rigidly applied rules (APA, 2013).

The overall prevalence of lifetime and 12-month OCD is 2.3% and 1.2%, respectively (Ruscio et al., 2010), with gender differences moderated by age. In adulthood, prevalence estimates are often found to be the same in men and women (Ruscio et al., 2010; Weissman et al., 1994), although it is worth noting that the Epidemiological Catchment Area (ECA) survey, one of the largest US studies investigating the prevalence of mental disorders, found that prevalence estimates for OCD were higher in women. In that study, the gender difference largely disappeared when other sociodemographic factors, such as marital status and age, were controlled for (Martin, 2003). Importantly, roughly two thirds of children with OCD are male, consistent with findings that OCD has an earlier onset among males (Lochner et al., 2004; Mathis et al., 2011).

OCD is associated with significant functional impairment including high rates of unemployment,

financial problems, and difficulties with social relationships. Social impairment and unemployment due to OCD have been found to be greater among men, and men with OCD are also more likely to be single (Mathis et al., 2011). The obsessions and compulsions associated with adult OCD can manifest in many different ways, and with gender differences. For example, in a Brazilian sample, men were more likely to have sexual and religious obsessions, with compulsions relating to ordering and symmetry, while women were more likely to have obsessions and compulsions relating to contamination, cleaning, and checking (Torresan et al., 2013). Similarly, a South African study found that men with OCD were significantly more likely than women to have harm-related obsessions and compulsions (Lochner et al., 2004). A recent study of a US community sample (N = 297) further suggests that OCD may be more heterogeneous among men than women. Specifically, men are more likely to endorse symptoms across a broad range of symptom dimensions (such as concerns about and rituals relating to contamination, symmetry, and harm or bad luck), whereas women are more likely to endorse symptoms within distinct symptom clusters (for example, only having contamination-related symptoms, or only having concerns about and rituals relating to symmetry; Raines et al., 2018). Research on gender differences in symptom severity is inconsistent, with some suggesting OCD symptoms are less severe for men (Torresan et al., 2013) and others finding no difference in this regard between men and women (Labad et al., 2008).

Like the anxiety disorders, OCD is highly co-morbid with other psychiatric disorders. The NCS-R found that 90% of adults who met the criteria for lifetime OCD also met the criteria for another lifetime psychiatric disorder, most often an anxiety disorder (Ruscio et al., 2010). Men with OCD are more likely than women to be diagnosed with SAD, tics, and substance use (Torresan et al., 2013) as well as bipolar disorder (Bogetto et al., 1999), whereas women with OCD are more likely to present with impulse-control and eating disorders (Mathis et al., 2011).

Men are significantly more likely than women to present with OCD at an earlier age, experience insidious onset, and have a chronic course (Mathis et al., 2011). Early onset OCD is characterized not only by male predominance, but also by other features such as greater likelihood of tics, certain kinds of obsessions and compulsions, and possibly a lower response rate to SSRIs (Box 9.2; Leckman et al., 2010). Studies of adult OCD have observed few differences between the genders in terms of treatment response, but one study investigating the response to clomipramine found that men were less likely than women to improve and more likely to experience a worsening of symptoms (Mundo et al., 1999). For psychotherapy response, very few studies have looked at gender as a predictive factor, and the few that exist are mostly underpowered. However, one study investigating the predictors of response to intensive residential treatment for severe OCD (involving both psychotherapy and medication) found that men were significantly less likely than women to respond (Stewart et al., 2006).

Theories to Explain Gender Differences in Anxiety Disorders and OCD

A broad range of theories have been put forward to account for gender differences in anxiety disorders and OCD. These range from those which emphasize biological factors such as hormonal differences, to those which emphasize sociocultural variables. Here we briefly outline some of this work. We note that an integrative psychobiological account remains to be fully delineated.

While several studies have investigated psychophysiological explanations for the differences in prevalence, clinical characteristics, and co-morbidity between men and women with anxiety disorders and OCD, findings have not always been consistent. For example, one meta-analysis of psychophysiological studies found that men had lower resting heart rates than women, but with no significant difference between men and women's heart rates during stressor challenge tasks (Stoney et al., 1987). In contrast, a number of studies have demonstrated that men have greater physiological reactivity in response to acute behavioural stressors when measuring skin conductance or blood pressure (McLean and Anderson, 2009). Men have also been found to exhibit greater HPA axis and autonomic reactivity compared to women in response to acute stressors (Kajantie and Phillips, 2006). Inconsistent findings may reflect differences in the methodology used and in definitions of physiological reactivity.

Hormonal explanations are also often cited to account for gender differences in anxiety disorders and OCD. For example, a number of studies have shown that testosterone protects against anxiety, for example by suppressing HPA axis reactivity. Therefore, higher levels of testosterone in men may contribute to the lower prevalence and severity of anxiety disorders (McHenry et al., 2014). Importantly, the menstrual cycle, pregnancy, and menopause are all closely associated with the clinical course of affective disorders among women and most likely contribute to the gender differences in prevalence, co-morbidity, and clinical characteristics of anxiety disorders and OCD (Altemus et al., 2016). However, the hormonal and other psychobiological mechanisms underlying these reproductive events are not fully understood, and further research is warranted.

A speculative argument from evolutionary psychology is that some female psychobiological characteristics that support reproduction may increase vulnerability to anxiety. For example, compared to males, females are consistently found to have higher levels of social cognition and capacity for attunement with others (Thompson and Voyer, 2014) – arguably adaptive behavioural characteristics that promote child development. At the same time, these characteristics may contribute to key attributes of anxiety, such as heightened sensitivity to separation, criticism, and rejection, therefore explaining the higher relative prevalence of anxiety disorders among women (Altemus et al., 2016).

Differences in gender role socialization could help explain some epidemiological gender differences in anxiety and OCD (Block, 1983). For example, in countries with more egalitarian gender roles, the gender difference in prevalence of anxiety disorders is narrower than in countries with more traditional gender roles (Seedat et al., 2009). Consistent with the traditional masculine gender role of managing distress alone rather than seeking social support, men may be less likely to seek health care treatment for anxiety disorders and OCD in general (Goodwin et al., 2002; Shear et al., 2000). Similarly, traditional gender roles may explain the results of studies demonstrating that men are more likely to cope with anxiety and OCD by supressing their fears through substance use, whereas women are more likely to cope by avoiding feared situations through patterns of agoraphobic avoidance (McLean and Anderson, 2009).

The symptoms of anxiety disorders and OCD may also be inconsistent with traditional masculine gender roles of strength and independence. This may contribute to explaining the greater distress experienced by men with these conditions. In particular, it has been argued that men with SAD experience more distress and impairment than women with SAD, as indicated by the higher rates of help-seeking among men with this disorder (Asher et al., 2017).

Differences in gender roles may also serve to reinforce traits associated with instrumentality in men (e.g. decisiveness and independence) and expressivity in women (e.g. gentleness and kindness). In relation to distress and anxiety, heightened instrumentality in men could be a useful protective tool for coping, and may contribute to explaining the lower rates of anxiety disorders among males. Accordingly, instrumentality has been shown to be negatively associated with anxiety, whereas there is no association between expressivity and anxiety (Moscovitch et al., 2005; Muris et al., 2005). It has been suggested that men may underreport anxiety or OCD symptoms due to 'un-masculine' associations with weakness and vulnerability (Pierce and Kirkpatrick, 1992). However, studies designed to encourage accurate self-reporting by using physiological measures of fear or anxiety have found no reporting bias between genders (McLean and Hope, 2010).

Similarly, theories of mastery could help to explain gender differences in the prevalence of anxiety and OCD (Box 9.3). Traditionally, boys have been raised with expectations of power and dominance in society, while girls have been raised with the message that they will have less control over their environment. As a result, boys are arguably given more opportunities to develop mastery, potentially immunizing them against the stress of tackling new or difficult situations. At the same time, girls raised to have less of a sense of mastery may be more likely to

---

Box 9.3 Theories to explain gender differences in anxiety disorders and OCD

- A range of theories have been proposed to explain gender differences in anxiety disorders and OCD, but further work is needed to delineate relevant mechanisms fully.
- Hormonal differences between males and females, most notably relating to the menstrual cycle, pregnancy, and menopause, may contribute to these differences.
- Masculine gender role socialization may contribute to the lower rates of help-seeking among men for anxiety and OCD. However, masculine gender roles may also promote protective characteristics such as instrumentality and mastery among men.

---

interpret stimuli as threatening (Chorpita and Barlow, 1998). In line with this theory, a large Australian community study (N = 7485) found that men had significantly higher levels of mastery (i.e. perceived control over one's future) than women, and that mastery mediated the relationship between gender and anxiety (Leach et al., 2008).

Conclusions

There are gender differences in the prevalence, clinical presentation, and course of some anxiety disorders and OCD. Although the reasons for these differences are not yet clear, it may be speculated that psychobiological and psychosocial factors play a role; nevertheless, further work is needed to delineate the relevant mechanisms fully, and to develop an integrated and comprehensive model to account for such differences, and to help clinicians to target interventions accordingly.

Further research may also help clarify mediators and moderators of gender differences in anxiety disorders and OCD. In particular, a range of data from research on gender differences in epidemiological, phenotypical, genetic, family, neuroimaging, neuropsychological, and intervention studies may contribute to our understanding. In addition, cross-cultural comparisons may help to shed light on the sociocultural risk and resilience factors that contribute to gender differences in these conditions (see Chapter 6). Such work may again ultimately assist in the development of more gender-specific and targeted therapeutic approaches for each gender.

References

Altemus M, Sarvaiya N, and Epperson CN (2016) Sex differences in anxiety and depression clinical perspectives. *Frontiers in Neuroendocrinology* 35 (3), 320–30.

APA (2013) *Diagnostic and Statistical Manual of Mental Disorders: DSM-5.* Arlington, VA: American Psychiatric Association.

Asher M and Aderka IM (2018) Gender differences in social anxiety disorder. *Journal of Clinical Psychology* (February), 1–12.

Asher M, Asnaani A., and Aderka I. M. (2017) Gender differences in social anxiety disorder: a review. *Clinical Psychology Review* 56(May), 1–12.

Barlow DH (2002) *Anxiety and Its Disorders: The Nature and Treatment of Anxiety and Panic.* 2nd ed. New York: Guilford Press.

Baxter AJ, Scott KM, Vos T, et al. (2013) Global prevalence of anxiety disorders: a systematic review and meta-regression. *Psychological Medicine* 43(5), 897–910.

Beesdo K, Knappe S, and Pine DS (2009) Anxiety and anxiety disorders in children and adolescents: developmental issues and implications for DSM-V. *Psychiatric Clinics of North America* 32(3), 483–524.

Beesdo-Baum K and Hilbert K (2015) Generalized Anxiety Disorder. In: DJ Stein and B Vythilingum (eds) *Anxiety Disorders and Gender.* 1st ed. Switzerland: Springer International Publishing, 1–29.

Block JH (1983) Differential premises arising from differential socialization of the sexes: some conjectures. *Child Development* 54 (6), 1335–54.

Bogetto F, Venturello S, Albert U, et al. (1999) Gender-related clinical differences in obsessive-compulsive disorder. *European Psychiatry* 14(8), 434–41.

Cairney J, McCabe L, Veldhuizen S, et al. (2007) Epidemiology of social phobia in later life. *American Journal of Geriatric Psychiatry* 15(3), 224–33.

Chorpita BF and Barlow DH (1998) The development of anxiety: the role of control in the early environment. *Psychological Bulletin* 124(1), 3–21.

Chou K-L, Liang K, and Mackenzie CS (2011) Binge drinking and Axis I psychiatric disorders in community-dwelling middle-aged and older adults. *The Journal of Clinical Psychiatry* 72(05), 640–7.

Clayton AH, Stewart RS, Fayyad R, et al. (2006) Sex differences in clinical presentation and response in panic disorder: pooled data from sertraline treatment studies. *Archives of Women's Mental Health* 9(3), 151–7.

Compton SN, Nelson AH, and March JS (2000) Social phobia and separation anxiety symptoms in community and clinical samples of children and adolescents. *Journal of the American Academy of Child & Adolescent Psychiatry* 39(8), 1040–6.

Cox BJ, Swinson RP, Shulman ID, et al. (1993) Gender effects and alcohol use in panic disorder with agoraphobia. *Behaviour Research and Therapy* 31(4), 413–16.

de Jonge P, Roest AM, Lim CCW, et al. (2016) Cross-national epidemiology of panic disorder and panic attacks in the world mental health surveys. *Depression and Anxiety* 33(12), 1155–77.

Deacon BJ, Abramowitz JS, Woods CM, et al. (2003) The Anxiety Sensitivity Index – revised: psychometric properties and factor structure in two nonclinical samples. *Behaviour Research and Therapy* 41(12), 1427–49.

Eaton WW, Kessler RC, Wittchen HU, et al. (1994) Panic and panic disorder in the United States. *American Journal of Psychiatry* 151 (3), 413–20.

Fehm L, Pelissolo A, Furmark T, et al. (2005) Size and burden of social phobia in Europe. *European Neuropsychopharmacology* 15(4), 453–62.

Goodwin R, Koenen K, Hellman F, et al. (2002) Helpseeking and access to mental health treatment for obsessive-compulsive disorder. *Acta Psychiatrica Scandinavica* 106(5), 143–9.

Grant JE and Odlaug BL (2015) Anxiety and related disorders in men. In: DJ Stein and B Vythilingum (eds) *Anxiety Disorders and Gender.* Switzerland: Springer International Publishing, 155–68.

Kajantie E and Phillips DIW (2006) The effects of sex and hormonal status on the physiological response to acute psychosocial stress. *Psychoneuroendocrinology* 31(2), 151–78.

Kessler RC, Chiu WT, Jin R, et al. (2006) The epidemiology of panic attacks, panic disorder, and agoraphobia in the National Comorbidity Survey Replication. *Archives of General Psychiatry* 63(4), 415.

Kessler RC, McGonagle KA, Zhao S, et al. (1994) Lifetime and 12-month prevalence of DSM-III-R psychiatric disorders in the United States. *Archives of General Psychiatry* 51(1), 8.

Kessler RC, Petukhova M, Sampson NA, et al. (2012) Twelve-month and lifetime prevalence and lifetime morbid risk of anxiety and mood disorders in the United States. *International Journal of Methods in Psychiatric Research* 21(3), 169–84.

Labad J, Menchon JM, Alonso P, et al. (2008) Gender differences in obsessive-compulsive symptom dimensions. *Depression and Anxiety* 25(10), 832–8.

Leach LS, Christensen H, Mackinnon AJ, et al. (2008) Gender differences in depression and anxiety across the adult lifespan: the role of psychosocial mediators. *Social Psychiatry and Psychiatric Epidemiology* 43(12), 983–98.

Leckman JF, Denys D, Simpson HB, et al. (2010) Obsessive-compulsive disorder: a review of the diagnostic criteria and possible subtypes and dimensional specifiers for DSM-V. *Depression and Anxiety* 27(6), 507–27.

Lochner C, Hemmings SMJ, Kinnear CJ, et al. (2004) Gender in obsessive-compulsive disorder: clinical and genetic findings. *European Neuropsychopharmacology* 14(2), 105–13.

MacKenzie CS, Reynolds K, Cairney J, et al. (2012) Disorder-specific mental health service use for mood and anxiety disorders: associations with age, sex, and psychiatric comorbidity. *Depression and Anxiety* 29(3), 234–42.

Martin P (2003) The epidemiology of anxiety disorders: a review. *Dialogues in Clinical Neuroscience* 5(3), 281–98.

Mathis MA de, Alvarenga P de, Funaro G, et al. (2011) Gender differences in obsessive-compulsive disorder: a literature review. *Revista Brasileira de Psiquiatria* 33(4), 390–9.

McHenry J, Carrier N, Hull E, et al. (2014) Sex differences in anxiety and depression: role of testosterone. *Frontiers in Neuroendocrinology* 35(1), 42–57.

McLean CP and Anderson ER (2009) Brave men and timid women? A review of the gender differences in fear and anxiety. *Clinical Psychology Review* 29(6), 496–505.

McLean CP, Asnaani A, Litz BT, et al. (2011) Gender differences in anxiety disorders: prevalence, course of illness, comorbidity and burden of illness. *Journal of Psychiatric Research* 45(8), 1027–35.

McLean CP and Hope DA (2010) Subjective anxiety and behavioral avoidance: gender, gender role, and perceived confirmability of self-report. *Journal of Anxiety Disorders* 24(5), 494–502.

Moscovitch DA, Hofmann SG, and Litz BT (2005) The impact of self-construals on social anxiety: a gender-specific interaction. *Personality and Individual Differences* 38(3), 659–72.

Mundo E, Bareggi SR, Pirola R, et al. (1999) Effect of acute intravenous clomipramine and antiobsessional response to proserotonergic drugs: is gender a predictive variable? *Biological Psychiatry* 45(3), 290–4.

Muris P, Meesters C, and Knoops M (2005) The relation between gender role orientation and fear and anxiety in nonclinic-referred children. *Journal of Clinical Child & Adolescent Psychology* 34(2), 326–32.

Ohayon MM and Schatzberg AF (2010) Social phobia and depression: prevalence and comorbidity. *Journal of Psychosomatic Research* 68(3), 235–43.

Pierce KA and Kirkpatrick DR (1992) Do men lie on fear surveys? *Behaviour Research and Therapy* 30(4), 415–18.

Raines AM, Oglesby ME, Allan NP, et al. (2018) Examining the role of sex differences in obsessive-compulsive symptom dimensions. *Psychiatry Research* 259, 265–9.

Roest AM, Vries YA, Lim CCW, et al. (2019) A comparison of DSM-5 and DSM-IV agoraphobia in the World Mental Health Surveys. *Depression and Anxiety* 16, da.22885.

Ruscio AM, Hallion LS, Lim CCW, et al. (2017) Cross-sectional comparison of the epidemiology of DSM-5 generalized anxiety disorder across the globe. *JAMA Psychiatry* 74(5), 465.

Ruscio AM, Stein DJ, Chiu WT, et al. (2010) The epidemiology of obsessive-compulsive disorder in the National Comorbidity Survey Replication. *Molecular Psychiatry* 15(1), 53–63.

Schmidt NB and Koselka M (2000) Gender differences in patients with panic disorder: evaluating cognitive mediation of phobic avoidance. *Cognitive Therapy and Research* 24(5), 533–50.

Seedat S, Scott KM, Angermeyer MC, et al. (2009) Cross-national associations between gender and mental disorders in the World Health Organization World Mental Health Surveys. *Archives of General Psychiatry* 66(7), 785–95.

Shear K, Feske U, and Greeno C (2000) Gender differences in anxiety disorders: clinical implications. In: E Frank (ed.) *Gender and Its Effects on Psychopathology*. Washington, DC: American Psychopathological Association, 151–65.

Sheikh JI, Leskin GA, and Klein DF (2002) Gender differences in panic disorder: findings from the national comorbidity survey. *American Journal of Psychiatry* 159(1), 55–8.

Simon NM, Zalta AK, Worthington JJ, et al. (2006) Preliminary support for gender differences in response to fluoxetine for generalized anxiety disorder. *Depression and Anxiety* 23(6), 373–6.

Starcevic V, Djordjevic A, Latas M, et al. (1998) Characteristics of agoraphobia in women and men with panic disorder with agoraphobia. *Depression and Anxiety* 8(1), 8–13.

Stein DJ, Kasper S, Andersen EW, et al. (2004) Escitalopram in the treatment of social anxiety disorder: analysis of efficacy for different clinical subgroups and symptom dimensions. *Depression and Anxiety* 20(4), 175–81.

Stein DJ, Lim CCW, Roest AM, et al. (2017) The cross-national epidemiology of social anxiety disorder: data from the World Mental Health Survey Initiative. *BMC Medicine* 15(1), 143.

Stewart SE, Yen C-H, Stack DE, et al. (2006) Outcome predictors for severe obsessive-compulsive patients in intensive residential treatment. *Journal of Psychiatric Research* 40(6), 511–19.

Stoney CM, Davis MC, and Matthews KA (1987) Sex differences in physiological responses to stress and in coronary heart disease: a causal link? *Psychophysiology* 24(2), 127–31.

Storch EA, Abramowitz J, and Goodman WK (2008) Where does obsessive-compulsive disorder belong in DSM-V? *Depression and Anxiety* 5(4), 336–47.

Thompson AE and Voyer D (2014) Sex differences in the ability to recognise non-verbal displays of emotion: a meta-analysis. *Cognition and Emotion* 28(7), 1164–95.

Torresan RC, Ramos-Cerqueira ATA, Shavitt RG, et al. (2013) Symptom dimensions, clinical course and comorbidity in men and women with obsessive-compulsive disorder. *Psychiatry Research* 209(2), 186–95.

Turgeon L, Marchand A, and Dupuis G (1998) Clinical features in panic disorder with agoraphobia. *Journal of Anxiety Disorders* 12(6), 539–53.

Vesga-López O, Schneier FR, Wang S, et al. (2008) Gender differences in generalized anxiety disorder: results from the National Epidemiologic Survey on Alcohol and Related Conditions (NESARC). *The Journal of Clinical Psychiatry* 69(10), 1606–16.

Weissman MM, Bland RC, Canino GJ, et al. (1994) The cross national epidemiology of obsessive compulsive disorder. *The Cross National Collaborative Group. The Journal of Clinical Psychiatry* 55 Suppl. 5–10.

Wittchen HU, Jacobi F, Rehm J, et al. (2011) The size and burden of mental disorders and other disorders of the brain in Europe 2010. *European Neuropsychopharmacology* 21(9), 655–79.

World Health Organization (2018) *International Statistical Classification of Diseases and Related Health Problems*. 11th revision. Available at: https://icd .who.int/browse11/l-m/en (accessed 26 February 2019).

Xu Y, Schneier F, Heimberg RG, et al. (2012) Gender differences in social anxiety disorder: results from the national epidemiologic sample on alcohol and related conditions. *Journal of Anxiety Disorders* 26(1), 12–19.

Yonkers KA, Bruce SE, Dyck IR, et al. (2003) Chronicity, relapse, and illness – course of panic disorder, social phobia, and generalized anxiety disorder: findings in men and women from 8 years of follow-up. *Depression and Anxiety* 17(3), 173–9.

Yonkers KA, Zlotnick C, Allsworth J, et al. (1998) Is the course of panic disorder the same in women and men? *The American Journal of Psychiatry* 155(5), 596–602.

Chapter

10

Post-Traumatic Stress Disorder in Men

Sonia Terhaag, David J. Pedder, Alyssa M. Sbisa, and David Forbes

Post-traumatic stress disorder (PTSD) is a psychiatric disorder that may develop following exposure to a potentially traumatic event. In developing our understanding of PTSD, identifying potential differences in prevalence, development, maintenance, and prognosis between sexes (Olff, 2017; Breslau, 2002) has been of great interest. Many theories and models have been developed to try to explain sex differences, and improve understanding, treatment, and recovery from this disorder. This chapter provides a snapshot of the current state of knowledge of PTSD with a special focus on the disorder in men, as well as providing insight into future directions and innovative approaches for studying and treating PTSD.

What Is PTSD?

PTSD is one of several disorders that may develop in response to a potentially traumatic event, which can range from one-time exposure to repeated exposures over many years. Types of traumatic events include physical and sexual assault, accidental injury, combat or warzone exposure, and sudden death or injury in others. Diagnostic criteria for PTSD have evolved since the disorder's introduction into the diagnostic nosology in 1980 in primary diagnostic manuals such as the World Health Organization's *International Classification of Diseases* (ICD), and the American Psychiatric Association's *Diagnostic and Statistical Manual of Mental Disorders*.

According to the DSM-5, PTSD is diagnosed using five main criteria:

(1) Experiencing a traumatic event that involves actual or real threat to self or others
(2) Re-experiencing of the trauma
(3) Avoidance
(4) Alterations in mood or cognitions
(5) Hyperarousal

Re-experiencing the trauma (2) includes intrusive memories, images/sounds/perceptions of the trauma that invade consciousness, dreams, and flashbacks of the event, and intense emotional or physical distressing reactions to reminders of the trauma. Avoidance (3) is often understood to be in reaction to (2) experiences, where the avoidance can take on a phobic quality. This includes intentional avoidance of places, people, objects, situations, thoughts, or feelings associated with the trauma. Criterion (4) includes changes in mood and thoughts (which are also found in depression and other disorders): low mood, loss of interest, social withdrawal and avoidance, inability to experience positive emotions, catastrophizing or exaggerated negative beliefs, cognitive distortions, and in some instances psychogenic amnesia. The last criterion (5) involves heightened alertness and arousal, such as feelings of irritability and anger, sleep difficulties, hypervigilance, difficulties with concentration, reckless/self-destructive behaviour, and an exaggerated startle response. Criterion (1) must be met for a diagnosis, as well as a combination of symptoms from each of the other four clusters. Symptoms must have been persistently present for at least one month, and the experience of symptoms must be causing distress or significantly interfere with daily functioning. Given the overlap of some of the symptoms with other anxiety and mood disorders (see Chapters 9 and 12), PTSD presentation is often very complex in both men and women, and co-morbidity is common.

Box 10.1 The nature of PTSD

- Post-traumatic stress disorder is a psychiatric disorder that develops in response to a potentially traumatic event, such as a motor vehicle accident, a natural disaster, interpersonal violence, or sudden death or injury
- Symptoms of PTSD are spread across four clusters, which include re-experiencing the event, avoidance related to the trauma, changes in mood and/or thoughts, and hyperarousal

Prevalence of PTSD

The reported lifetime prevalence rate of PTSD in adult males ranges from 3 to 13% across published studies (Ditlevsen and Elklit, 2012, McLean et al., 2011). Research has consistently indicated that the prevalence of PTSD in men is approximately half that of women (Tolin and Foa, 2006), although the magnitude of this difference fluctuates across the lifespan and can further vary based on trauma exposure and type of trauma.

Trauma Exposure

Despite men having significantly lower prevalence rates of PTSD compared to women, they are more likely to be exposed to potentially traumatic events. For instance, in the United States, 61% of men had experienced at least one traumatic incident during their lifetime, compared to 51% of women (Kessler et al., 1995). Another study in Australian adults found similar rates of PTSD, with 64.6% of men and 49.5% of women reporting at least one traumatic incident (Creamer et al., 2001). In understanding rates of repeated exposure, the study revealed that of these men, 38% had experienced only one trauma event, 28% experienced two events, and 34% had experienced three or more events (Creamer et al., 2001).

In attempting to understand the sex differences in prevalence rates, it is important to consider trauma types. Men report higher rates of most trauma types compared to women (Chapman et al., 2012; Creamer et al., 2001; Kessler et al., 1995; Tolin and Foa, 2006). For instance, men report a higher likelihood of exposure to combat or witnessing someone being killed (37.8% of men vs 16.1% of women); involvement in threatening accidents (28.3% of men vs 13.6% of women); and exposure to natural disasters (19.9% of men vs 12.7% of women; Creamer et al., 2001). Comparatively, men report lower rates of exposure to sexual violence (e.g., rape or molestation) than women (3.8% vs 12.9%; Creamer et al., 2001). As sexual violence of this nature is most strongly associated with PTSD onset, this might explain some of the gender differences in PTSD rates, with men less likely to experience and/or report these events (Creamer et al., 2001).

Having said this, even when the type of trauma event is controlled for, gender differences in PTSD rates remain consistent, with men continuing to report half the rate of PTSD for women (Kessler et al., 1995). By controlling for type of trauma exposure in a meta-analysis, Tolin and Foa (2006) found that men were less likely to meet criteria for PTSD and reported less severity of PTSD symptoms compared to women for all types of trauma. Even in trauma types that men are more likely to experience (nonsexual assault, combat, accidental injury, witnessing someone badly injured or killed), men are less likely to meet criteria for PTSD and report less severe symptomatology (Tolin and Foa, 2006). Of note, for childhood sexual abuse no gender differences in PTSD rates have been found, despite men experiencing less exposure than women (Tolin and Foa, 2006).

Co-morbidity and Related Conditions

Men with PTSD commonly also meet diagnostic criteria for co-occurring mental health disorders and related conditions (Hourani et al., 2016). Up to 88% of men with PTSD meet criteria for at least one other mental health disorder (Kessler et al., 1995). Within a 12-month period, up to 51.6% of men with PTSD also met criteria for a major depressive episode compared to 3.8% without PTSD, and 40.2% of men with PTSD met criteria for generalized anxiety disorder compared to 1.7% without PTSD (Creamer et al., 2001).

High prevalence rates of co-morbid substance use disorders are also a common feature in the context of PTSD in men, more so than in women (Galatzer-Levy et al., 2013). Within a 12-month period, 37.6% of men with PTSD also met criteria for alcohol use disorder compared to 8.5% without PTSD, indicating that men with PTSD are 6.5 times more likely to report co-morbid alcohol use disorder (Creamer et al., 2001). Also within a 12-month period, 22.6% of men with PTSD met criteria for drug use disorder compared to 3.9% without PTSD, indicating men with PTSD are 7.2 times more likely to have a co-morbid drug use disorder (Creamer et al., 2001). For men in the military, problematic alcohol use and depression are the strongest predictors of PTSD (Hourani et al., 2016).

Similar to substance use, anger and irritability are common symptoms in men with PTSD. Anger and irritability are cornerstone symptoms of PTSD, and problematic rates of these particular symptoms have been noted in men with PTSD (Jakupcak and Tull, 2005). Specifically, anger, aggression, and violence have been found to increase in men with PTSD compared to men without PTSD, such as being more than

- The PTSD prevalence rates of men are half that of women
- Men are more likely to be exposed to traumatic events than women
- Alcohol and other drug use disorders are commonly co-occurring in men with PTSD
- Anger, irritability, and violence are increased in men with PTSD compared to men without PTSD

twice as likely to engage in acts of aggression and violence in intimate relationships. This pattern is replicated and further increased in male veterans, where higher levels of anger are associated with PTSD, more so than in any other mental health disorder. Anger scores have also been found to be higher in male veterans with PTSD than female veterans with PTSD (Castillo et al., 2002). Given that the co-morbidity of anger, aggression, and substance use is higher in men than women, men are more likely to exhibit externalizing disorders (e.g., substance use disorders or conduct disorder) in the context of PTSD, whereas women are more likely to exhibit internalizing disorders (e.g., anxiety or depression; Kessler et al., 2005).

Development of PTSD over the Lifespan

The distribution of PTSD rates differs across the lifespan, with findings suggesting that PTSD prevalence among men increases to peak at middle age, and then decreases steadily. In a meta-analysis by Tolin and Foa (2006), this gender difference in the pattern of PTSD prevalence was already observable in childhood, with boys less likely to meet criteria for PTSD than girls. Men in their early 40s demonstrate the highest prevalence of PTSD, whereas men in their early 70s demonstrate the lowest (Ditlevsen and Elklit, 2012). A recent National Comorbidity Survey supports this by finding the highest lifetime prevalence of PTSD is in individuals 45–59 years old and the lowest in those over 60 (Kessler et al., 2005). The greatest difference between men and women is in early adulthood (21- to 25-year-olds), where men are three times less likely than women to have PTSD (Ditlevsen and Elklit, 2012). Data also show that men report a less chronic course of the disorder than

women (Breslau et al., 1998; Kessler et al., 1995). In order to elucidate these differential prevalence rates across the lifespan, this section considers the biological, environmental, and social factors that contribute to the development and maintenance of PTSD in men.

Biological Underpinnings

Over the last twenty years, research has demonstrated the importance of neuroendocrine factors in PTSD. Studies have shown PTSD is related to complex dysregulation of the hypothalamic–pituitary–adrenal and hypothalamic–pituitary–gonadal axes. Meta-analysis of sixty-six studies found that lower levels of stress steroid hormones, such as cortisol, are related to PTSD, with men exhibiting higher levels of hair cortisol concentrations (HCC) compared to women (Stalder et al., 2017). Further, a study examining pre- and post-deployment HCC in male soldiers determined low cortisol was predictive of a higher rate of PTSD symptomatology (Steudte-Schmiedgen et al., 2015).

Other hormones like testosterone have been shown to be associated with PTSD, and although several studies have explored this relationship, the direction of the association is not entirely clear. In samples of men with PTSD, analysis of plasma (Spivak et al., 2003), serum (Karlović et al., 2012), and cerebrospinal fluid (Mulchahey et al., 2001) have found no difference, with higher and lower levels of testosterone, respectively. In a male military cohort, however, increased testosterone levels from pre- to post-deployment predicted development of PTSD symptoms at one and two years (Reijnen et al., 2015). Relatedly, a recent meta-analysis (Passos et al., 2015) found that certain inflammatory markers are associated with PTSD. Interleukin (IL)-1β, IL-6, and interferon-γ levels were higher in patients with PTSD than in healthy controls. While these analyses did not stratify for sex, previous studies have shown increased pro-inflammatory cytokines (i.e., TNF-α, IL-6) in men with combat-related PTSD (Passos et al., 2015).

The bulk of the literature supports strong associations between biological risk factors and PTSD, although further study in this field is required. For example, a recent meta-analysis has shown age moderates biological markers of PTSD, including cortisol, heart rate, and systolic blood pressure (Morris et al., 2016). Understanding moderators of biological markers could assist in recognizing subsamples of individuals at increased risk of developing PTSD. Research efforts are ongoing to untangle the complex relationship between biological markers, such as hormones and inflammatory markers, and PTSD. While these findings are developing a better understanding of the biological underpinnings of PTSD, its implications for PTSD and sex specifically are not yet clear.

Prior Interpersonal Trauma

Previous exposure to interpersonal trauma, including childhood abuse, is a risk factor for the development of PTSD (Brewin et al., 2000). A recent review of over 30,000 adults from 20 different countries has shown that experience of interpersonal violence during childhood or adulthood (e.g., witnessed violence at home as a child, being beaten by a caregiver as a child, or beaten by someone else other than a romantic partner) also increases vulnerability of developing PTSD following a subsequent traumatic experience (Liu et al., 2017). In male Vietnam veterans, Bremner et al. (1993) discovered higher rates of childhood physical abuse in those with combat-related PTSD than in combat veterans without the disorder. Similarly, Coker et al. (2005) showed that a history of childhood abuse was significantly associated with higher PTSD scores in men who were victims of intimate partner violence.

Occupational Exposures

The relationship between combat exposure and PTSD is well established. Not only is a PTSD diagnosis approximately two times higher in veterans than the general population, but other factors, including number of deployments and intensity of combat, influence susceptibility (Boasso et al., 2015). In a sample of over 300,000 veterans who had sought health care at Veterans Affairs in the USA, men were found to have higher rates of PTSD diagnosis than women (Maguen et al., 2010); however, sex differences in PTSD are absent when level of military trauma exposure is similar (Woodhead et al., 2012).

Similarly, first-responder occupations (i.e., police officers, paramedics, firefighters, search and rescue personnel) are considered a risk factor in the development of PTSD given the repeated and cumulative nature of traumatic stressors and exposure experienced by people in these occupations. Given that generally men represent a much greater proportion of the first-responder workforce (Berger et al., 2012), it is important to consider the experience of PTSD in men in this context. A review of over 20,000 rescue workers found the prevalence of PTSD to be 10%, substantially higher than the 1.3–3.5% reported in the general population across several countries (Berger et al., 2012). Studies examining gender differences in rescue workers and first responders have generally found women to exhibit a higher prevalence of PTSD (Bowler et al., 2010), reflecting similar trends to those seen in the general population. However, one study examining disaster responders found men had a greater likelihood for probable PTSD than women (Loo et al., 2016). A study of police responders to the 9/11 World Trade Center terrorist attack showed higher prevalence of PTSD symptoms in females; however, this gender difference was absent at the two-year follow-up (Bowler et al., 2012), suggesting a different pattern of onset in male and female first responders. Overall, this highlights that while rates of PTSD are generally higher in those working in high-exposure occupations, to some extent this closes the gender gap in prevalence.

Social and Cultural Factors

Social and cultural factors, such as sexual orientation, ethnicity, and social support also impact on PTSD in both men and women, as they influence whether someone is exposed to a trauma initially, and how they respond to it consequently. Gay and bisexual men experience higher risk of PTSD onset than heterosexual men due in part to greater exposure to interpersonal violence, traumatic events, and an earlier age of trauma exposure (e.g., childhood maltreatment; Roberts et al., 2010). Further, the trajectory of lifetime rates of PTSD in men shows variability by culture. Nordic samples have shown the highest prevalence of PTSD occurs in women during their early 40s and in men during their early 50s (Ditlevsen and Elklit, 2010), while an Australian study found lower lifetime rates in elderly women (Creamer and Parslow, 2008); and German research found increased rates in individuals over 60 years of age (Maercker et al., 2008). In a study across low-income post-conflict countries, equal rates of PTSD were found in men and women in Ethiopia, lower rates among men in Algeria and Cambodia, and higher rates in men in Gaza (de Jong et al., 2001). While cultural determinants of mental health are extremely complex and beyond the scope of this chapter, these findings across cultures do highlight that there is important variation across cultures in response to trauma.

Social support is a well-established protective factor against the development of psychiatric disorders. Divorced, separated, and widowed male veterans are at greater risk for a PTSD diagnosis than married ones, indicating that social support serves as a protective factor during the peri- and post-trauma period (Creamer et al., 2001). Further, research has shown that perception of social support in male veterans and injury survivors is negatively associated with PTSD (King et al., 2006; Nickerson et al., 2017), meaning that as perceptions of support increase, symptoms of PTSD are proportionately lower. Although research continues to find social support is more strongly related to the development of PTSD symptoms in women compared to men (Andrews et al., 2003), very little is known about the specific factors underlying this difference. One possible explanation is that PTSD and social support have a bidirectional relationship, where PTSD can drive away social support by way of symptoms such as being angry and irritable, closed off to others and avoiding reminders which may include hobbies, places, and people (Nickerson et al., 2017). Further research is necessary to examine gender differences and the various facets of the construct of social support, especially in the context of cultural influences, in the development and maintenance of PTSD.

Box 10.3 PTSD over the male lifespan

- PTSD prevalence in males increases with age until it peaks in middle age and then declines: men in their early 40s demonstrate the highest prevalence and men in their early 70s the lowest
- Alterations in cortisol, testosterone, and inflammatory markers are associated with PTSD in men
- Previous exposure to traumatic events, first-responder occupation, combat exposure, and lack of social support are associated with increased risk for developing PTSD

Gender Differences in PTSD Expression and Recovery

Expression of PTSD Symptoms

A potential explanation for lower rates of PTSD in men compared to women may be differences in expression of symptoms following traumatic events (Tolin and Foa, 2006). Compared to women, men tend to report more hypervigilance, reckless self-destructive behaviour, violence, anger, irritability, and nightmares, whilst reporting less negative self-beliefs, avoidance, restricted affect, and sleep disturbance (see Carragher et al., 2016 for a summary).

The patterns of symptoms expressed by males and females may be reinforced through gender role expectations, where men are socialized to externalize negative emotions and women taught to internalize them, aligning with 'acceptable' masculine and feminine gender roles and behaviours (Foster et al., 2004, Tolin and Foa, 2006). Cultures that emphasize traditional gender roles by discouraging emotional expression in men reveal greater differences in PTSD rates with lower prevalence of PTSD in men compared to women (Norris et al., 2001). Such findings are associated with men exhibiting higher levels of maladaptive coping compared to women, in trying to manage trauma symptoms (Carmassi et al., 2014).

Gender differences also exist in cognitions following traumatic events and in relation to how men and women appraise their traumatic stress symptoms. Men perceive traumatic events as less aversive than women experiencing the same event, resulting in lower vulnerability to PTSD risk for men (Norris et al., 2002). Men are also less likely than women to process the event as a subjective threat and less likely to report a subsequent loss of personal control or dissociation (Olff et al., 2007). Tolin and Foa (2002) found gender differences in patterns of cognitive processing, memory of the event, and the effect of trauma on cognitive schemas. Men are also less likely than women to blame themselves for the trauma and less likely to have negative beliefs about themselves, or believe the world is a dangerous and unsafe place. In turn, men are less likely than women to attempt to avoid thoughts and feelings associated with the trauma (25.0% vs 56.4%; Sonne et al., 2003), which would consequently be associated with better adjustment and processing of the experience, and lower prevalence rates.

Assessment and Diagnosis

Given the gender differences in expression of PTSD symptoms, it has been posited that men may be less likely to meet the DSM-5 PTSD diagnostic criteria as they are heavily grounded on internalizing symptomatology. For instance, the symptoms commonly experienced by men following traumatic events (e.g., anger, substance use) may not be sufficiently covered by current PTSD criteria, whereas symptoms more likely expressed by women (e.g., avoidance, fear) are central to the PTSD diagnosis (Tolin and Foa, 2006). Additionally, there is the possibility of misdiagnosis of PTSD and complex trauma in clinical and research settings. Given the association between PTSD and personality disorders in complex trauma, men may be under- or overdiagnosed with antisocial personality disorder, and women with borderline personality disorder (Olff et al., 2007).

Furthermore, men may demonstrate a lack of willingness to acknowledge and report symptoms associated with PTSD (e.g., emotional distress) as this may not align with what they consider to be socially acceptable masculine behaviour (e.g., not wanting to appear weak; Tolin and Foa, 2006). Such underreporting of symptoms in men may reduce the reliability of self-report procedures in assessing PTSD prevalence rates in men and women, and further complicates the issue of assessment and diagnosis of PTSD in men.

Help-Seeking and Support

In line with the potential reduced reporting or disclosure of PTSD symptoms among men, it is also useful to examine help-seeking behaviours in men with PTSD. When men access social support, they report comparable levels of social support and support satisfaction to women (Andrews et al., 2003). However, they are generally less likely to seek out support, both formal and informal, and this mitigates the benefit potentially derived from sources of support. For example, in a sample of Vietnam veterans, men were less likely to disclose a traumatic event of childhood sexual abuse, and the timing of the disclosure had no impact on PTSD symptoms, whereas women had increased symptom severity with delayed disclosure (Ullman and Filipas, 2005).

Moreover, the experience men can have with help-seeking can further impact on symptoms and behaviours. In men experiencing intimate partner violence, positive help-seeking experiences were associated with reduced problematic alcohol use, but negative help-seeking experiences were associated with increased PTSD symptom severity (Douglas and Hines, 2011). Furthermore, men were less likely than women to report that PTSD severely impacted their social functioning (74.4% vs 97.4%), albeit there were no gender differences in impairments to occupational functioning (Sonne et al., 2003).

On a positive note, and given the high proportion of men in military samples, research has found that male and female military members with PTSD are equally likely to access mental health services and treatment (Hourani et al., 2016). However, more men with PTSD sought mental health support for co-morbid substance use problems, whereas more women sought support for co-morbid depression (Hourani et al., 2016). Furthermore, the predictors for accessing mental health services varied according to gender. Combat exposure, recent medical illness, and history of sexual abuse were the strongest predictors for men in utilizing mental health services, whereas depression and problematic alcohol use were the strongest predictors for women (Hourani et al., 2016). Social support from within the military for men was associated with lower levels of PTSD, while support from outside the military (i.e., from family and friends) had no effect on PTSD symptoms (Smith et al., 2013).

> **Box 10.4 How men experience and report PTSD symptoms**
>
> - Men report greater hypervigilance and self-destructive behaviour than women, and less avoidance and negative self-beliefs following trauma exposure
> - Men perceive traumatic events as less averse than women
> - Men may under report PTSD symptoms partly due to expectations with traditional gender roles and behaviours (e.g., not appearing as weak)
> - Men are less likely to seek out formal and informal support, except for in the military where men and women with PTSD are equally likely to seek mental health services

Treatment, Recovery, and Prognosis

Psychological Treatments

Over time, many interventions, including treatment and prevention, have been developed in response to greater understanding of the aetiology and symptomatology of PTSD. First-line evidence-based psychological interventions include mainstay cognitive-behavioural trauma-focused treatments such as Prolonged Exposure (PE), Cognitive Processing Therapy (CPT), and Eye Movement Desensitization and Reprocessing (EMDR). Overall, evidence suggests that there are gender differences in response to traditional PTSD treatments. A meta-analysis of the available evidence suggests that women generally experience greater reductions in PTSD symptom outcomes compared to men following trauma-focused interventions (Wade et al., 2016). It is important to note, however, that the body of literature regarding PTSD treatment in men predominantly examines psychological treatment for the effects of wartime trauma; as previously noted, men are significantly more likely to experience military/wartime-related trauma exposure (Mills et al., 2011). As such, many treatments that focus specifically on men are in the context of wartime exposure and/or combat. In contrast, much less evidence is available for PTSD treatment in the context of sexual trauma in men compared to women. Further research is warranted to establish whether gender differences in treatment response are evident and consistent across trauma types. Findings thus far are varied, ranging from large gender differences (Galovski et al., 2013) to none (Beck et al., 2009, Ehlers et al., 2003), depending on type of trauma. Further, although traditional treatments such as CPT and PE are good at addressing internalizing aspects of PTSD, they may fall short in addressing externalized symptoms of the disorder, often encountered in the military context and among men. Therefore, treatment protocols need to be developed and tested for externalizing problems (e.g., anger and aggression) in the context of PTSD, as they would be particularly relevant and applicable in treating men (Cash et al., 2018).

Pharmacological Treatments

In terms of pharmacological interventions, there is no PTSD-specific agent, and the most evidence-based first-line pharmacological interventions are those also used for treating anxiety and depression (see Chapters 9 and 12), namely selective serotonin reuptake inhibitors (SSRIs) and serotonin-norepinephrine reuptake inhibitors (SNRIs; Marshall et al., 2001; Hoskins et al., 2015). Compared to men, women are more than 1.5 times more likely to be prescribed pharmacological treatment for PTSD (Harpaz-Rotem et al., 2008), even after adjusting for psychiatric comorbidity (Bernardy et al., 2013). This highlights considerable need for the exploration of gender differences in responsiveness to pharmacological treatments, and what the potential underlying mechanisms may be. To date, explanations of the gender differences in prescription of medications for PTSD focus only on symptomatology, such as women being more likely to report symptoms such as sleep disturbance.

Treatment Innovations

Beyond traditional therapeutic treatment approaches to PTSD, rapid technological advancements in the last two decades have led to fascinating new modalities and approaches to traditional treatments, with some holding great promise for the treatment of PTSD in men. They may offer new solutions to issues seen in men with PTSD, such as the high dropout rate or reluctance to seek treatment (Blain et al., 2010; Murphy and Busuttil, 2015). These exciting new advances centre on telehealth and virtual reality.

Telehealth includes delivery of traditional treatments (such as CPT and PE) through a technological medium such as phone, online, or electronic feedback systems. Research suggests that there is good uptake, efficacy, and retention for this PTSD treatment modality in men. In particular, early findings suggest that telehealth delivery makes treatments no less effective compared to in-person therapies for PTSD (Yuen et al., 2015), and has great potential for being able to reach those seeking treatment who may otherwise experience barriers such as geographical remoteness.

Virtual reality (VR) involves a computer-generated environment and is especially applicable to exposure-based treatments. For example, it may involve undergoing PE treatment with a simulated environment that resembles the traumatic exposure. Given that this experience is immersive, it has the potential to be much more potent than the individual having to remember their traumatic experience to practice exposure. Research of VR in the treatment of PTSD so far suggests that it is an effective approach, particularly in military contexts (Rothbaum et al., 2010). A systematic review of the VR-based exposure treatment literature suggests that overall it is comparably efficacious to traditional treatments. It may be particularly useful in the treatment of those who are resistant to traditional exposure treatment, although the research to date does suggest similar attrition rates to traditional exposure therapy (Gonçalves et al., 2012). As VR-based exposure treatment is relatively new, the evidence base requires expansion with methodologically rigorous clinical trials that standardize the application of this treatment modality to allow comparison, and that have sample sizes large enough to allow statistical comparison in treatment response between male and female participants.

These new treatment modalities may have additional potential benefits for men, with research suggesting men prefer technology-based approaches to traditional mental health care (Wilson et al., 2008). This may be especially true in military contexts, given the high degree of stigma still associated with mental health issues in this environment, which acts as a barrier to seeking treatment (Hoge et al., 2004).

Recovery and Prognosis

Most research suggests that many people recover from PTSD. A meta-analysis of spontaneous remission in PTSD suggests that between 8 to 89% of those with PTSD recover without treatment, and that this is determined by type of traumatic event only (Nexhmedin et al., 2014). Many individuals improve further with the help of PTSD treatments, and new advances in technology continue to improve access, uptake, and outcomes from PTSD treatment for both men and women. However, despite these encouraging outcomes, a proportion of those with PTSD continue to struggle with symptomatology. PTSD increases risk for suicide (compared to those without PTSD), even after controlling for other mental health disorders (Gradus et al., 2010; Krysinska and Lester, 2010). Further, as men generally evidence smaller recovery effect sizes following treatment (Weeks et al., 2013), it is imperative that research efforts continue to find new ways to improve recovery and prognosis and factor gender into these endeavours.

Box 10.5   Treatment of PTSD and prognosis

- Traditional treatment approaches for PTSD include cognitive-behavioural therapies and exposure-based therapies such as Prolonged Exposure (PE); and these treatments tend to be effective for men
- Pharmacotherapy for PTSD is based primarily on the use of SSRIs, which can be effective in those who may not respond to traditional treatment approaches
- New innovative treatments and modalities are being developed and show promise for application to PTSD treatment. For example, virtual reality exposure therapy has been shown to be effective and well tolerated by men with PTSD
- Recovery and prognosis for PTSD is generally good with treatment for most, although a significant proportion will struggle with chronic PTSD

Conclusions

This chapter reviews the current state of knowledge on PTSD in men, with evidence suggesting that while men are at lower risk of developing the disorder throughout the lifespan compared to women, there are important aspects of their experience that are especially problematic and interfere with treatment and prognosis. In particular, men are more likely to be exposed to potentially traumatic events and experience higher degrees of co-morbidity. Problematic anger and aggression, as well as substance use disorders, commonly co-occur with PTSD, especially among men. Potential explanations underpinning these gender differences include biological mechanisms, such as reduced physiological responsiveness to stressful events, societal norms around expression of emotional symptoms, cultural explanations, as well as how PTSD is assessed and diagnosed. Men are less likely to seek formal and informal support for PTSD and, when they do take up treatment, they generally do not respond as well as women. New innovations in treatment, such as telehealth modalities and virtual reality, provide exciting new avenues that may be especially applicable and useful in the context of PTSD treatment among men. The goal for continued research in this area should include a focus on improving early identification and intervention for men and women with PTSD, and to further improve treatments, old and new, to reduce the detrimental effect of trauma and PTSD on mental health and well-being.

References

Andrews, B., Brewin, C. R., and Rose, S. 2003. Gender, social support, and PTSD in victims of violent crime. *Journal of Traumatic Stress*, 16, 421.

Beck, J. G., Coffey, S. F., Foy, D. W., Keane, T. M., and Blanchard, E. B. 2009. Group cognitive behavior therapy for chronic posttraumatic stress disorder: an initial randomized pilot study. *Behavior Therapy*, 40, 82–92.

Berger, W., Coutinho, E. S. F., Figueira, I., Marques-Portella, C., Luz, M. P., Neylan, T. C., Marmar, C. R., and Mendlowicz, M. V. 2012. Rescuers at risk: a systematic review and meta-regression analysis of the worldwide current prevalence and correlates of PTSD in rescue workers. *Social Psychiatry and Psychiatric Epidemiology*, 47, 1001–11.

Bernardy, N. C., Lund, B. C., Alexander, B., Jenkyn, A. B., Schnurr, P. P., and Friedman, M. J. 2013. Gender differences in prescribing among veterans diagnosed with posttraumatic stress disorder. *Journal of General Internal Medicine*, 28 Suppl 2, S542–S548.

Blain, L. M., Galovski, T. E., and Robinson, T. 2010. Gender differences in recovery from posttraumatic stress disorder: a critical review. *Aggression and Violent Behavior*, 15, 463–74.

Boasso, A. M., Steenkamp, M. M., Nash, W. P., Larson, J. L., and Litz, B. T. 2015. The relationship between course of PTSD symptoms in deployed US Marines and degree of combat exposure. *Journal of Traumatic Stress*, 28, 73–8.

Bowler, R. M., Han, H., Gocheva, V., Nakagawa, S., Alper, H., Digrande, L., and Cone, J. E. 2010. Gender differences in probable posttraumatic stress disorder among police responders to the 2001 World Trade Center terrorist attack. *American Journal of Industrial Medicine*, 53, 1186–96.

Bowler, R. M., Harris, M., LI, J., Gocheva, V., Stellman, S. D., Wilson, K., Alper, H., Schwarzer, R., and Cone, J. E. 2012. Longitudinal mental health impact among police responders to the 9/11 terrorist attack. *American Journal of Industrial Medicine*, 55, 297–312.

Bremner, J. D., Southwick, S. M., Johnson, D. R., Yehuda, R., and Charney, D. S. 1993. Childhood physical abuse and combat-related posttraumatic stress disorder in Vietnam veterans. *American Journal of Psychiatry*, 150(2), 235–9.

Breslau, N. 2002. Gender differences in trauma and posttraumatic stress disorder. *Journal of Gender-Specific Medicine*, 5, 34–40.

Breslau, N., Kessler, R. C., Chilcoat, H. D., Schultz, L. R., Davis, G. C., and AndreskI, P. 1998. Trauma and posttraumatic stress disorder in the community: the 1996 Detroit Area Survey of Trauma. *Archives of General Psychiatry*, 55, 626–32.

Brewin, C. R., Andrews, B., and Valentine, J. D. 2000. Meta-analysis of risk factors for posttraumatic stress disorder in trauma-exposed adults. *Journal of Consulting and Clinical Psychology*, 68, 748–66.

CarmassI, C., Akiskal, H., Bessonov, D., Massimetti, G., Calderani, E., Stratta, P., Rossi, A., and Dell, L. 2014. Gender differences in DSM-5 versus DSM-IV-TR PTSD prevalence and criteria comparison among 512 survivors to the L' Aquila earthquake. *Journal of Affective Disorders*, 160, 55–61.

Carragher, N., Sunderland, M., Batterham, P. J., Calear, A. L., Elhai, J. D., Chapman, C., and Mills, K. 2016. Discriminant validity and gender differences in DSM-5 posttraumatic stress disorder symptoms. *Journal of Affective Disorders*, 190, 56–67.

Cash, R., Varker, T., Mchugh, T., Metcalf, O., Howard, A., Lloyd, D., Costello, J., Said, D., and Forbes, D. 2018. Effectiveness of an Anger Intervention for Military Members with PTSD: A Clinical Case Series. *Military Medicine*, 183(9–10), e286–90.

Castillo, D. T., Baca, J. C. D., Conforti, K., Qualls, C., and Fallon, S. K. 2002. Anger in PTSD: general psychiatric and gender differences on the BDHI. *Journal of Loss and Trauma*, 7, 119–28.

Chapman, C., Mills, K., Slade, T., Mcfarlane, A. C., Bryant, R., Creamer, M., Silove, D., and Teesson, M. 2012. Remission from post-traumatic stress disorder in the general population. *Psychological Medicine*, 42, 1695–1703.

Coker, A. L., Weston, R., Creson, D. L., Justice, B., and Blakeney, P. 2005. PTSD symptoms among men and women survivors of intimate partner violence: the role of risk and protective factors. *Violence and Victims*, 20, 625.

Creamer, M., Burgess, P., and Mcfarlane, A. C. 2001. Post-traumatic stress disorder: findings from the Australian National Survey of Mental Health and Well-being. *Psychological Medicine*, 31, 1237–47.

Creamer, M. and Parslow, R. 2008. Trauma exposure and posttraumatic stress disorder in the elderly: a community prevalence study. *The American Journal of Geriatric Psychiatry*, 16, 853–6.

Ditlevsen, D. N. and Elklit, A. 2010. The combined effect of gender and age on post traumatic stress disorder: do men and women show differences in the lifespan distribution of the disorder? *Annals of General Psychiatry*, 9, 32.

Ditlevsen, D. N. and Elklit, A. 2012. Gender, trauma type, and PTSD prevalence: a re-analysis of 18 nordic convenience samples. *Annals of General Psychiatry*, 11, 26.

Douglas, E. M. and Hines, D. A. 2011. The helpseeking experiences of men who sustain intimate partner violence: an overlooked population and implications for practice.

Journal of Family Violence, 26, 473–85.

Ehlers, A., Clark, D. M., Hackmann, A., McManus, F., Fennell, M., Herbert, C., and Mayou, R. 2003. A randomized controlled trial of cognitive therapy, a self-help booklet, and repeated assessments as early interventions for posttraumatic stress disorder. *Archives of General Psychiatry*, 60 (10), 1024–32. doi: 10.1001/archpsyc.60.10.1024

Foster, J. D., Kuperminc, G. P., and Price, A. W. 2004. Gender differences in posttraumatic stress and related symptoms among inner-city minority youth exposed to community violence. *Journal of Youth and Adolescence*, 33, 59–69.

Galatzer-Levy, I. R., Nickerson, A., Litz, B. T., and Marmar, C. R. 2013. Patterns of lifetime PTSD comorbidity: a latent class analysis. *Depression and Anxiety*, 30, 489–96.

Galovski, T. E., Blain, L. M., Chappuis, C., and Fletcher, T. 2013. Sex differences in recovery from PTSD in male and female interpersonal assault survivors. *Behaviour Research and Therapy*, 51, 247–55.

Gonçalves, R., Pedrozo, A. L., Freire Coutinho, E. S., Figueira, I., and Ventura, P. 2012. Efficacy of virtual reality exposure therapy in the treatment of PTSD: a systematic review. *PLoS ONE*, 7, 1–7.

Gradus, J. L., Qin, P., Lincoln, A. K., Miller, M., Lawler, E., Sørensen, H. T., and Lash, T. L. 2010. Posttraumatic stress disorder and completed suicide. *American Journal of Epidemiology*, 171, 721–7.

Harpaz-Rotem, I., Rosenheck, R. A., Mohamed, S., and Desai, R. A. 2008. Pharmacologic treatment of posttraumatic stress disorder among privately insured americans. *Psychiatric Services*, 1184.

Hoge, C. W., Koffman, R. L., Castro, C. A., Messer, S. C., Mcgurk, D., and Cotting, D. I. 2004. Combat duty in Iraq and Afghanistan, mental health problems, and barriers to care. *The New England Journal of Medicine*, 13.

Hoskins, M., Pearce, J., Bethell, A., Dankova, L., Bisson, J. I., Barbui, C., Tol, W. A., Van Ommeren, M., De Jong, J., Seedat, S., and Chen, H. 2015. Pharmacotherapy for post-traumatic stress disorder: systematic review and meta-analysis. *British Journal of Psychiatry*, 206, 93–100.

Hourani, L., Williams, J., Bray, R. M., Wilk, J. E., and Hoge, C. W. 2016. Gender differences in posttraumatic stress disorder and help seeking in the US Army. *Journal of Women's Health*, 25, 22–31.

Jakupcak, M. and Tull, M. T. 2005. Effects of trauma exposure on anger, aggression, and violence in a nonclinical sample of men. *Violence and Victims*, 20, 589.

de Jong, J. T., Komproe, I. H., Van Ommeren, M., El Masri, M., Araya, M., Khaled, N., van De Put, W., and Somasundaram, D. (2001). Lifetime events and posttraumatic stress disorder in 4 postconflict settings. *JAMA*, 286(5), 555–62. doi:10.1001/jama.286.5.555

Karlović, D., Serretti, A., Vrkić, N., Martinac, M., and Marčinko, D. 2012. Serum concentrations of CRP, IL-6, TNF-α and cortisol in major depressive disorder with melancholic or atypical features. *Psychiatry Research*, 198, 74–80.

Kessler, R. C., Berglund, P., Demler, O., Jin, R., Merikangas, K. R., and Walters, E. E. 2005. Lifetime prevalence and age-of-onset distributions of DSM-IV disorders in the National Comorbidity Survey replication. *Archives of General Psychiatry*, 62, 593–602.

Kessler, R. C., Sonnega, A., Bromet, E., Hughes, M., and Nelson, C. B. 1995. Posttraumatic stress disorder in the National Comorbidity Survey. *Archives of General Psychiatry*, 52, 1048–60.

King, D. W., Taft, C., King, L. A., Hammond, C., and Stone, E. R. 2006. Directionality of the association between social support and posttraumatic stress disorder: a longitudinal investigation. *Journal of Applied Social Psychology*, 36, 2980–92.

Krysinska, K. and Lester, D. 2010. Post-traumatic stress disorder and suicide risk: a systematic review. *Archives of Suicide Research*, 14, 1–23.

Liu, H., Petukhova, M. V., Sampson, N. A., Aguilar-Gaxiola, S., Alonso, J., Andrade, L. H., Bromet, E. J., De Girolamo, G., Haro, J. M., and Hinkov, H. 2017. Association of DSM-IV posttraumatic stress disorder with traumatic experience type and history in the World Health Organization World Mental Health Surveys. *JAMA Psychiatry*, 74, 270–81.

Loo, G. T., Dimaggio, C. J., Gershon, R. R., Canton, D. B., Morse, S. S., and Galea, S. 2016. Coping behavior and risk of post-traumatic stress disorder among federal disaster responders. *Disaster Medicine and Public Health Preparedness*, 10, 108–17.

Maercker, A., Forstmeier, S., Wagner, B., Glaesmer, H., and Brähler, E. 2008. Post-traumatic stress disorder in Germany. Results of a nationwide epidemiological study. *Der Nervenarzt*, 79, 577–86.

Maguen, S., Ren, L., Bosch, J. O., Marmar, C. R., and Seal, K. H. 2010. Gender differences in mental health diagnoses among Iraq and Afghanistan veterans enrolled in veterans affairs health care. *American Journal of Public Health*, 100, 2450–6.

Marshall, R. D., Beebe, K. L., Oldham, M., and Zaninelli, R. 2001. Efficacy and safety of paroxetine treatment for chronic PTSD: a fixed-dose, placebo-controlled study. *American Journal of Psychiatry*, 158, 1982.

Mclean, C. P., Asnaani, A., Litz, B. T., and Hofmann, S. G. 2011. Gender differences in anxiety disorders: prevalence, course of illness, comorbidity and burden of illness. *Journal of Psychiatric Research*, 45, 1027–35.

Mills, K. L., Mcfarlane, A. C., Slade, T., Creamer, M., Silove, D., Teesson, M., and Bryant, R. 2011. Assessing the prevalence of trauma exposure in epidemiological surveys. *Australian and New Zealand Journal of Psychiatry*, 45, 407–15.

Morris, M. C., Hellman, N., Abelson, J. L., and Rao, U. 2016. Cortisol, heart rate, and blood pressure as early markers of PTSD risk: a systematic review and meta-analysis. *Clinical Psychology Review*, 49, 79–91.

Mulchahey, J. J., Ekhator, N. N., Zhang, H., Kasckow, J. W., Baker, D. G., and Geracioti, T. D. 2001. Cerebrospinal fluid and plasma testosterone levels in post-traumatic stress disorder and tobacco dependence. *Psychoneuroendocrinology*, 26, 273–85.

Murphy, D. and Busuttil, W. 2015. PTSD, stigma and barriers to help-seeking within the UK Armed Forces. *Journal of the Royal Army Medical Corps*, 161, 322–6.

Nexhmedin, M., Wicherts, J. M., Lobbrecht, J., and Priebe, S. 2014. Remission from post-traumatic stress disorder in adults: a systematic review and meta-analysis of long term outcome studies. *Clinical Psychology Review*, 34, 249–55.

Nickerson, A., Creamer, M., Forbes, D., Mcfarlane, A. C., O'Donnell, M. L., Silove, D., Steel, Z., Felmingham, K., Hadzi-Pavlovic, D., and Bryant, R. A. 2017. The longitudinal relationship between post-traumatic stress disorder and perceived social support in survivors of traumatic injury. *Psychological Medicine*, 115.

Norris, F. H., Friedman, M. J., Watson, P. J., Byrne, C. M., Diaz, E., and Kaniasty, K. 2002. 60,000 disaster victims speak: Part I. An empirical review of the empirical literature, 1981–2001. *Psychiatry: Interpersonal and Biological Processes*, 65, 207–39.

Norris, F. H., Perilla, J. L., and Murphy, A. D. 2001. Postdisaster stress in the United States and Mexico: a cross-cultural test of the multicriterion conceptual model of posttraumatic stress disorder. *Journal of Abnormal Psychology*, 110, 553.

Olff, M. 2017. Sex and gender differences in post-traumatic stress disorder: an update. *European Journal of Psychotraumatology*, 8.

Olff, M., Langeland, W., Draijer, N., and Gersons, B. P. 2007. Gender differences in posttraumatic stress disorder. *Psychological Bulletin*, 133, 183.

Passos, I. C., VAsconcelos-Moreno, M. P., Costa, L. G., Kunz, M., Brietzke, E., Quevedo, J., Salum, G., Magalhães, P. V., Kapczinski, F., and Kauer-Sant'anna, M. 2015. Inflammatory markers in post-traumatic stress disorder: a systematic review, meta-analysis, and meta-regression. *The Lancet Psychiatry*, 2, 1002–12.

Reijnen, A., Geuze, E., and Vermetten, E. 2015. The effect of deployment to a combat zone on testosterone levels and the association with the development of posttraumatic stress symptoms: a longitudinal prospective Dutch military cohort study. *Psychoneuroendocrinology*, 51, 525–33.

Roberts, A. L., Austin, S. B., Corliss, H. L., Vandermorris, A. K., and Koenen, K. C. 2010. Pervasive trauma exposure among US sexual orientation minority adults and risk of posttraumatic stress disorder. *American Journal of Public Health*, 100, 2433–41.

Rothbaum, B. O., Rizzo, A. S., and Difede, J. 2010. Virtual reality exposure therapy for combat-related posttraumatic stress disorder. *Annals of the New York Academy of Sciences*, 1208, 126–32.

Smith, B. N., Vaughn, R. A., Vogt, D., King, M. W., and Shipherd, J. C. 2013. Main and interactive effects of social support in predicting mental health symptoms in men and women following military stressor exposure. *Anxiety, Stress and Coping*, 26, 52–69.

Sonne, S. C., Back, S. E., Zuniga, C. D., Randall, C. L., and Brady, K. T. 2003. Gender differences in individuals with comorbid alcohol dependence and post-traumatic stress disorder. *American Journal on Addictions*, 12, 412–23.

Spivak, B., Maayan, R., Mester, R., and Weizman, A. 2003. Plasma testosterone levels in patients with combat-related posttraumatic stress disorder. *Neuropsychobiology*, 47, 57–60.

Stalder, T., Steudte-Schmiedgen, S., Alexander, N., Klucken, T., Vater, A., Wichmann, S., Kirschbaum, C., and Miller, R. 2017. Stress-related and basic determinants of hair cortisol in humans: a meta-analysis. *Psychoneuroendocrinology*, 77, 261–74.

Steudte-Schmiedgen, S., Stalder, T., Schönfeld, S., Wittchen, H.-U., Trautmann, S., Alexander, N., Miller, R., and Kirschbaum, C. 2015. Hair cortisol concentrations and cortisol stress reactivity predict PTSD symptom increase after trauma exposure during military deployment. *Psychoneuroendocrinology*, 59, 123–33.

Tolin, D. F. and Foa, E. B. 2002. Gender and PTSD: A cognitive model. In: R. P. O. Kimerling and J. Wolfe (eds) *Gender and PTSD*. New York: Guilford Press.

Tolin, D. F. and Foa, E. B. 2006. Sex differences in trauma and posttraumatic stress disorder: a quantitative review of 25 years of research. *Psychological Bulletin*, 132, 959.

Ullman, S. E. and Filipas, H. H. 2005. Gender differences in social reactions to abuse disclosures, post-abuse coping, and PTSD of child sexual abuse survivors. *Child Abuse and Neglect*, 29, 767–82.

Wade, D., Varker, T., Kartal, D., O'Donnell, M., Forbes, D., and Hetrick, S. 2016. Gender difference in outcomes following trauma-focused interventions for posttraumatic stress disorder: systematic review and meta-analysis. *Psychological Trauma: Theory, Research, Practice, and Policy*, 8, 356–64.

Weeks, W., Watts, B. V., Young, Y., Schnurr, P. P., Friedman, M. J., Mayo, L., and Weeks, W. B. 2013. Meta-analysis of the efficacy of treatments for posttraumatic stress disorder. *Journal of Clinical Psychiatry*, 74, E541–E550.

Wilson, J. A. B., Onorati, K., Mishkind, M., Reger, M. A., and Gahm, G. A. 2008. Soldier attitudes about technology-based approaches to mental health care. *Cyberpsychology and Behavior: The Impact of the Internet, Multimedia and Virtual Reality on Behavior and Society*, 11, 767–9.

Woodhead, C., Wessely, S., Jones, N., Fear, N. T., and Hatch, S. L. 2012. Impact of exposure to combat during deployment to Iraq and Afghanistan on mental health by gender. *Psychological Medicine*, 42, 1985–96.

Yuen, E. K., Gros, D. F., Price, M., Zeigler, S., Tuerk, P. W., Foa, E. B., and Acierno, R. 2015. Randomized controlled trial of home-based telehealth versus in-person prolonged exposure for combat-related ptsd in veterans: preliminary results. *Journal of Clinical Psychology*, 71, 500–12.

Suicide and Self-Harm in Young Men

Philip Hazell

This chapter delineates sex differences in suicide and self-harm, considering epidemiological and clinical data sources from across diverse settings. A focus is then placed upon young men in particular, with an exploration of what places them at risk of such acts. Finally, implications for prevention and management are addressed.

Terminology

Suicide is the deliberate taking of one's own life. In many countries cause of death, and therefore classification as suicide, must be determined by coronial enquiry. Until the mid-twentieth century, under Common Law, suicide and attempted suicide were punishable felonies. The United Kingdom repealed the law with the Suicide Act of 1961 (UK Government, 1961). There remain other discriminatory regulations. For example, most life insurance policies do not pay a death benefit if someone commits suicide during the first thirteen months of being insured. Some policies have even longer exclusion periods (Canstar, 2018).

Aiding and abetting suicide (as in medically assisted suicide) remains a crime in most jurisdictions. To confuse matters, one legal definition of suicide requires that the person was 'in the possession and enjoyment of his mental faculties', while self-killing by an insane person is not suicide (The Law Dictionary, 2018). Suicide data reported for epidemiological purposes do not make this distinction. A determination of suicide is made if the deceased gave a clear indication of their intent (for example via a suicide note or an online video) or where the circumstances of the death make suicide extremely likely. Hanging and asphyxiation are the least ambiguous causes of suicide death. Poisoning, firearm suicides, falling from a height and drowning could be accidental. To evade detection some murders are disguised as suicide. Suicide contracts, where one

individual allows another person to end their life before that person kills themselves, are a rare variant of aiding and abetting that may raise the suspicion of murder-suicide. A suicide cluster refers to a 'group of suicides or suicide attempts, or both, that occur close together in time and space than would normally be expected on the basis of statistical prediction or community expectation' (O'Carroll et al., 1988). Although there is some indication that suicide clusters should involve at least three suicide cases, there is lesser agreement about their closeness in space and time (Kõlves and Yu, 2018).

Self-harm is an act with a non-fatal outcome in which an individual deliberately did one or more of the actions shown in Box 11.1.

While the term self-harm is agnostic to suicide intent, most self-harm is of low lethality and most people who engage in self-harm are not at increased risk for suicide, at least in the short term.

Other terms may be used to describe self-harming behaviour, depending on the context. *Non-suicidal self-injury* is restricted to external injury, and where there is no suicide intent. *Parasuicide* is self-harm aimed at realizing changes that the subject desires via the actual or expected physical consequences of the self-harm. *Attempted suicide* is a more specific subcategory of parasuicide characterized by a strong intention to die. *Self-injurious behaviour* is a term

---

Box 11.1 Actions related to self-harm

- Initiation of behaviour (for example, self-cutting, jumping from a height), which they intended to cause self-harm
- Ingestion of a substance in excess of the prescribed or generally recognized therapeutic dose
- Ingestion of a recreational or illicit drug that was an act that the person regarded as self-harm
- Ingestion of a non-ingestible substance or object

---

used to describe repetitive and stereotyped self-harming in people with intellectual disability and associated neurodevelopmental disorders.

Epidemiology

Rates of suicide vary considerably between countries. In 2012, the highest standardized suicide rates (greater than 15 deaths per 100,000 population per year) occurred in Eastern Africa, the Indian subcontinent, and member states of the former Soviet Union. The lowest suicide rates (fewer than five deaths per 100,000 per year) occurred in North and Southern Africa, Central America, the Arabian peninsula, and parts of South East Asia (WHO, 2014). Data quality of suicide mortality is variable, and it is probable that estimates from Africa and parts of Asia in particular are unreliable. In most high-income countries (HIC) suicide rates across the lifespan are greater for males than females. In Australia, for example, in the period 2014–2016 deaths from suicide were 2.8 times more common in males than females in the age group 15–24 years (Australian Institute of Health and Welfare, 2018). Gender differences in suicide rates are less marked in lower- and middle-income countries (LMIC) than in HIC (WHO, 2014). The gender ratios for youth in LMIC are close to one (see Figure 11.1).

The leading method of suicide worldwide is pesticide poisoning, which accounts for about 30% of all suicide deaths (Gunnell et al., 2007). In most HIC hanging and vehicular exhaust predominate, followed by firearms and poisoning (Centers for Disease Control and Prevention, 2004, Cantor and Neulinger, 2000, Beautrais, 2000). An exception is the USA, where firearms are the most common suicide method (Centers for Disease Control and Prevention, 2004). Suicide by jumping is a relatively uncommon method of suicide in most countries (Gunnell and Nowers, 1997), although jumping from a height is the primary method of choice for suicide completers in Hong Kong (Hau, 1993). A variation on jumping from a height is jumping (usually from a platform or bridge) into the path of an oncoming train (Taylor et al., 2016).

One explanation for the different gender pattern in LMIC is ready access to and use of agricultural chemicals as a means of self-poisoning among females. Suicide by intentional pesticide ingestion primarily occurs in rural areas of LMIC in Africa, Central America, South-East Asia, and the Western Pacific.

Data about self-harm typically come from two sources: hospital data concerning emergency department presentations and hospitalization, and self-report

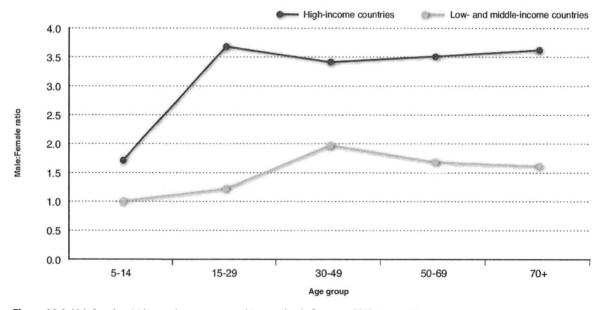

Figure 11.1 Male:female suicide rates by age group and income-level of country, 2012. Reprinted from WHO, *Preventing Suicide: A Global Imperative*, page 21, Copyright World Health Organization (2014). http://apps.who.int/iris/bitstream/handle/10665/131056/9789241564779_eng.pdf;jsessionid= 99BE8B241E27CFE2B3FBA8A2B9A0A06C?sequence=1 (accessed 6 December 2018)

data obtained from population surveys. Both sources are an unreliable indicator of the true prevalence of self-harm. Only a minority of people who self-harm (about 10%) seek medical attention, and health service coding systems miss or misclassify some instances of self-harm. Some behaviours that are more common in men, such as self-battery by hitting a hard object with the fist, may not be classified as self-harm, yet the correlates are the same as for recognized forms of self-harm such as cutting. Self-report data are vulnerable to recall bias. In addition, if the survey is anonymous there is no means to verify or clarify information.

Rates of hospital-treated self-harm are lower for men than women. For example, among 15–24-year-olds in Australia in the period 2010–2011, 143.1 per 100,000 (95% CI 137.4–149.1) males were treated in hospital for self-harm compared with 344.9 per 100,000 (95% CI 335.7–354.3) females (Carter et al., 2016). In community surveys self-harm is also typically reported by fewer males than females. For example, amongst a sample of approximately 15,000 people aged 15–16 years, 5% of males and 10% of females had engaged in self-harm in the previous year (Madge et al., 2008). A meta-analysis showed that across studies men were significantly less likely to report a history of non-suicidal self-injury than women (Bresin and Schoenleber, 2015). Moderator analyses showed that the gender difference was larger for referred samples, compared to community samples. In contrast, a meta-analysis restricted to studies conducted in China found that among college students, non-suicidal self-injury was more common in males than females (OR 1.56, 95% CI 1.30 to1.87) (Yang and Feldman, 2017).

Among hospital samples, poisoning is the most common form of self-harm, while the most commonly reported methods of self-harm in community surveys are cutting, burning, and biting (Carter et al., 2016). It is logical that hospitals will see people who have engaged in medically harmful forms of self-harm.

Factors Associated with Suicidal Behaviour and Self-Harm

Suicide is associated with a multitude of risks, spanning individual, familial, community and societal domains, as summarized in Box 11.2. Mental health problems most frequently related to suicidal behaviours include: mood disorders, such as major

> **Box 11.2 Factors associated with suicide**
> - Mental health problems, including mood disorders, psychotic disorders, eating disorders, anxiety and stress-related disorders
> - Substance-use problems
> - Chronic medical problems, notably if associated with chronic pain
> - Previous self-harm or suicide attempt
> - Stressful life events, notably interpersonal issues, financial problems
> - Social isolation, unemployment
> - Psychological characteristics, including aggression and impulsivity

depression and bipolar disorder; schizophrenia and other psychotic disorders; substance-related disorders; personality disorders (especially borderline and antisocial personality disorder); eating disorders; anxiety/somatoform disorders, including post-traumatic stress disorder; and adjustment disorder. A previous suicide attempt is the strongest risk factor for completed suicide. In the months preceding an attempted or completed suicide, individuals often experience stressors and negative life events. Stressors can include estrangement from partner and children, bereavement, chronic physical illness, unemployment, bully victimization, financial problems, and shame upon the exposure of failure or illegal activity. Psychological characteristics or vulnerabilities, such as aggression and impulsivity, poor problem-solving skills, perfectionism, worry, and rumination might exacerbate the impact of other risk factors (Dhingra et al., 2016). Hopelessness, a state of negative expectancies concerning oneself and one's future, is one of the strongest predictors of suicidal ideation and behaviour. The desire to escape from psychological suffering and psychological pain is a common motive for suicide.

In a large European study, the motives for self-harm amongst 15–16-year-olds were (in descending order of frequency): to get relief from a terrible state of mind, to die, to punish oneself, to show others one's level of desperation, to find out if one was loved, to gain revenge, to gain attention, and to frighten someone (Madge et al., 2008). A systematic review found that a childhood experience of neglect, maltreatment, or sexual abuse was a frequently reported association with later self-harm (Fliege et al., 2009). Other correlates included a childhood experience of maternal ill health, somatic complaints, aggressiveness, internalizing and externalizing symptoms, and (in males) poor school performance. Proximal factors include the experience of more negative emotions in daily life, dissociative symptoms, and alexithymia. People who self-harm also seem to more often experience stressful life events and to have fewer coping skills to manage them (Fliege et al., 2009).

Putative Mechanisms for Gender Differences

Higher suicide rates among young males (living in HIC) are attributed to the use of higher lethality means such as firearms and hanging (Bridge et al., 2006). In turn young men may have greater access to such means owing to firearm ownership, or skills in knot tying derived from traditionally male past-times. Less concern about body disfigurement in men than women may also influence the choice of suicide method (Hawton, 2000). Related to method is the intensity of intent. Suicidal ideation remains more common among women than men, but when men have suicidal thoughts they seem to be held with greater intensity. Even when the same method is used, such as poisoning, men take higher doses than women (Freeman et al., 2017). Men may fixate on a suicide plan more readily than women. There is an association between researching suicide topics on the internet and suicide rates for males but not females (Chandler, 2018). People with autistic traits (for which men are overrepresented) have higher rates of suicidal behaviour than other individuals (Zahid and Upthegrove, 2017). It is feasible that fixation mediates the relationship between autistic traits and suicidality.

Of the mental disorders associated with suicide, substance abuse and antisocial personality occur more commonly in men than women, but this is offset by a higher incidence in women of depression, eating disorders, and borderline personality disorder. Intoxication is a proximal risk factor associated with suicidal behaviour. Studies have found that men are more likely than women to have drunk alcohol in the hours before a suicide attempt (The Guardian, 2018).

Young males have a greater propensity to aggression, which is linked with suicidality and to other causes of death, such as homicide (Rice, 2015). But young males are also more likely than females to die from non-violent causes (Australian Institute of Health and Welfare, 2018); the reason is unclear.

Active factors such as risk-taking behaviour in men account for some of the gender variance, but so do passive factors such as avoidance of preventive health care (Rice, 2015).

Males are known to have more difficulty seeking professional help when experiencing emotional problems (Moller-Leimkuhler, 2002). Young men who die from suicide have less contact with healthcare agencies in the preceding year than young women (Gontijo Guerra and Vasiliadis, 2016). Goyne (2018) has proposed that males of Anglo-Irish-Scottish heritage in particular are engendered with a fierce sense of self-reliance that renders help-seeking an anathema. Goyne writes,

> Admitting to a fault, showing emotion, seeking help, backing down under threat, revealing pain, being overly friendly, having a mental problem, being even slightly effeminate, having concerns about sexuality, needing support, losing in competition, trying too hard (especially as a student), falling in love, caring too much, even smiling too often, can be construed as signs of weakness, potentially resulting in a loss of face or feelings of shame. Because men are expected to handle problems with rugged independence, when they need help they cannot ask for it without exacerbating the negative emotions that brought them to need help in the first place. Indeed, young men caught in this vicious cycle might eventually regard suicide as preferable to the dilemma and shame of admitting a weakness they neither understand nor know how to manage.

There is also the uncomfortable proposition that young men are viewed as expendable (Holter, 2002) and behave as such. The argument goes that because the capacity for women to procreate is rate-limited they must be protected. In contrast, the capacity for men to procreate is limited only by the number of available partners. Men are replaceable. The impact of the First World War on the populations of participating nations provides an illustration. Of the 16 or 17 million people who died as a result of military action, or secondary causes such as disease and famine, about 80% were male. Birth rates during the war dropped dramatically in participating nations, but rebounded to above baseline levels in the years following (Vandenbroucke, 2012). Military strategists anticipate this. No nation would enter a conflict if the known outcome was a protracted decline in the birth rate.

Other social factors such as unemployment have been considered but then rejected as plausible causes for gender differences in suicide rates (Hawton, 1998). That said, a Danish case register study found a small association between unemployment and suicide in males but not females (Qin et al., 2000). In the same study, having a child under the age of 2 years was protective for females, but not males (Qin et al., 2000).

Men may respond less well to treatments directed to mental disorders associated with suicide risk, such as depression. In an effectiveness trial of the selective serotonin reuptake inhibitor citalopram involving 2876 people, women were 33% more likely to achieve a full remission of their depression despite the fact that women in the study were more severely depressed than the men when the study began. The gender difference in treatment response was not accounted for by adherence, time to response, or side effects (Young et al., 2009). Pharmacokinetic factors offer a plausible explanation for differential responses to antidepressant treatment (Marsh, 2010). There are gender differences in antidepressant drug absorption, distribution, metabolism, and elimination, all of which lead to higher steady-state plasma levels of antidepressant drugs in women. Gastric emptying and small bowel and colonic transit times are slower for women than men. Women have a lower lean muscle to adipose tissue ratio leading to a greater volume of drug distribution. Finally, there are gender differences in hepatic metabolism (Marsh, 2010). For a further consideration of depression in males, the reader is referred to Chapter 12.

Under some circumstances men also respond less well than women to psychological therapies directed to depression. In a trial of Cognitive Behaviour Therapy (CBT)-oriented multimodal therapy directed to people with depression and chronic pain, treatment effect sizes were significantly greater for women than men (ES 0.96 v ES 0.65, t = 2.757, df = 296, p = 0.006) (Pieh et al., 2012). Another study found that men responded better to interpretive psychotherapy, while women responded better to supportive therapy (Ogrodniczuk et al., 2001). At the least, commonly delivered forms of psychotherapy such as CBT may need modification to be acceptable and effective for men (Spendelow, 2015).

A systematic review of psychosocial treatments directed at reducing the repetition of self-harm found few clinical trials had sufficient male participants to permit meaningful subgroup analyses based on gender. Of the few studies in which comparisons were possible, significant effects were found for women but not for men (Hawton et al., 2016).

Implications for Prevention and Treatment

Suicide prevention is an aspiration that is finding traction in many jurisdictions around the globe. For example, the Australian National Health and Medical Research Council Centre for Excellence in Suicide Prevention and the Black Dog Institute have formulated an evidence-based programme for implementation in New South Wales, Australia, that comprises nine elements (NHMRC Centre for Research Excellence in Suicide Prevention and Black Dog Institute, 2015):

- appropriate and continuing aftercare following suicide attempts
- high-quality psychological treatments delivered in person or online
- gatekeeper training in workplaces and community organizations
- community suicide prevention programmes
- reducing access to means
- responsible suicide reporting by media
- school-based peer support and mental health literacy programmes
- general practitioner programmes
- training of frontline staff

This programme does not specifically target males, and the need for specific strategies to prevent suicide in men has been championed by organizations such as the Australian Institute for Male Health and Studies, although their output to date has been aspirational rather than prescriptive (Australian Institute of Male Health and Studies, 2017). The aims of the organization are shown in Box 11.3.

Box 11.3 Goals to prevent suicide in men (Australian Institute of Male Health and Studies, 2017)

- disseminate targeted literature
- build community capacity
- develop male peer-support training programmes
- educate health professionals, provide counselling and mental health support for men
- promote networking and inter-agency collaborative endeavours
- develop and disseminate National Guidelines for male suicide prevention, and
- conduct basic and applied research

Evaluation of past suicide prevention endeavours has yielded mixed results with respect to impact on male suicide rates. A depression-training programme for general practitioners implemented in Gotland led to reduced suicide rates among females but not males (Rihmer et al., 1995). In contrast, a multi-level suicide prevention initiative conducted in the Szolnok region of Hungary resulted in a reduction in suicide rates for both men and women (Szekely et al., 2013). The authors attributed the success of the programme in men to the use of an anonymous emergency hotline, and the public health campaign to promote help-seeking.

One public health strategy has been to enlist male-dominated sporting codes to promote a message that destigmatizes mental illness and encourages help-seeking among men. Examples include the dedication of a round of an Australian Football competition to 'mental health and suicide prevention' (Ringland, 2017) and the dedication of a whole season of English football to the same cause (Daily Mail, 2018). A related strategy is to have elite sportsmen publicly disclose their experience of mental health problems, or to acknowledge the role mental illness may have played in the death of colleagues (Channel 4, 2012). Whether these approaches have a favourable effect on male suicide rates is yet to be demonstrated (Goyne, 2018). The experience from public awareness campaigns in other contexts has not been encouraging for males. For example, public awareness campaigns have been successful in improving the detection of breast cancer in women (O'Mahony et al., 2017; Soomro, 2017) but not prostate cancer in men (Thomsen et al., 2016).

Young men are less likely than women to engage with support services, but such services are also less likely to engage with young men. This could be because men tend to show their distress through aggression, intoxication, or avoidance, which engender neither sympathy nor a desire to help. A study of 1305 consecutive referrals to a psychiatric emergency service in the USA found men were hospitalized at a lower rate than women (OR 0.70, 95%CI 0.53 to 0.93). In the same study, use of restraint in the emergency service was associated with a lower likelihood of hospitalization (OR 0.35, 95% CI 0.22 to 0.55), as was intoxication with alcohol (OR 0.76, 95% CI 0.58 to 0.99) or amphetamine (OR 0.50, 95% CI 0.34 to 0.72). These authors attributed the latter findings to short-term problems that resolve in the emergency

department (ED) with medication or brief respite, but one wonders whether there was a missed opportunity to identify and address enduring problems such as depression. When depressive symptoms *have* been identified, analysis of a nationally representative dataset of ED presentations from the USA found men were *more* likely than women to be hospitalized (OR 1.22, 95% CI 1.04 to 1.43) (Rost et al., 2011). A consensus conference has canvassed the possibility of gender-specific approaches to the screening and management of mental health problems in the ED, but the ideas have yet to be developed (Ranney et al., 2014). Issues for further consideration include whether gender specific factors should influence:

- risk stratification and hospitalization decisions, in general, and for suicide risk in particular
- the approach to lethal means restriction
- the likelihood of outpatient follow-up and ED recidivism, and
- the tailoring of within-ED interventions to increase compliance with recommended treatment regimens

In terms of treatment for depression, the lower response rate to antidepressant medication in males compared to females, in conjunction with pharmacokinetic data, suggests that recommended doses for males should be adjusted upward. Prescriber education and psycho-education for the patient should address gender-specific side effects such as erectile dysfunction and ejaculatory delay.

Empirically informed psychological therapies tailored to men in terms of content and mode of delivery are needed (Seidler et al., 2018). Such therapies could usefully borrow from Dialectical Behaviour Therapy and include strategies for managing therapy-interfering behaviours.

Gender differences in internet search behaviour (Chandler, 2018) corroborate the idea that the internet could be a way to overcome inhibition of emotional expressiveness for males facing issues related with depression. There is also an opportunity to redirect men who search suicide on the internet to online support services.

Face-to-face psychological treatment could also be modified to facilitate the engagement of male patients. There is an assumption that owing to its pragmatic and structured approach, CBT should suit males (Spendelow, 2015) but evidence already presented in this chapter contradicts that view. It is not often acknowledged, but most psychotherapists are female and have recently graduated from clinical masters' programmes (American Psychological Association, 2017; Diamond, 2011). For some young men this may be a barrier to engagement (Diamond, 2011). Another therapist, or another therapy, may be a better fit. Spendelow (2015) reviewed strategies recommended by others to facilitate psychological therapies with men, especially those who hold traditional masculinized attitudes. These suggestions include those shown in Box 11.4.

The final recommendation (make the physical treatment environment 'male friendly' by, for example, supplying newspapers) might be updated to 'provide access to Wi-Fi in the waiting area'.

Conclusions

In HIC, more young males than females die from suicide, and they demonstrate greater intent when they attempt suicide. Gender differences are less marked in LMIC. Male characteristics such as aggression, a greater propensity to fixate on some issues while dismissing others, a reluctance to seek help and a poorer response to certain mental health interventions may contribute to vulnerability to suicide, but it is hard to see why such factors would be less operative for males living in LMIC than in HIC. Males also have a higher rate of problematic alcohol use than females, but the difference is evident in both HIC and LMIC (Rehm, 2006). An alternative possibility is that factors that protect against suicide among females in HIC are less operative in LMIC. Such factors may include access to high-quality health and

> **Box 11.4** Strategies to facilitate psychological therapies in men (Spendelow, 2015)
> - normalize ambivalence about therapy and acknowledge differences between psychotherapy and masculinity
> - emphasize collaboration or a 'power sharing' model of treatment including the use of regular therapist self-disclosure
> - use non-clinical language where possible (e.g., call sessions 'coaching' rather than therapy)
> - consider being physically active during sessions (e.g., getting out of chairs, walking around)
> - make the environment 'male friendly'

mental health care (including toxicology services in the event of poisoning), as well as income support for single mothers. Because they are more likely to use self-poisoning as a means of self-harm, young women are over-represented in hospital data. In the community gender differences in self-harm are less marked, and in some instances reversed.

Strategies to reduce the incidence of suicide and self-harm are – in most instances – less effective in men than women. The disparity is likely a result both of hard-wired differences and also the way in which men are socialized. Over and above generic prevention strategies, promising leads for lowering suicide rates in young men include gender-specific approaches to the assessment and management of mental health crises, and tailored psychological therapies that facilitate engagement and persistence with treatment. Restricting access to firearms continues to be an important public health strategy.

References

American Psychological Association. 2017. *Summary Report, Graduate Study in Psychology 2017: Student Demographics* [online]. American Psychological Association. Available at: www.apa.org/education/grad/survey-data/2017-student-demographics.aspx [Accessed 7 January 2019].

Australian Institute of Male Health and Studies. 2017. *National Guidelines for Male Suicide Prevention Program Design – 2017* [online]. Canberra: Australian Government. Available at: http://malesuicidepreventionaustralia.com.au/wp-content/uploads/2017/02/Guidelines_Program_Design_Jan2017.pdf [Accessed 27 December 2018].

Australian Institute of Male Health and Studies. 2018. *Deaths in Australia* [online]. Canberra: Australian Government. Available at: www.aihw.gov.au/reports/life-expectancy-death/deaths-in-australia/data [Accessed 6 December 2018].

Beautrais, A. L. 2000. Methods of youth suicide in New Zealand: trends and implications for prevention. *Aust N Z J Psychiatry*, 34, 413–19.

Bresin, K. and Schoenleber, M. 2015. Gender differences in the prevalence of nonsuicidal self-injury: A meta-analysis. *Clin Psychol Rev*, 38, 55–64.

Bridge, J. A., Goldstein, T. R., and Brent, D. A. 2006. Adolescent suicide and suicidal behavior. *J Child Psychol Psychiatry*, 47, 372–94.

Canstar. 2018. *Does life insurance cover suicide?* [online]. Available at: www.canstar.com.au/life-insurance/life-insurance-cover-suicide [Accessed 14 December 2018].

Cantor, C. and Neulinger, K. 2000. The epidemiology of suicide and attempted suicide among young

Australians. *Aust N Z J Psychiatry*, 34, 370–87.

Carter, G., Page, A., Large, M., Hetrick, S., Milner, A. J., Bendit, N., Walton, C., Draper, B., Hazell, P., Fortune, S., Burns, J., Patton, G., Lawrence, M., Dadd, L., Robinson, J., and Christensen, H. 2016. Royal Australian and New Zealand College of Psychiatrists clinical practice guideline for the management of deliberate self-harm. *Aust N Z J Psychiatry*, 50, 939–1000.

Centers for Disease Control and Prevention 2004. Methods of suicide among persons aged 10–19 years – United States, 1992–2001. *MMWR Morb Mortal Wkly Rep*, 53, 471–4.

Chandler, V. 2018. Google and suicides: what can we learn about the use of internet to prevent suicides? *Public Health*, 154, 144–50.

Channel 4. 2012. Rugby stars tackle mental health 'stigma' [online]. Available at: www.channel4.com/ news/rugby-super-league-final-mental-health [Accessed 27 December 2018].

Daily Mail. 2018. Football clubs join suicide prevention campaign [online]. Available at: www .dailymail.co.uk/wires/pa/article-5970435/Football-clubs-join-suicide-prevention-campaign.html [Accessed 27 December 2018].

Dhingra, K., Boduszek, D., and O'Connor, R. C. 2016. A structural test of the Integrated Motivational-Volitional model of suicidal behaviour. *Psychiatry Res*, 239, 169–78.

Diamond, S. A. 2011. *On the 'Feminization' of Psychotherapy: Does Your Therapist's Gender Really Matter? Does the Sex of Psychotherapists Really Matter?* [online]. Available at: www .psychologytoday.com/us/blog/evil-deeds/201105/the-feminization-psychotherapy-does-your-therapists-gender-really-matter [Accessed 7 January 2019].

Fliege, H., Lee, J. R., Grimm, A., and Klapp, B. F. 2009. Risk factors and correlates of deliberate self-harm behavior: a systematic review. *J Psychosom Res*, 66, 477–93.

Freeman, A., Mergl, R., Kohls, E., Szekely, A., Gusmao, R., Arensman, E., Koburger, N., Hegerl, U., and Rummel-Kluge, C. 2017. A cross-national study on gender differences in suicide intent. *BMC Psychiatry*, 17, 234.

Gontijo Guerra, S. and Vasiliadis, H. M. 2016. Gender differences in youth suicide and healthcare service use. *Crisis*, 37, 290–8.

Goyne, A. 2018. Suicide, Male Honour and the Masculinity Paradox: Its Impact on the ADF [online]. Canberra: Department of Defence. Available at: www.defence.gov.au/ adc/adfj/Documents/issue_203/ ADF%20Journal%20203_Article_ Goyne.pdf [Accessed 7 January 2019].

The Guardian. 2018. Why are men more likely than women to take their own lives? [online]. Available at: www.theguardian.com/science/ 2015/jan/21/suicide-gender-men-women-mental-health-nick-clegg [Accessed 20 December 2018].

Gunnell, D., Eddleston, M., Phillips, M. R., and Konradsen, F. 2007. The global distribution of fatal pesticide self-poisoning: systematic review. *BMC Public Health*, 7, 357.

Gunnell, D. and Nowers, M. 1997. Suicide by jumping. *Acta Psychiatr Scand*, 96, 1–6.

Hau, K. T. 1993. Suicide in Hong Kong 1971–1990: age trend, sex ratio, and method of suicide. *Soc Psychiatry Psychiatr Epidemiol*, 28, 23–7.

Hawton, K. 1998. Why has suicide increased in young males? *Crisis*, 19, 119–24.

2000. Sex and suicide. Gender differences in suicidal behaviour. *Br J Psychiatry*, 177, 484–5.

Hawton, K., Witt, K. G., Taylor Salisbury, T. L., Arensman, E., Gunnell, D., Hazell, P., Townsend,

E., and Van Heeringen, K. 2016. Psychosocial interventions for self-harm in adults. *Cochrane Database Syst Rev*, Cd012189.

Holter, O. G. 2002. A theory of gendercide. *J Genocide Res*, 4, 11–38.

Kõlves, K. and Yu, W. K. 2018. *Review of Suicide Clusters and Evidence-Based Prevention Strategies in School-Aged Children*. Brisbane, Australia: Australian Institute for Suicide Research and Prevention.

The Law Dictionary. 2018. What is suicide? [online]. Available at: https://thelawdictionary.org/suicide [Accessed 24 December 2018].

Madge, N., Hewitt, A., Hawton, K., De Wilde, E. J., Corcoran, P., Fekete, S., Van Heeringen, K., de Leo, D., and Ystgaard, M. 2008. Deliberate self-harm within an international community sample of young people: comparative findings from the Child and Adolescent Self-Harm in Europe (CASE) Study. *J Child Psychol Psychiatry*, 49, 667–77.

Marsh, W. K. 2010. Sex-related differences in antidepressant response: when to adjust treatment. *Current Psychiatry*, 9, 25–30.

Moller-Leimkuhler, A. M. 2002. Barriers to help-seeking by men: a review of sociocultural and clinical literature with particular reference to depression. *J Affect Disord*, 71, 1–9.

NHMRC Centre for Research Excellence in Suicide Prevention and Black Dog Institute. 2015. *Proposed Suicide Prevention Framework for NSW*. Sydney: Mental Health Commission of NSW.

O'Carroll, P. W., Mercy, J. A., and Steward, J. A. A. C. F. D. C. 1988. CDC recommendations for a community plan for the prevention and containment of suicide clusters. *Morb Mortal Wkly Rep*, 37(Suppl 6), 1–12.

O'Mahony, M., Comber, H., Fitzgerald, T., Corrigan, M. A., Fitzgerald, E.,

Grunfeld, E. A., Flynn, M. G. and Hegarty, J. 2017. Interventions for raising breast cancer awareness in women. *Cochrane Database Syst Rev*, 2, Cd011396.

Ogrodniczuk, J. S., Piper, W. E., Joyce, A. S., and McCallum, M. 2001. Effect of patient gender on outcome in two forms of short-term individual psychotherapy. *J Psychother Pract Res*, 10, 69–78.

Pieh, C., Altmeppen, J., Neumeier, S., Loew, T., Angerer, M., and Lahmann, C. 2012. Gender differences in response to CBT-orientated multimodal treatment in depressed patients with chronic pain. *Psychiatr Prax*, 39, 280–5.

Qin, P., Agerbo, E., Westergard-Nielsen, N., Eriksson, T., and Mortensen, P. B. 2000. Gender differences in risk factors for suicide in Denmark. *Br J Psychiatry*, 177, 546–50.

Ranney, M. L., Locci, N., Adams, E. J., Betz, M., Burmeister, D. B., Corbin, T., Dalawari, P., Jacoby, J. L., Linden, J., Purtle, J., North, C., and Houry, D. E. 2014. Gender-specific research on mental illness in the emergency department: current knowledge and future directions. *Acad Emerg Med*, 21, 1395–402.

Rehm, J., Chisholm, D., Room, R., Lopez, A. D. 2006. Alcohol [online]. Washington, DC: The International Bank for Reconstruction and Development / The World Bank. Available at: www.ncbi.nlm.nih.gov/books/NBK11720/ [Accessed 7 January 2019].

Rice, T. R. 2015. Violence among young men: the importance of a gender-specific developmental approach to adolescent male suicide

and homicide. *Int J Adolesc Med Health*, 27, 177–81.

Rihmer, Z., Rutz, W. and Pihlgren, H. 1995. Depression and suicide on Gotland. An intensive study of all suicides before and after a depression-training programme for general practitioners. *J Affect Disord*, 35, 147–52.

Ringland, E. 2017. Local AFL clubs come together to tackle high suicide rates [online]. Available at: www.suicidepreventioncollaborative.org.au/whats-happening-2/news/local-afl-clubs-come-together-to-tackle-high-suicide-rates [Accessed 27 December 2018].

Rost, K., Hsieh, Y. P., Xu, S., and Harman, J. 2011. Gender differences in hospitalization after emergency room visits for depressive symptoms. *J Womens Health (Larchmt)*, 20, 719–24.

Seidler, Z. E., Rice, S. M., Ogrodniczuk, J. S., and Oliffe, J. L. 2018. Engaging men in psychological treatment: a scoping review. *Am J Mens Health*, 12, 1882–900.

Soomro, R. 2017. Is breast cancer awareness campaign effective in Pakistan? *J Pak Med Assoc*, 67, 1070–3.

Spendelow, J. S. 2015. Cognitive-behavioral treatment of depression in men: tailoring treatment and directions for future research. *Am J Mens Health*, 9, 94–102.

Szekely, A., Konkoly Thege, B., Mergl, R., BIrkas, E., Rozsa, S., Purebl, G., and Hegerl, U. 2013. How to decrease suicide rates in both genders? An effectiveness study of a community-based intervention (EAAD). *PLoS One*, 8, e75081.

Taylor, A. K., Knipe, D. W., and Thomas, K. H. 2016. Railway suicide in England and Wales 2000–2013: a time–trends analysis. *BMC Public Health*, 16, 270.

Thomsen, F. B., Mikkelsen, M. K., Hansen, R. B., and Brasso, K. 2016. The Movember campaign: impact on referral patterns and diagnosis of prostate cancer. *Scand J Public Health*, 44, 228–32.

UK Government. 1961. *The Suicide Act* [online]. London: The National Archives. Available at: www.legislation.gov.uk/ukpga/Eliz2/9–10/60/section/3 [Accessed 20 December 2018].

Vandenbroucke, G. 2012. *On a Demographic Consequence of the First World War* [online]. Available at: https://voxeu.org/article/demographic-consequence-first-world-war [Accessed 6 December 2018].

WHO. 2014. *Preventing Suicide: A Global Imperative*. Geneva: World Health Organization.

Yang, X. and Feldman, M. W. 2017. A reversed gender pattern? A meta-analysis of gender differences in the prevalence of non-suicidal self-injurious behaviour among Chinese adolescents. *BMC Public Health*, 18, 66.

Young, E. A., Kornstein, S. G., Marcus, S. M., Harvey, A. T., Warden, D., Wisniewski, S. R., Balasubramani, G. K., Fava, M., Trivedi, M. H., and John Rush, A. 2009. Sex differences in response to citalopram: a STAR*D report. *J Psychiatr Res*, 43, 503–11.

Zahid, S. and UPthegrove, R. 2017. Suicidality in autistic spectrum disorders. *Crisis*, 38, 237–46.

Chapter

12

Depression

Guy Goodwin

Depression was famously described as a wimp of a word by William Styron. A Pulitzer-prize winning author, his own experience of depression was described in a memoir, *Darkness Visible*, about thirty years ago. It took a brave man to speak in public about mental illness at the time. Depression is a word that has 'slithered innocuously through our language like a slug, leaving little trace of its intrinsic malevolence, and preventing by its very insipidity, a general awareness of the horrible intensity of the illness when it is out of control' (Styron, 2010). Styron gave us a definitive account of a man enduring a severe depressive episode. It highlighted his own vulnerability by virtue of family history, the professional and personal disappointments that preceded its onset, and its excruciating and lengthy course and subsequent recovery. He illuminated the obvious link between the agony of depression and the impulse to commit suicide. It encapsulates, at the level of the individual, what severe depression is like for an intelligent, creative man. Systematic research at the population level largely confirms this individual experience. It also demonstrates modest differences from the rates and patterns of illness described in women.

When we refer to depression it is now usually conceptualized as a constellation of particular symptoms that persist over an interval of time. The more severe and numerous the symptoms and the longer the interval, the worse the functional consequences for the individual. 'Major depression' is defined as five or more of the symptoms shown in Box 12.1, persisting for at least two weeks. It is quite a low bar, but applied systematically it has allowed us to quantify the incidence, prevalence, and apparent aetiology of depressive episodes in large samples, and to compare males with females.

This construct defines a major depressive episode, which occurs in a life course that may be unipolar or bipolar. It derives from the approach to classification of psychiatric disorder that is now familiar from both

the traditions of the *Diagnostic and Statistical Manual* (DSM) of the American Psychiatric Association and the *International Classification of Diseases* (ICD) of the World Health Organization. The use of so-called operational criteria dates from DSM-III in 1980. Prior to that, descriptions of abnormal mental states were both more impressionistic and interwoven with interpretation. Thus, in DSM-II, the central formulation of psychiatric practice with outpatients was that symptoms were a manifestation of neurosis. On this view depression was an automatic and unconscious defence mechanism against 'anxiety'. Textbooks for psychiatrists, such as those of Mayer-Gross, Roth, and Slater, barely covered 'the neuroses'. Prior to DSM-III and the development of systematic interviews like the Present State Examination, reliable research into patient populations and the impact of treatments was effectively non-existent, especially for non-psychotic illness. Psychotic illnesses were somewhat

---

Box 12.1 DSM-5 criteria for a major depressive episode (APA, 2013)

There must be depressed mood or a loss of interest or pleasure in daily activities for more than two weeks. Specific symptoms, at least five of these nine, must be present nearly every day. There is impaired function: social, occupational, educational. All compared with a normal baseline and present for at least two weeks.

(1) depressed mood
(2) markedly diminished interest or pleasure
(3) significant weight loss
(4) insomnia or hypersomnia
(5) psychomotor agitation or retardation
(6) fatigue or loss of energy
(7) worthlessness or excessive/inappropriate guilt
(8) diminished ability to think or concentrate, or indecisiveness
(9) recurrent thoughts of death, suicidal ideation

better served by traditional diagnosis and less confused by psychodynamic interpretation.

Phenomenology and Symptom Patterns

A depressed individual complains of a range of subjective and objective difficulties. These changes from their customary mental and physical state are conventionally described as symptoms. As already described, the core items in a major depression episode (MDE) are low mood and lack of interest. Neither DSM or ICD systems have suggested a difference between men and women in their respective definitions of an episode of major depression, which implies no sex-specific symptoms or experience.

However, the major depressive disorder (MDD) construct is itself problematic. In the STAR-D study, of 3703 depressed outpatients there were 1030 unique symptom profiles, of which 83.9% were endorsed by five or fewer subjects. The most common symptom profile had a frequency of just 1.8% (Fried and Nesse, 2015). Efforts to identify latent classes of symptoms have also been disappointing (van Loo et al., 2012). Since these analyses have taken men and women with MDEs together, it is interesting that sex has not emerged as a data-driven correlate of any particular pattern.

However, modest sex differences have been described in large systematic studies that have compared the frequency of individual symptoms. For example, Smith and colleagues studied 199 males and 399 females with a history of MDD and characterized retrospectively their 'worst ever' episode (Smith et al., 2008). There were no significant differences between the sexes for agitated activity, weight gain, poor appetite, loss of energy/tiredness, poor concentration, early morning wakening, suicidal ideation, loss of pleasure, and dysphoria. However, females more frequently reported diminished libido, excessive sleep, diurnal variation of mood, and excessive self-reproach. Males reported 'initial insomnia' more frequently than females.

Direct comparison of symptom rates in another reasonably large sample of individuals with a *current* MDE also suggested minor differences between men and women; however, in nearly 1115 participants, almost all such differences were less than 10% (Schuch et al., 2014). Furthermore, these differences did not replicate the 'worst ever' pattern. The only clinically significant finding appeared to be 10% higher rates of weight gain and of a corresponding

diagnosis of atypical depression in women. Atypical depression was also present during the worst ever episode in 31.6% of females, compared to 21.1% of the males. It was identified when at least two of the three symptoms of excessive physical fatigue, overeating, and over-sleeping were present in the episode (Angst et al., 2006). The different rate of atypical depression profiles between the sexes is worth bearing in mind, modest though the difference is. The metabolic syndrome and inflammation are more related to the atypical depression subtype, whereas hypercortisolemia appears more specific for melancholic depression (Penninx et al., 2013). There is an emerging hypothesis (Uher et al., 2014) that this may eventually direct treatment choices but it remains to be established by prospective clinical trials.

In summary, the differences described above capture differences in average effects *between* sexes that are modest compared with the variation in presentations and outcome *within* either sex.

Neurobiology

The great variation in symptom patterns in depression cries out for some unifying approach to diagnosis based on underlying mechanisms. This has driven the development, by the US National Institute for Mental Health, of the approach know as RDoC or Research Domains Criteria. It assumes that underlying the variable symptom patterns of all psychiatric syndromes there may be more reliable biotypes. The details are beyond the scope of this chapter, but in the case of depression, biotypes have been proposed recently, based on functional magnetic resonance imaging (fMRI) in a large multisite sample ($n = 1188$) (Drysdale et al., 2017). Four biotypes were defined on the basis of distinct patterns of dysfunctional connectivity in limbic and frontostriatal networks. They were associated with differing clinical-symptom profiles and predicted responsiveness to transcranial magnetic stimulation therapy in a small subset. While this study illustrates the principle, there has already been a failure of independent replication (Dinga et al., 2019), hence theory so far runs ahead of practice.

It follows that in the absence of qualitative differences in clinical presentation, possible neurobiological underpinning of any difference between the sexes is equally not yet understood. Animal studies suggest that there may be differential regulation of appetite, sex, and stress response between males and females (Bale and Epperson, 2015). This implies inter-actions, during maturation, between the hypothalamic–pituitary–adrenal (HPA) axis, poster-ior pituitary hormones, gonadal steroids, monoa-mines, and gamma-aminobutyric acid (GABA) transmission. These rich possibilities are poorly matched by the clinical data. Most studies of neuro-biology in MDD per se do not usually even distin-guish between males and females and no differences have been reliably described. The issue of declining testosterone with increasing age in males will be con-sidered below, and is also addressed in Chapter 23.

The Incidence and Prevalence of MDD in Men and Women

It is widely accepted that men are less likely to develop a major depressive episode than women. This differ-ence is consistently described in both clinical and com-munity samples and it is substantial. A representative US study – the National Co-morbidity Survey Replication or NCS-R (Kessler et al., 2005) – surveyed over 9000 English-speaking respondents, and quanti-fied the lifetime risk of 'any mood disorder' to be 1.5 times higher for women. The difference is not seen for bipolar disorder (see Chapter 14). These findings have been essentially repeated in other community samples (Table 12.1) and may be even more discrepant in clinical samples.

There is a sense that carving out an entity like MDD creates a distinct category that is artificial. It may fail to take account of co-morbidity and the obvious overlaps with anxiety disorders, which could increase rates of diagnosis in women (see Chapter 9). Additionally, diagnoses heavily weighted to male chil-dren and adolescents (ADHD, autism, conduct dis-order) may somehow take precedence and reduce the detection of co-morbid depression (see Chapters 2 and 3). However, given that the broad similarities between the depressive syndrome in men and women are more striking than the differences, community-based interview studies using operational criteria should give fair estimates of incidence and prevalence. Therefore, it is unlikely that lower depression rates in men are an artifact of DSM-driven methodology. Other explanations that are offered are based on a different interpretation of what depression is in men; behavioural and impulse control disorders (indeed, general psychopathology) are more common in

men, and could be some kind of depressive equiva-lent. This looks increasingly improbable as one absorbs the family and twin studies to be described below. An explanation for lower male rates in com-munity samples must be sought in the aetiology of major depressive disorder.

The Aetiology of Major Depression

The earliest studies of the origins of major depression in the community were conducted in women by George Brown and Tirrell Harris (Brown and Harris, 1986). Their model of depression conjectured that there exist 'vulnerability factors', notably early mater-nal loss, lack of a confiding relationship, greater than three children under the age of 14 at home, and unemployment, which increase the risk for depression. The timing of the onset of depressive episodes can be accounted for by the occurrence of what they described as independent life events – losses, disappointments – that provoke the episode. This formulation has proved very influential. It has had a primary purpose (to explain the aetiology of depression scientifically) and a secondary purpose in that it helps individual patients to understand their predicament and why it has arisen. The major limitation of the original observations was the failure to control for (or even consider) genetic factors. Much work in the social sciences still does not do so. It also, obviously, omitted to study men.

Nevertheless, this way of thinking about the causes of depression has proved fruitful from a heuristic perspective, not least for understanding depression in men. It has benefitted immeasurably from combin-ing simple observational and historical data, as estab-lished by Brown and Harris, with genetically informative designs. In particular it has been founded on large studies of twins led by Kenneth Kendler. Such studies depend on the fact that monozygotic or identical twins have essentially identical genetic inher-itance, while dizygotic twins share 50% of each other's genes. Twins share a common environment in utero and usually after birth. Therefore, they provide ideal comparison groups for teasing out what appear to be genetic from environmental causes in any disorder. In general, the greater the difference between monozy-gotic and dizygotic outcomes, the more likely a gen-etic explanation becomes. Such explanations have been unwelcome to some ways of thinking about psychiatric problems and human behaviour more generally. Hence, twin studies have been regularly

Table 12.1 Gender ratios for depressive disorders. Table taken from a review (Kuehner, 2017)*

	Location	Age (years)	Number of participants	Diagnostic criterion	Gender ratio (women:men)
Lifetime prevalence					
WMHS: Seedat et al.[10]	worldwide	..	73,000	DSM-IV major depressive disorder	1:9
WMHS: Seedat et al.[10]	worldwide	..	73,000	DSM-IV dysthymia	1:9
WMHS: Bromet et al.[12] (89,000 participants worldwide)	high-income countries	≥18	..	DSM-IV major depressive disorder	1:8
WMHS: Bromet et al.[12] (89,000 participants worldwide)	low-income and middle-income countries	≥18	..	DSM-IV major depressive disorder	2:1
NESARC: Hasin et al.[12]	USA	≥18	43000	DSM-IV major depressive disorder	2:0
NCS-R: Kessler et al.[13]	USA	≥18	9000	DSM-IV major depressive disorder	1:7
NEMESIS: de Graaf et al.[14]	Netherlands	18–64	7000	DSM-IV major depressive disorder	2:1
NEMESIS: de Graaf et al.[14]	Netherlands	18–64	7000	DSM-IV dysthymia	3:4
12-month prevalence					
EBC/ECNP study: Wittchen et al.[15] (25 studies)	Europe	≥14	..	DSM-IV major depressive disorder	2:3
NESARC: Hasin et al.[12]	USA	≥18	43,000	DSM-IV major depressive disorder	2:0
NCS-R: Kessler et al.[13]	USA	≥18	9000	DSM-IV major depressive disorder	1:4
DEGS1-MH: Jacobi et al.[15]	Germany	18–74	5300	DSM-IV major depressive disorder	2:5
DEGS1-MH: Jacobi et al.[15]	Germany	18–74	5300	DSM-IV dysthymia	1:9

Odds ratios for major depressive disorder and dysthymia in epidemiological studies of adults since 2003. WMHS = WHO. World Mental Health Survey. DSM-IV = *Diagnostic and Statistical Manual of Mental Disorders*, 4th ed. NESARC = National Epidemiologic Survey on Alcohol and Related Conditions. NCS-R = National Comorbidity Survey Replication. NEMESIS = Netherlands Mental Health Survey and Incidence Study. EBC = European Brain Council. ECNP = European College of Neuropsychopharmacology. DEGS1 MH = German Health Interview and Examination Survey for Adults.
The superscripted numbers are references in the original paper.
* For individual studies refer to references in this review.

criticized as being somehow fatally flawed, usually on spurious grounds. They are now supported by increasingly large molecular genetic studies where the direction of causation cannot be contested and the results are statistically beyond dispute. There are no examples yet where the heritability conclusions from twin studies have not been supported by genome wide association (GWA) studies. In a real sense this helps retrospectively to reinforce confidence in the aetiological findings of studies in twins.

A major US twin study of 3790 complete male–male, female–female, and male–female twin pairs, showed that a lifetime diagnosis of MDD is equally heritable in men and women (heritability 39%), and most genetic risk factors influenced liability to MDD similarly in both sexes (Kendler and Prescott, 1999). The question was subsequently revisited in a much larger sample of 42,161 twins (15,493 complete pairs) in the national Swedish Twin Registry (Kendler et al., 2006b). The heritability of liability to major depression turned out to be similar to the earlier study for women (42%) but lower for men (29%). Modelling suggested that some genetic risk factors for major depression are sex-specific in their effect, but there was no evidence that genetic and environmental risk factors in major depression had changed in birth cohorts spanning nearly six decades.

A fine-grained model of the developmental pathways to major depression in men has been derived from a detailed study of 2935 adult male twins, interviewed twice over a 2–4-year period (Kendler et al., 2006a). It was possible to predict a depressive episode over 1 year follow up from a range of risk factors. The overall model explained about 50% of the risk and was similar to that derived for women in a previous study. Childhood parental loss and low self-esteem emerged as more potent variables in men compared with women. Genetic risks exerted a broader range of interactions in men than in women. Externalizing symptoms did not provide a more prominent pathway to MDD in men than in women, as had previously been suggested.

Personality and Individual Differences

Old-style psychodynamic formulations of neurosis confounded personality and illness episodes. DSM-III proposed a separate axis for personality disorder. Thus an illness like MDD was said to be an Axis I problem while an abnormal personality should be thought of as an independent (Axis II) variable. In the models of psychopathology generated from twin studies, individual differences in personality are measured as continuous variables, rather than disorders, and they contribute to the risk of depression. Trait neuroticism, in particular, appears to mediate the impact of adverse life events on the risk for a depressive episode in both men and women. This is elegantly demonstrated in Figure 12.1. This shows that a given level of neuroticism interacts with an increasing burden of adversity to increase the risk of a depressive episode. The overall pattern is again similar in both sexes, but the impact of minor stresses may be slightly lower in men than in women.

Mean levels of neuroticism tend to be lower in men and trait extraversion higher. These differences

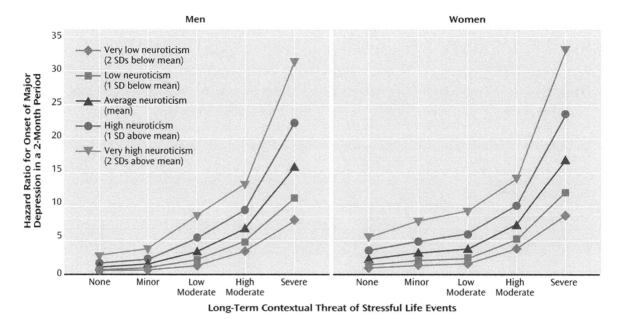

Figure 12.1 The interaction between vulnerability and adversity in men and women (Kendler et al., 2004)

provide an obvious starting point for thinking about gender differences in aetiology. Evolutionary theorists have suggested that neuroticism represents an optimized trait (Allen and Badcock, 2006). Heightened reactivity to negative outcomes may have had a survival benefit in a hostile and unpredictable environment. It may therefore have been selected up to the point where the disadvantages outweigh the advantages (Nettle, 2004). The different biological and social roles of males and females in evolution may have determined different optimal levels for the sexes. Certainly the first genetic locus showing variation that correlated with 'neuroticism' in mice was also the first identified in the human population (Fullerton et al., 2003). The consequence is that women have on average moderately higher N (neuroticism) than men. However, they will clearly be increasingly over-represented at extreme and disadvantageous levels of neuroticism compared with males. This probably explains much of the difference in rates of depression between men and women. It is reinforced by the increasing realization that life events are also often a consequence of personality-driven choices and so in a sense have a genetic component (Jeronimus et al., 2014).

Maintenance of MDD

Recurrence rates and the impact of risk factors in recurrent MDD have also been examined in a modest sized subset of the Virginia twin population (van Loo et al., 2018). The patterns for men and women were similar. Co-morbid anxiety, early traumas, and family history were associated with a higher probability for relapse in both sexes. Any gender differences were subtle and the study was not powered to be definitive. In men, risk factors related to early and recent adverse life events and socioeconomic problems appeared to be less important than for women. In both sexes, later recurrences in the illness course appeared to be associated with weaker or no-provoking life events. This effect has been likened metaphorically to 'priming' in the illness course of epilepsy (Kendler et al., 2000). Other longitudinal studies of remission, recurrence, or a chronic course of depression have failed to show differences between males and females (Kuehner, 2017).

The incidence of completed suicide at all ages is higher in men than in women in most regions and countries (Bertolote and Fleischmann, 2002; and see

Chapter 11). Correspondingly, the excess mortality in depressed individuals compared with the general population is clearly higher among men than women (Cuijpers et al., 2014). In Denmark, this excess mortality for patients diagnosed by a psychiatrist (hence referred to and treated in secondary rather than primary care) translated into a reduced life expectancy of 14.0 years in men and 10.1 years in women (calculating from age 15) (Laursen et al., 2016). The increased mortality was highest for death due to suicide and accidents but the absolute number of deaths was highest for natural causes. Poor physical health and failure to seek treatment will have contributed to this observation. It is further evidence that current interventions for depression in men leave much to be desired. For a discussion on suicide in young men, the reader is referred to Chapter 11.

Molecular Genetics

Variation in the human genome is essentially present from conception. Accordingly, any association between genetic variation and human behaviour or illness must be unidirectional. While twin studies have seemed to require a genetic explanation (as already described), study of phenotypes always carries some risk of reverse causation. The idea that social causes are primary in determining human behaviour has been and remains politically attractive to a left-leaning academia in the social sciences and humanities. The early molecular genetic studies of psychiatric disorders fuelled scepticism because they were underpowered and generated a disconcerting number of false positives. This has changed dramatically since the first definitive study of schizophrenia, published in 2014, which demonstrated over 100 single nucleotide polymorphisms (SNPs) significantly associated with a DSM-IV diagnosis (Schizophrenia Working Group of the Psychiatric Genomics Consortium, 2014). The Cross-Disorder Group of the Psychiatric Genomics Consortium estimated SNP-based heritability of MDD at approximately 21% (Cross-Disorder Group of the Psychiatric Genomics et al., 2013). An identical figure for genome-wide common variants was derived from another study of Han Chinese women (Peterson et al., 2017). Moreover, there is evidence for overlap between SNPs associated with neuroticism and MDD (Genetics of Personality et al., 2015). Finally, neuroticism itself has been shown to be reliably associated with over 100 genetic variants

(Nagel et al., 2018). Definitive findings on the molecular pathways underlying the key developmental variables and whether there are important biological differences will soon be available. The most interesting questions may be how far Gene x Environment interaction will be comprehensible.

In summary, there have been reliable comparisons between the aetiological pathways to MDD in men and women. We can now be confident that they are underpinned by genetically determined risks. No important differences between men and women have yet emerged, but the increasing precision of our understanding suggests we may yet find we can explain the modest differences that do appear to exist, from twin studies.

Response to Treatment

Medication

Successful treatment implies choice of a particular drug at a particular dose. Whether sex should guide choice remains an open question. It is perhaps also deceptively easier to ask than to answer because it is complicated by age, menopausal status in women, and drug tolerability. There are currently no clear guideline recommendations favouring a particular strategy for women over men. In the recent update of the BAP guidelines for the treatment of depression, sex was barely discussed in first-stage treatment options (Cleare et al., 2015). The largest study to examine the response in MDD to a single antidepressant (citalopram) was STAR-D (Trivedi et al., 2006; Young et al., 2009). Male sex was associated with a 5% lower remission rate (24.1%) than female (29.4%). This effect was much less than that seen with large differences in education and insurance status. In a similar systematic study, the negative effects of early (4–7y) abuse and neglect were also much more profound (a near 70% difference in favourable outcome) (Williams et al., 2016).

Testosterone and the Ageing Male

Testosterone is the principal androgen in men and is essential for the development and maintenance of secondary male characteristics. It is broadly accepted that when testosterone levels decrease, patients can experience physical and psychological effects, which can compromise their general well-being, sexuality, and fertility (Hackett et al., 2017).

Testosterone levels fall with age and the rate of fall is highly variable. It was observed twenty years ago that there was an apparent relationship between mood and hormone level (Barrett-Connor et al., 1999). In 856 men, aged 50–89 years, self-reported depressed mood was significantly and inversely associated with bioavailable testosterone and dihydrotestosterone, independent of age, weight change, and physical activity. Bioavailable testosterone levels were 17% lower for the twenty-five men with categorically defined depression than levels observed in all other men. It was reasonably suggested that treatment with testosterone might improve depressed mood in older men who have low levels of bioavailable testosterone. Subsequent trials in patients with depression have tended to be small scale. A systematic review ten years ago of seven trials of testosterone treatment for a current episode of MDD concluded that it may have an antidepressant effect in depressed patients, especially those with hypogonadism or HIV/AIDS and elderly subpopulations. Thus, overall response rate in testosterone treated patients was 54%, compared with placebo at 33%. The route by which testosterone is administered may play a role in treatment response because the gel formulation appeared to be superior to intra-muscular (Zarrouf et al., 2009).

A larger number of studies are now available that have looked at the impact of testosterone replacement in hypogonadal men more generally: outcomes were more related to well-being than major depression per se (Elliott et al., 2017). The findings suggest a class effect of testosterone administration in improving quality of life, depressive symptoms, erectile function, and libido, with no statistically significant increase in the risk of adverse reactions or events (although most studies have been short term). The use of testosterone in older men appears to have increased dramatically in recent years apparently as a 'hormone replacement therapy' that was assumed to carry few risks. In the USA, it tripled between 2001 and 2011. The US Food and Drug Administration (FDA) then issued a safety bulletin on January 31, 2014, following reports of a possible association between testosterone therapy and the risk of myocardial infarction and stroke. Since then the use of testosterone and the incidence of new use has fallen dramatically. At its peak in 2013, about 3% of men over 30 years were being prescribed testosterone by their physicians (Baillargeon et al., 2018).

As things stand, the BAP guideline on treating depressive disorders with antidepressants recommended that testosterone should be considered as a next-step option after antidepressant treatment has failed in hypogonadal men (Cleare et al., 2015). It is questionable how often this option is even considered by psychiatrists in many countries.

A recent practice guideline provides a useful update on the challenge of testosterone deficiency (TD) (Hackett et al., 2017). For psychiatrists, it is important to recognize that the commonest form in men older than 50 years, so-called secondary TD, is often co-morbid with obesity and metabolic syndrome. Oral glucocorticoids, opioids, and dopamine antagonists can also suppress testosterone levels.

For a further discussion on testosterone in older men, the reader is referred to Chapter 23.

Psychological Treatment

Evidence-based psychological treatments for an episode of major depression include cognitive behaviour therapy (CBT), behavioural activation, and inter-personal psychotherapy. In general, these approaches are more appropriate for patients with less severe depression, who are able to concentrate and remember to change behaviour as the psychotherapy directs. Guidelines (e.g. www.nice.org .uk/guidance/gid-cgwave0725/documents/short-version-of-draft-guideline) do not make different recommendations for men and women. Prevention of relapse may be facilitated by a CBT or a mindfulness-based approach.

'Male Depression'

There has been speculation that the lower rates of MDD in men are due to a failure to capture male depression and that the elevated rates of alcohol/substance misuse, violence, and suicide are actually evidence in favour of undiagnosed and untreated depression. According to this view, women may 'act in' because they are more likely to express their feeling and focus on their own inadequacies, while men 'act out'. Thus, depression in men may be expressed through anger and self-destructiveness (Kilmartin,

2005). This view harks back to a pre-DSM form of diagnosis by interpretation. It obviously also ignores the fact that the core symptoms of MDD (its phenomenology) in men are very similar to MDD in women, and so is the heritability.

There may be cultural and personal attitudes and preferences that inhibit men from seeking help. In one focus group study of men with a history of depression (Rochlen et al., 2010), three main themes emerged. First, men felt at odds with their experiences of depression and beliefs about appropriate ways to seek help. Second, men outlined alternative symptom profiles that could interfere with the recognition of depression and willingness to seek help. Finally, men expressed a range of positive and negative reactions toward depression treatment and treatment providers.

Conclusions

Men and women get depressed in the same way and broadly through the same mechanisms of vulnerability and incident life events. Treatments are similar, as are short-term outcomes. Major depression is an illness and it compounds other causes of chronic disability. A world health survey (Moussavi et al., 2007) concluded,

> Depression produces the greatest decrement in health compared with the chronic diseases angina, arthritis, asthma, and diabetes. The co-morbid state of depression incrementally worsens health compared with depression alone, with any of the chronic diseases alone, and with any combination of chronic diseases without depression. These results indicate the urgency of addressing depression as a public-health priority to reduce disease burden and disability, and to improve the overall health of populations.

Men generally enjoy worse physical health than women. The important interactions between physical ill-health and depressive illness particularly disadvantage men and disproportionately shorten their lives. Men are also more likely than women to take their own lives. Improving research and the effective treatment of major depression remains a neglected problem worldwide.

References

Allen, N. B. and Badcock, P. B. 2006. Darwinian models of depression: a review of evolutionary accounts of mood and mood disorders. *Prog*

Neuropsychopharmacol Biol Psychiatry, 30, 815–26.

Angst, J., Gamma, A., Benazzi, F., Silverstein, B., Ajdacic-Gross, V., Eich, D., and Rossler, W. 2006. Atypical depressive syndromes in

varying definitions. *Eur Arch Psychiatry Clin Neurosci*, 256, 44–54.

Baillargeon, J., Kuo, Y. F., Westra, J. R., Urban, R. J., and Goodwin, J. S. 2018. Testosterone prescribing in the United States, 2002–2016. *JAMA*, 320, 200–2.

Bale, T. L. and Epperson, C. N. 2015. Sex differences and stress across the lifespan. *Nature Neuroscience*, 18 (10), 1413–20.

Barrett-Connor, E., Von Muhlen, D. G., and Kritz-Silverstein, D. 1999. Bioavailable testosterone and depressed mood in older men: the Rancho Bernardo Study. *J Clin Endocrinol Metab*, 84, 573–7.

Bertolote, J. M. and Fleischmann, A. 2002. Suicide and psychiatric diagnosis: a worldwide perspective. *World Psychiatry*, 1, 181–5.

Brown, G. W. and Harris, T. 1986. Stressor, vulnerability and depression: a question of replication. *Psychol Med*, 16, 739–44.

Cleare, A., Pariante, C. M., Young, A. H., Anderson, I. M., Christmas, D., COWEN, P. J., Dickens, C., Ferrier, I. N., Geddes, J., Gilbody, S., Haddad, P. M., Katona, C., Lewis, G., Malizia, A., Mcallister-Williams, R. H., Ramchandani, P., Scott, J., Taylor, D., Uher, R., and Members of the Consensus, M. 2015. Evidence-based guidelines for treating depressive disorders with antidepressants: a revision of the 2008 British Association for Psychopharmacology guidelines. *J Psychopharmacol*, 29, 459–525.

Cross-Disorder Group of the Psychiatric Genomics, C., Lee, S. H., Ripke, S., Neale, B. M., Faraone, S. V., Purcell, S. M., Perlis, R. H., Mowry, B. J., Thapar, A., Goddard, M. E., Witte, J. S., Absher, D., AGartz, I., Akil, H., Amin, F., Andreassen, O. A., Anjorin, A., Anney, R., Anttila, V., Arking, D. E., Asherson, P., Azevedo, M. H., Backlund, L., Badner, J. A., Bailey, A. J., Banaschewski, T., BArchas, J. D., Barnes, M. R., Barrett, T. B., Bass, N., Battaglia, A., Bauer, M., Bayes, M., Bellivier, F., Bergen, S. E., Berrettini, W., Betancur, C., BEttecken, T., Biederman, J., Binder, E. B., Black, D. W.,

Blackwood, D. H., Bloss, C. S., Boehnke, M., Boomsma, D. I., Breen, G., Breuer, R., Bruggeman, R., Cormican, P., Buccola, N. G., Buitelaar, J. K., Bunney, W. E., Buxbaum, J. D., Byerley, W. F., Byrne, E. M., Caesar, S., Cahn, W., Cantor, R. M., Casas, M., Chakravarti, A., Chambert, K., Choudhury, K., Cichon, S., Cloninger, C. R., Collier, D. A., Cook, E. H., Coon, H., Cormand, B., Corvin, A., Coryell, W. H., Craig, D. W., Craig, I. W., Crosbie, J., Cuccaro, M. L., Curtis, D., Czamara, D., Datta, S., Dawson, G., Day, R., DE Geus, E. J., Degenhardt, F., Djurovic, S., Donohoe, G. J., Doyle, A. E., Duan, J., Dudbridge, F., Duketis, E., Ebstein, R. P., Edenberg, H. J., Elia, J., Ennis, S., Etain, B., Fanous, A., Farmer, A. E., Ferrier, I. N., Flickinger, M., Fombonne, E., Foroud, T., Frank, J., Franke, B., et al. 2013. Genetic relationship between five psychiatric disorders estimated from genome-wide SNPs. *Nat Genet*, 45, 984–94.

Cuijpers, P., Vogelzangs, N., Twisk, J., Kleiboer, A., Li, J., and Penninx, B. W. 2014. Is excess mortality higher in depressed men than in depressed women? A meta-analytic comparison. *J Affect Disord*, 161, 47–54.

Dinga, R., Schmaal, L., Penninx, B. W., van Tol, M. J., Veltman, D. J., van Velzen, L., Mennes, M., van der Wee, N. J., and Marquand, A. F. 2019. Evaluating the evidence for biotypes of depression: methodological replication and extension of Drysdale et al. (2017). *NeuroImage: Clinical*, 22, 101796.

Drysdale, A. T., Grosenick, L., Downar, J., Dunlop, K., Mansouri, F., Meng, Y., Fetcho, R. N., Zebley, B., Oathes, D. J., Etkin, A., Schatzberg, A. F., Sudheimer, K., Keller, J., Mayberg, H. S., Gunning, F. M., Alexopoulos, G. S., Fox M. D., Pascual-Leone, A., Voss, H. U., Casey, B. J., Dubin, M. J., and Liston, C. 2017. Resting-state connectivity biomarkers define

neurophysiological subtypes of depression. *Nat Med*, 23, 28–38.

Elliott, J., Kelly, S. E., Millar, A. C., Peterson, J., Chen, L., Johnston, A., Kotb, A., Skidmore, B., Bai, Z., Mamdani, M., and Wells, G. A. 2017. Testosterone therapy in hypogonadal men: a systematic review and network meta-analysis. *BMJ Open*, 7, e015284.

Fried, E. I. and Nesse, R. M. 2015. Depression is not a consistent syndrome: an investigation of unique symptom patterns in the STAR*D study. *J Affect Disord*, 172, 96–102.

Fullerton, J., Cubin, M., TiwarI, H., Wang, C., Bomhra, A., Davidson, S., Miller, S., Fairburn, C., Goodwin, G., Neale, M. C., Fiddy, S., Mott, R., Allison, D. B., and Flint, J. 2003. Linkage analysis of extremely discordant and concordant sibling pairs identifies quantitative-trait loci that influence variation in the human personality trait neuroticism. *Am J Hum Genet*, 72, 879–90.

Genetics of Personality, De Moor, M. H., Van Den Berg, S. M., Verweij, K. J., Krueger, R. F., Luciano, M., Arias Vasquez, A., Matteson, L. K., Derringer, J., Esko, T., Amin, N., Gordon, S. D., Hansell, N. K., Hart, A. B., Seppala, I., Huffman, J. E., Konte, B., Lahti, J., Lee, M., Miller, M., Nutile, T., Tanaka, T., Teumer, A., Viktorin, A., Wedenoja, J., Abecasis, G. R., Adkins, D. E., Agrawal, A., Allik, J., Appel, K., Bigdeli, T. B., Busonero, F., Campbell, H., Costa, P. T., Davey Smith, G., Davies, G., De Wit, H., Ding, J., Engelhardt, B. E., Eriksson, J. G., Fedko, I. O., Ferrucci, L., Franke, B., Giegling, I., Grucza, R., Hartmann, A. M., Heath, A. C., Heinonen, K., Henders, A. K., Homuth, G., Hottenga, J. J., Iacono, W. G., Janzing, J., Jokela, M., Karlsson, R., Kemp, J. P., Kirkpatrick, M. G., Latvala, A., Lehtimaki, T., Liewald, D. C., Madden, P. A., Magri, C., Magnusson, P. K., Marten, J.,

Maschio, A., Medland, S. E., Mihailov, E., Milaneschi, Y., Montgomery, G. W., Nauck, M., Ouwens, K. G., Palotie, A., Pettersson, E., Polasek, O., Qian, Y., Pulkki-Raback, L., Raitakari, O. T., Realo, A., Rose, R. J., Ruggiero, D., Schmidt, C. O., Slutske, W. S., Sorice, R., Starr, J. M., St Pourcain, B., Sutin, A. R., Timpson, N. J., Trochet, H., Vermeulen, S., Vuoksimaa, E., Widen, E., Wouda, J., Wright, M. J., Zgaga, L., Porteous, D., Minelli, A., Palmer, A. A., Rujescu, D., Ciullo, M., Hayward, C., et al. 2015. Meta-analysis of Genome-wide Association Studies for Neuroticism, and the Polygenic Association with Major Depressive Disorder. *JAMA Psychiatry*, 72, 642–50.

Hackett, G., Kirby, M., Edwards, D., Jones, T. H., Wylie, K., Ossei-Gerning, N., David, J., and Muneer, A. 2017. British Society for Sexual Medicine Guidelines on adult testosterone deficiency, with statements for UK practice. *J Sex Med*, 14, 1504–23.

Jeronimus, B. F., Riese, H., Sanderman, R., and Ormel, J. 2014. Mutual reinforcement between neuroticism and life experiences: a five-wave, 16-year study to test reciprocal causation. *J Pers Soc Psychol*, 107, 751–64.

Kendler, K. S., Gardner, C. O., and Prescott, C. A. 2006a. Toward a comprehensive developmental model for major depression in men. *Am J Psychiatry*, 163, 115–24.

Kendler, K. S., Gatz, M., Gardner, C. O., and Pedersen, N. L. 2006b. A Swedish national twin study of lifetime major depression. *Am J Psychiatry*, 163, 109–14.

Kendler, K. S., Kuhn, J., and Prescott, C. A. 2004. The interrelationship of neuroticism, sex, and stressful life events in the prediction of episodes of major depression. *Am J Psychiatry*, 161, 631–6.

Kendler, K. S. and Prescott, C. A. 1999. A population-based twin study of lifetime major depression in men and women. *Arch Gen Psychiatry*, 56, 39–44.

Kendler, K. S., Thornton, L. M., and Gardner, C. O. 2000. Stressful life events and previous episodes in the etiology of major depression in women: an evaluation of the 'kindling' hypothesis. *Am J Psychiatry*, 157, 1243–51.

Kessler, R. C., Berglund, P., Demler, O., Jin, R., Merikangas, K. R., and Walters, E. E. 2005. Lifetime prevalence and age-of-onset distributions of DSM-IV disorders in the National Comorbidity Survey Replication. *Arch Gen Psychiatry*, 62, 593–602.

Kilmartin, C. 2005. Depression in men: communication, diagnosis and therapy. *The Journal of Men's Health and Gender*, 2, 95–99.

Kuehner, C. 2017. Why is depression more common among women than among men? *Lancet Psychiatry*, 4, 146–58.

Laursen, T. M., Musliner, K. L., Benros, M. E., Vestergaard, M., and Munk-Olsen, T. 2016. Mortality and life expectancy in persons with severe unipolar depression. *J Affect Disord*, 193, 203–7.

Moussavi, S., Chatterji, S., Verdes, E., Tandon, A., Patel, V., and Ustun, B. 2007. Depression, chronic diseases, and decrements in health: results from the World Health Surveys. *Lancet*, 370, 851–8.

Nagel, M., Jansen, P. R., StringeR, S., Watanabe, K., De Leeuw, C. A., Bryois, J., Savage, J. E., Hammerschlag, A. R., Skene, N. G., Munoz-Manchado, A. B., Andme Research, T., White, T., Tiemeier, H., Linnarsson, S., Hjerling-Leffler, J., Polderman, T. J. C., Sullivan, P. F., Van Der Sluis, S., and Posthuma, D. 2018. Meta-analysis of Genome-wide Association Studies for neuroticism in 449,484 individuals identifies novel genetic loci and pathways. *Nat Genet*, 50, 920–7.

Nettle, D. 2004. Evolutionary origins of depression: a review and reformulation. *J Affect Disord*, 81, 91–102.

Penninx, B. W., Milaneschi, Y., Lamers, F., and Vogelzangs, N. 2013. Understanding the somatic consequences of depression: biological mechanisms and the role of depression symptom profile. *BMC Med*, 11, 129.

Peterson, R. E., Cai, N., Bigdeli, T. B., Li, Y., Reimers, M., Nikulova, A., Webb, B. T., Bacanu, S. A., Riley, B. P., Flint, J., and Kendler, K. S. 2017. The genetic architecture of major depressive disorder in Han Chinese women. *JAMA Psychiatry*, 74, 162–8.

Rochlen, A. B., Paterniti, D. A., Epstein, R. M., Duberstein, P., Willeford, L., and Kravitz, R. L. 2010. Barriers in diagnosing and treating men with depression: a focus group report. *Am J Mens Health*, 4, 167–75.

Schizophrenia Working Group of the Psychiatric Genomics Consortium. 2014. Biological insights from 108 schizophrenia-associated genetic loci. *Nature*, 511, 421–7.

Schuch, J. J., Roest, A. M., Nolen, W. A., Penninx, B. W., and De Jonge, P. 2014. Gender differences in major depressive disorder: results from the Netherlands study of depression and anxiety. *J Affect Disord*, 156, 156–63.

Smith, D. J., Kyle, S., Forty, L., Cooper, C., Walters, J., Russell, E., Caesar, S., Farmer, A., Mcguffin, P., Jones, I., Jones, L., and Craddock, N. 2008. Differences in depressive symptom profile between males and females. *J Affect Disord*, 108, 279–84.

Styron, W. 2010. *Darkness Visible: A Memoir of Madness*. New York: Open Road Media.

Trivedi, M. H., Rush, A. J., Wisniewski, S. R., Nierenberg, A. A., Warden, D., Ritz, L., Norquist, G., Howland, R. H., Lebowitz, B., Mcgrath, P. J., Shores-Wilson, K., Biggs, M. M., Balasubramani, G. K., Fava, M., and

Team, S. D. S. 2006. Evaluation of outcomes with citalopram for depression using measurement-based care in STAR*D: implications for clinical practice. *Am J Psychiatry*, 163, 28–40.

Uher, R., Tansey, K. E., Dew, T., Maier, W., Mors, O., Hauser, J., Dernovsek, M. Z., Henigsberg, N., Souery, D., Farmer, A., and Mcguffin, P. 2014. An inflammatory biomarker as a differential predictor of outcome of depression treatment with escitalopram and nortriptyline. *Am J Psychiatry*, 171, 1278–86.

Van Loo, H. M., Aggen, S. H., Gardner, C. O., and Kendler, K. S. 2018. Sex

similarities and differences in risk factors for recurrence of major depression. *Psychol Med*, 48, 1685–93.

Van Loo, H. M., De Jonge, P., Romeijn, J. W., Kessler, R. C., and Schoevers, R. A. 2012. Data-driven subtypes of major depressive disorder: a systematic review. *BMC Med*, 10, 156.

Williams, L. M., Debattista, C., Duchemin, A. M., Schatzberg, A. F., and Nemeroff, C. B. 2016. Childhood trauma predicts antidepressant response in adults with major depression: data from the randomized international study

to predict optimized treatment for depression. *Transl Psychiatry*, 6, e799.

Young, E. A., Kornstein, S. G., Marcus, S. M., Harvey, A. T., Warden, D., Wisniewski, S. R., BAlasubramani, G. K., Fava, M., Trivedi, M. H., and John Rush, A. 2009. Sex differences in response to citalopram: a STAR*D report. *J Psychiatr Res*, 43, 503–11.

Zarrouf, F. A., Artz, S., Griffith, J., Sirbu, C., and Kommor, M. 2009. Testosterone and depression: systematic review and meta-analysis. *J Psychiatr Pract*, 15, 289–305.

Chapter

13

Postnatal Depression in Men

Karen-Leigh Edward and Richard Fletcher

This chapter provides an overview of paternal postnatal depression (PPND). The chapter begins by defining the concept of PPND, situating the disorder in the context of clinical depression or major depressive disorder (MDD). Reference is made to the emergence of this previously considered *rare* disturbance to men's health. The potential risk factors for men in terms of PPND are highlighted in the bio-psycho-social domains. The impact of PPND for the family and the couple's relationship are discussed. Strategies for the prevention and management of PPND are presented, with specific details provided for active and passive approaches that clinicians can engage in when working with men who experience PPND.

The Concept of Paternal Postnatal Depression

Depression, otherwise known as clinical depression or major depressive disorder (MDD), is a serious mood disorder (see also Chapter 12). The US *Diagnostic and Statistical Manual of Mental Disorders* (DSM-5) (APA, 2013) stipulates that to meet criteria for MDD, the individual must experience five or more symptoms during the same two-week period (at least one of the symptoms being either a depressed mood or loss of interest/pleasure). Other symptoms include: weight loss, slowing down of thought and physical movement, fatigue, feelings of worthlessness, poor concentration, suicidal thoughts or recurrent thoughts of death. Depression is common and is identified as one of the top burdens of disease measured as Disability Adjusted Life Years (DALYs). In the past decade, depression has been identified in the top-ten causes of DALYs for both men and women between the ages of 15 and 44 years (WHO, 2011; IHME, 2018).

Mood changes are often a concern for people in the transition to parenthood. While prenatal and postnatal depression is well researched in women,

paternal postnatal depression (PPND) is less well known. It is important to note that depression can occur at any time in the perinatal period for both women and men, where 'perinatal' refers to both the prenatal (represents pregnancy) and postnatal stage (up to 12 months postpartum). PPND has historically been considered quite rare, but is gaining increased recognition. A recent meta-analysis provides a clear picture of an increase in research into paternal depression in the last thirty or so years (Cameron et al., 2016). Evidence suggests PPND is associated with a personal history of depression in the prenatal period, where prenatal depression with or without anxiety is considered a strong predictor for PPND (Edward et al., 2015). Much research during the twenty-first century points to the onset of PPND often following depression in the mother, with a prevalence rate of approximately 8–10% overall (Edmondson et al., 2010; Dudley et al., 2001; Figueiredo and Conde, 2011; Hanington et al., 2012; Pinheiro et al., 2006; Veskrna, 2010; Wee et al., 2011). Attitudes to PND differ between men and women: women generally hold the belief that PND has its roots in biological aetiology rather than psychosocial triggers (Edward et al., 2015), whilst men often believe PND does not relate to males at all. Meta-analysis (Cameron et al., 2016) provides compelling evidence that the highest rates of paternal depression are observed in the early period (3–6 months postpartum). Box 13.1 details biopsychosocial parameters pertinent to fathers during this early transition period into parenthood. These factors are an important consideration for healthcare professionals when working with men who are becoming a father.

Effects on Children and Family

Paternal postnatal depression is associated with an elevated risk of behavioural and developmental problems in children of the depressed father. For

> **Box 13.1** Some bio-psycho-social factors associated with an elevated risk for PPND for men (Kim and Swain, 2007; Da Costa et al., 2019)
>
> - A personal history of depression
> - Maternal PND
> - Older age
> - Poor sleep quality
> - Low testosterone level
> - Low cortisol level
> - Social stressors such as finances/employment
> - Lack of support outside the family unit
> - Incongruity between the reality and expectations of becoming a father
> - Poor social functioning
> - Poor marital communication
> - Impaired bonding with the infant
> - Feelings of being excluded in the perinatal period (i.e., before birth, during birth, following birth)

example, paternal depressive symptoms are a risk factor for excessive infant crying and fussiness (van den Berg et al., 2009; Davé et al., 2005), bonding disorder (Edhborg et al., 2005; Parfitt et al., 2013; Kerstis et al., 2016), compromised parenting patterns affecting children's development (Sethna et al., 2012; Sethna et al., 2015), and the development of oppositional defiant disorder and poor social and emotional outcomes in children (Meadows et al., 2007; Fletcher et al., 2011).

In the postnatal period, mothers and fathers must jointly manage the demands of a new baby, while renegotiating their roles and relationship. The impact of PPND may be seen in the way that fathers carry out their parenting role and their interactions with their infant, as well as in the ways that the father and mother negotiate tasks and responsibilities in the context of their parenting roles. Compared to non-depressed fathers, those with depressive symptoms during the first year of infancy are less likely to play with or read to their children and more likely to be verbally critical, to be withdrawn and to use spanking as a method of discipline (Davis et al., 2011; Sethna et al., 2015).

These behaviours are consistent with the evidence of increased anger and irritability as particular features of male depression (Cavanagh et al., 2017), underlining how PPND might negatively influence the parenting of mothers. Antenatal paternal depression has been shown to predict maternal postnatal depression (Paulson et al., 2016) and mothers whose partners are depressed are less likely to tell stories to their infants. Common challenges, such as developing infants' sleep routine, which require coordination and cooperation between parents, will be more difficult if either partner is depressed. Although generally mothers carry the bulk of caring responsibilities, including night feeds and care for the infant, an unsettled infant can impact on fathers' well-being and on the couple's relationship. A 'vicious cycle' can emerge where infant night waking leads to poor parental sleep which in turn is linked to fathers' (and mothers') depressive symptoms, fathers' disengagement with caring and low co-parenting quality (Cook et al., 2017; Saxbe et al., 2016; McDaniel and Teti, 2012).

Strategies for the Prevention and Management of Paternal Postnatal Depression

Screening for PND in mothers is commonplace, and is indeed considered best practice in healthcare in the perinatal period (last month of pregnancy to five weeks postpartum). However, routine screening of fathers in not usual. The Edinburgh Postnatal Depression Scale (EPDS) is a widely accessible and commonly used screening tool for postnatal depression in mothers. However, the cut off point for fathers is lower than for mothers, i.e., if fathers scored >7 they are advised to speak with their general practitioner about any symptoms of distress or depression that they may be experiencing (see Table 13.1) (Matthey, 2008).

There are a number of strategies that healthcare providers can use for the prevention and management of PPND and these strategies may be active, passive, or undertaken at an organizational level.

Active Strategies

Opportunities for screening fathers for PPND can be at various points during the perinatal period. For example, during the prenatal visits for the mother, treating clinicians can engage fathers in verbal discussion about their experience of impending parenthood. These times also afford an opportunity to ask the father about any depressive symptoms and highlight support services that may be available to him and the family should he experience any symptoms. During

Table 13.1 Scale cut-off points for men for the EPDS and other depression screening scales (Edward et al., 2015)

Year	Reference and country	n men (women)	Methods	Postnatal timeframe	Standardized tools/scales used	Scale cut-off Men (Women)
1994	Ballard et al. United Kingdom	200	comparative	6 weeks post-birth 6 months	EPDS	≥13
2001	Dudley et al. Australia	92 (92)	cross-sectional with interview	birth-12 months	EPDS	>12 (>12)
2001	Matthey et al. Australia	157(157)	longitudinal	antenatal 6 weeks 12 weeks 12 months	EPDS BDI GHQ	>12 >9 >7
2002	Skari et al. Norway	122 (127)	prospective, longitudinal cohort study	0–4 days post-birth 6 weeks 6 months	GHQ-28	≥6 (≥6)
2004	Pinheiro et al. Brazil	386 (386)	cross-sectional	6–12 weeks post-birth	BDI	>10
2005	Edhborg et al. Sweden	106 (106)	cross-sectional	1 week post-birth 2 months	PBQ EPDS	≥12 1st factor ≥17 2nd factor ≥10 3rd factor ≥9/10 (≥9/10)
2008	Edhborg Sweden	113 (155)	cross-sectional	birth 1 week 2 months	EPDS	≥9/10 (≥9/10)
2009	Gao et al. China	130 (130)	cross-sectional	6–8 weeks post-birth	EPDS	≥13 (≥13)
2010	Nishimura and Ohashi Japan	133 (178)	cross-sectional	4 weeks post-birth	EPDS CES-D	≥7/8 (≥8/9) ≥16
2011	Escriba`-Aguir and Artazcoz Spain	409 (420)	longitudinal	3rd trimester 3 months post-birth 12 months	EPDS	≥11 (12/13)
2011	Mao et al. China	376 (376)	cross-sectional	birth 6–8 weeks post-birth	EPDS	≥13 (≥13)
2012	Pio De Almeida et al. Brazil	173 (222)	cross-sectional	post-birth (exact time not specified)	EPDS	≥13 (≥13)

Abbreviations: BDI=Beck Depression Inventory; CES-D=Center for Epidemiologic Studies Depression Scale; EPDS=Edinburgh Postnatal Depression Scale; GHQ=General Health Questionnaire; GHQ-28=General Health Questionnaire-28; PBQ=Postpartum Bonding Questionnaire.

and in the period immediately after the birth, hospital stay information – such as discharge instructions – can provide important guidance on where and when to seek help for mothers and fathers should they be experiencing problems such as depressive symptoms. During the admission (and at the antenatal hospital visits for birth classes or preadmission preparation for the mother), screening for depressive symptoms can be undertaken for both the mother and father. Screening opportunities can also present themselves postnatally during consultations with clinicians or during regular infant well-being examinations.

In addition, primary care providers can readily engage fathers-to-be or new fathers in conversation about fatherhood and offer mental health screening. As detailed above, the Edinburgh Postnatal Depression Scale (EPDS) is a reliable and valid tool for PND in both fathers and mothers. In fathers, the threshold scores are slightly lower than in mothers (see Table 13.1). Other tools are also able to be used to assess depressive symptoms in the perinatal period for both mothers and fathers and include the Beck Depression Inventory (BDI), Center for Epidemiologic Studies Depression Scale (CES-D), General health Questionnaire-28 (GHQ), and Postpartum Bonding Questionnaire (PBQ). However, it should be noted that threshold scores for males and females may differ with each of these tools/scales and may be impacted by issues such as sleep disturbance commonly associated with having a young child. Table 13.1 – adapted from Edward et al. (2015) – provides cut off points for men and women for the EPDS and other depression rating scales, in the postpartum period.

Passive Strategies

An example of passive communication and a preventative intervention to raise awareness of PPND is use of signage (e.g. posters in the waiting room). Brochures and handouts to take home are also commonplace in healthcare, and these can be used as information tools for fathers as well as mothers. Information specifically for fathers may be included as an addition to the information mothers routinely receive from maternity service providers, primary health, and other relevant health services. Furthermore, digital spaces offer further opportunities where connections, supports, and information can be provided to men about PPND. Connecting people by using online forums as virtual 'support groups' has become a feature in health in recent times, and indeed online forums are already available for women who are in the postpartum period (Teaford et al., 2019). These social connections allows people to share information, garner social support, and – through a virtual space – reduce feelings of isolation. Virtual spaces also offer the

potential for anonymity, which is an advantage for individuals who find 'seeking help' difficult. It is well known that symptoms of depression are exacerbated by social isolation, accordingly connecting people can provide much-needed support as well as acting as a source of information for fathers at risk of developing PPND.

Materials, whether printed or digital, will be more effective in reaching fathers if the design and text are tailored to them. It cannot be assumed that labelling information 'for parents' will attract fathers as well as mothers (Bateson et al., 2017). As marketing professionals have discovered, reaching fathers requires a specific, visible emphasis on the role that fathers play in family life (Snoad, 2012). In consideration of these last few points, materials will be more likely to be read by fathers that include images of men, with or without their partners and babies, and which use the word 'father' as well as partner or parent.

Administrative Strategies

Administrative strategies for the prevention and management of PPND encompass policies, procedures, and practices, and are mainly concerned with the provision of a policy to inform practices, which may relate to any or all of the following clinical practices and/or outcomes:

- Routine screening for mothers *and* fathers using the EPDS (or other relevant scale)
- Standard antenatal education services for parents, which includes mental health education and information regarding relevant resources/supports that parents can use
- Routine and standardized postnatal parenting classes for mothers *and* fathers
- Formalized communication processes between maternity and mental health and/or primary health service providers where fathers may be linked for follow-up care if depressive symptoms are detected through routine screening

In healthcare, communication is essential between the service user and the service provider. However, maternity services care is generally woman-centred, and there is a growing imperative for maternity services to become more father-inclusive (Rominov et al., 2017), particularly since in developed nations over 90% of fathers attend the birth of their baby (Singh and Newburn, 2003).

What Care Providers Should Know

Care providers should be mindful of, and responsive to, the incidence and the effects of PPND. Specifically, the consequences for family (infants and children), the impact on the relationship with the mother, strategies to use in better engaging men in prevention, and education of depression in the perinatal period. Connecting men with other fathers (whether this occurs face to face or in a virtual space) can also be of benefit and should be explored as an option for fathers.

It is well accepted maternal PND is a strong predictor of PPND; what is not as well known is that when a mother is experiencing PND the rate of depression in fathers increases to between 24 and 50% (Musser et al., 2013). This figure is alarming, yet maternal healthcare providers are not generally aware of the elevated risk for fathers, as they are centred on the care of the mother and infant, and screening for depressive symptoms is directed toward the mother. In organizations where routine screening for depressive symptoms occurs, the service often does not have the organizational processes in place to facilitate staff providing services or referral for fathers.

Both maternal and paternal mental health have implications for the broader family unit, such as the risk for developmental problems of children, dysfunctional coping strategies that may be employed by fathers in attempts to cope with depressive symptoms (e.g. substance misuse, expressions of anger or frustration and withdrawal from the family and others). An important consideration in the prevention and treatment of PND in mother and fathers is help-seeking behaviours. The help-seeking behaviours of men are usually different to women. Therefore it is important that care providers facilitate opportunities to reach out to fathers to prevent, detect, and manage depressive symptoms as they transition into fatherhood or experience the advent of another addition to his family. Self-screening using he EPDS by fathers with their partners may provide an opportunity for detecting and preventing depressive symptoms while also overcoming the barrier of gender differences in help-seeking behaviours (Edward et al., 2019).

Fathers' lack of contact with the health services and systems of support should not be underestimated. The 'usual arrangements' for new fathers in Australia is captured by the description in Box 13.2.

> **Box 13.2** A case vignette depicting 'usual care' for a father with PNDD (Fletcher et al., 2006)
>
> When Michelle and Anthony attend Michelle's general practitioner after a positive pregnancy test, Anthony expresses his support but asks few questions. When asked about the couple's intentions for pregnancy care, Anthony's quick glance towards Michelle flags his uncertainty. For the following visits, Michelle attends the clinic alone. Anthony does participate in the ultrasound consultation and he joins in when prompted during the antenatal classes, but he accepts that the emphasis throughout is appropriately on the mother and ensuring a successful birth. During the birth, he wonders if he is in the way and is grateful in the end that the mother and baby are healthy. After the birth, when the home visiting nurse arrives, Anthony goes to make coffee and misses most of the discussion. His return to work precludes him attending the doctor's check-ups for mother and baby.

Care providers can make clear that fathers are viewed as important for the infant's well-being rather than simply as a support person for the mother or a provider for the family. This may include inquiring about the father when mothers present without their partner and providing information to fathers or via the mother that is specific for fathers (see websites in Box 13.3). Since most new parents will be unaware that fathers may also experience postnatal depression (Smith et al., 2019), raising awareness of paternal postnatal depression among both mothers and fathers is important.

On a broader scale, establishing routine screening of fathers across services that support families in the perinatal period, will increase the detection of depression in this population (Fletcher et al., 2016). Clinicians seeing fathers for other health issues can also inquire about the role of children in the presentation as part of consultations to identify mental health issues that may not have been spontaneously raised by the father during the consultation (Fletcher et al., 2013). In clinical practice, the development of referral pathways and tailored treatment regimens are key to facilitate care. Further research addressing subgroups in the population of depressed fathers, such as low-income, rural, or those with co-morbidities, is required (O'Brien et al., 2017).

Partnering with Fathers in the Perinatal Period

While maternity staff (such as midwives) usually acknowledge the importance of engaging with fathers (Rominov et al., 2017; Coutinho et al., 2016), there remain barriers to this being successfully achieved in practice. Fathers are often in a kind of 'undefined space' in maternity services where they are important, but are clearly not 'the patient' (Steen et al., 2012). Some barriers include the educational preparedness of staff related to working with fathers; timing of appointments where these may exclude fathers; the quality of the couple's relationship; the man's receptiveness to maternity service supports; and language and cultural barriers.

Partnering with fathers in the perinatal period can be achieved at any point during the perinatal period. Partnering with the patient and the family (in this case the mother and the father) facilitates the opportunity for shared decision-making, health education, and the mobilization of resources to support the birth journey in a timely way. Father-inclusive partnering strategies include communication through care plans, web-based information and support links, and flexibility of appointments to allow for fathers to attend. Box 13.3 provides a set of websites that provide useful information and support for fathers with PPND.

Conclusions

Whilst postnatal depression is well understood and routinely screened for in new mothers, it remains

> **Box 13.3** Useful websites for fathers with PPND
>
> (1) Depression and anxiety in new fathers available from www.beyondblue.org.au/who-does-it-affect/men/what-causes-anxiety-and-depression-in-men/new-fathers
> (2) Fathers and depression available from www.pregnancbirthbaby.org.au/fathers-and-depression
> (3) How is dad going? Available from www.panda.org.au/info-support/how-is-dad-going
> (4) Paternal depression available from www.news-medical.net/health/Paternal-Depression.aspx
> (5) Sad Dads available from www.parents.com/parenting/dads/sad-dads/

under-recognized in fathers. Maternal postnatal depression predicts paternal postnatal depression, and it can have profound implications for the entire family unit. In particular, depressed, emotionally unavailable, and angry fathers can have a powerful detrimental effect on their partners and offspring, with PPND being associated with an elevated risk of behavioural and developmental problems in children. Screening for postnatal depression is commonplace for mothers, but often not for fathers, even though the same screening tools can be applied to both parents. There are a number of active and passive strategies that can be used by clinicians to engage and partner with fathers in the perinatal period more effectively.

References

APA 2013. *Diagnostic and Statistical Manual of Mental Disorders (DSM-5)*. Arlington, VA: American Psychiatric Publishing.

Bateson, K., Darwin, Z., Galdas, P. and Rosan, C. 2017. Engaging fathers: acknowledging the barriers. *Journal of Health Visiting*, 5(3), 126–32.

Cameron, E. E., Sedov, I. D., and Tomfohr-Madsen, L. M. 2016. Prevalence of paternal depression in pregnancy and the postpartum: an updated meta-analysis. *Journal of Affective Disorders*, 206, 189–203.

Cavanagh, A., Wilson, C. J., Kavanagh, D. J., and Caputi, P. 2017. Differences in the expression of symptoms in men versus women with depression: a systematic review and meta-analysis. *Harvard Review of Psychiatry*, 25(1), 29–38.

Cook, F., Giallo, R., Petrovic, Z., Coe, A., Seymour, M., Cann, W., and Hiscock, H. 2017. Depression and anger in fathers of unsettled infants: a community cohort study. *Journal of Paediatrics and Child Health*, 53 (2), 131–5.

Coutinho, E. C., Antunes, J. G. V. C., Duarte, J. C., Parreira, V. C., Chaves, C. M. B., and Nelas, P. A. B. 2016. Benefits for the father from their involvement in the labour and birth sequence. *Procedia – Social and Behavioral Sciences*, 217, 435–42.

Da Costa, D., Danieli, C., Abrahamowicz, M., Dasgupta, K., Sewitch, M., Lowensteyn, I., and Zelkowitz, P. 2019. A prospective study of postnatal depressive symptoms and associated risk factors in first-time fathers. *Journal of Affective Disorders*, 249, 371–7.

Davé, S., Nazareth, I., Sherr, L., and Senior, R. 2005. The association of paternal mood and infant temperament: a pilot study. *British Journal of Developmental Psychology*, 23(4), 609–21.

Davis, R. N., Davis, M. M., Freed, G. L., and Clark, S. J. 2011. Fathers' depression related to positive and negative parenting behaviors with 1-year-old children. *Pediatrics*, 127(4), 612–18.

Dudley, M., Roy, K., Kelk, N., and Bernard, D. 2001. Psychological correlates of depression in fathers and mothers in the first postnatal year. *Journal of Reproductive and Infant Psychology*, 19(3), 187–202.

Edhborg, M., Matthiesen, A.-S., Lundh, W., and Widström, A.-M. 2005. Some early indicators for depressive symptoms and bonding 2 months postpartum – a study of new mothers and fathers. *Archives of Women's Mental Health*, 8(4), 221–31.

Edmondson, O. J. H., Psychogiou, L., Vlachos, H., Netsi, E., and Ramchandani, P. G. 2010. Depression in fathers in the postnatal period: assessment of the Edinburgh Postnatal Depression Scale as a screening measure. *Journal of Affective Disorders*, 125(1–3), 365–8.

Edward, K.-l., Castle, D., Mills, C., Davis, L., and Casey, J. 2015. An integrative review of paternal depression. *American Journal of Men's Health*, 9(1), 26–34.

Edward, K.-l., Giandinoto, J.-A., Stephenson, J., Mills, C., Mcfarland, J., and Castle, D. J. 2019. Self-screening using the Edinburgh postnatal depression scale for mothers and fathers to initiate early help seeking behaviours. *Archives of Psychiatric Nursing*, 33(4), 421–7.

Figueiredo, B. and Conde, A. 2011. Anxiety and depression in women and men from early pregnancy to 3-months postpartum. *Archives of Women's Mental Health*, 14(3), 247–55.

Fletcher, R., Dowse, E., and St George, J. 2016. Screening dads for depression in Australian early parenting centres. *Australian Nursing and Midwifery Journal*, 24(5), 36.

Fletcher, R. J., Feeman, E., Garfield, C., and Vimpani, G. 2011. The effects of early paternal depression on children's development. *Medical Journal of Australia*, 195(11–12), 685–9.

Fletcher, R. J., Maharaj, O. N. N., Fletcher Watson, C. H., May, C., Skeates, N., and Gruenert, S. 2013. Fathers with mental illness: implications for clinicians and health services. *The Medical Journal of Australia*, 199(3), S34–S36.

Fletcher, R. J., Matthey, S., and Marley, C. G. 2006. Addressing depression and anxiety among new fathers. *Medical Journal of Australia*, 185(8), 461–3.

Hanington, L., Heron, J., Stein, A., and Ramchandani, P. 2012. Parental depression and child outcomes – is marital conflict the missing link? *Child: Care, Health and Development*, 38(4), 520–9.

IHME. 2018. *Findings from the Global Burden of Disease Study 2017*. Seattle, WA: IHME.

Kerstis, B., Aarts, C., Tillman, C., Persson, H., Engström, G., Edlund, B., Öhrvik, J., Sylvén, S., and Skalkidou, A. 2016. Association between parental depressive symptoms and impaired bonding with the infant. *Archives of Women's Mental Health*, 19(1), 87–94.

Kim, P. and Swain, J. E. 2007. Sad dads: paternal postpartum depression. *Psychiatry (Edgmont (Pa.: Township))*, 4(2), 35–47.

Matthey, S. 2008. Using the Edinburgh Postnatal Depression Scale to screen for anxiety disorders. *Depression and Anxiety*, 25(11), 926–31.

McDaniel, B. T. and Teti, D. M. 2012. Coparenting quality during the first three months after birth: the role of infant sleep quality. *Journal of Family Psychology*, 26(6), 886.

Meadows, S. O., McLanahan, S. S., and Brooks-Gunn, J. 2007. Parental depression and anxiety and early childhood behavior problems across family types. *Journal of Marriage and Family*, 69(5), 1162–77.

Musser, A. K., Ahmed, A. H., Foli, K. J., and Coddington, J. A. 2013. Paternal postpartum depression: what health care providers should know. *Journal of Pediatric Health Care*, 27(6), 479–85.

O'Brien, A. P., McNeil, K. A., Fletcher, R., Conrad, A., Wilson, A. J., Jones, D., and Chan, S. W. 2017. New fathers' perinatal depression and anxiety – treatment options: an integrative review. *American Journal of Men's Health*, 11(4), 863–76.

Parfitt, Y., Pike, A., and Ayers, S. 2013. The impact of parents' mental health on parent–baby interaction: A prospective study. *Infant Behavior and Development*, 36(4), 599–608.

Paulson, J. F., Bazemore, S. D., Goodman, J. H., and Leiferman, J. A. 2016. The course and interrelationship of maternal and paternal perinatal depression. *Archives of Women's Mental Health*, 19(4), 655–63.

Pinheiro, R. T., Magalhaes, P. V. S., Horta, B. L., Pinheiro, K. A. T., Da Silva, R. A., and Pinto, R. H. 2006. Is paternal postpartum depression associated with maternal postpartum depression? Population-based study in Brazil. *Acta Psychiatrica Scandinavica.*, 113(3), 230–2.

Rominov, H., Giallo, R., Pilkington, P. D., and Whelan, T. A. 2017. Midwives' perceptions and experiences of engaging fathers in perinatal services. *Women and Birth*, 30(4), 308–18.

Saxbe, D. E., Schetter, C. D., Guardino, C. M., Ramey, S. L., Shalowitz, M. U., Thorp, J., Vance, M., and Eunice Kennedy Shriver National Institute for Child Health and Human Development Community Child Health Network. 2016. Sleep quality predicts persistence of parental postpartum depressive symptoms and transmission of depressive symptoms from mothers to fathers. *Annals of Behavioral Medicine*, 50(6), 862–75.

Sethna, V., Murray, L., Netsi, E., Psychogiou, L., and Ramchandani, P. G. 2015. Paternal depression in the postnatal period and early father–infant interactions. *Parenting*, 15(1), 1–8.

Sethna, V., Murray, L., and Ramchandani, P. 2012. Depressed fathers' speech to their 3-month-old infants: a study of cognitive and mentalizing features in paternal speech. *Psychological Medicine*, 42(11), 2361–71.

Singh, D. and Newburn, M. 2003. What men think of midwives. *Midwives – London*, 6, 70–5.

Smith, T., Gemmill, A. W., and Milgrom, J. 2019. Perinatal anxiety and depression: awareness and attitudes in Australia. *International Journal of Social Psychiatry*, 65(5), 378–87.

Snoad, L. 2012. Fathers the central figure in family brand campaigns. *Marketing Week*, 35(17), 20.

Steen, M., Downe, S., Bamford, N., and Edozien, L. 2012. Not-patient and not-visitor: a metasynthesis fathers' encounters with pregnancy, birth and maternity care. *Midwifery*, 28(4), 422–31.

Teaford, D., McNiesh, S., and Goyal, D. 2019. New mothers' experiences with online postpartum forums. *MCN: The American Journal of Maternal/Child Nursing*, 44(1), 40–5.

van den Berg, M. P., van der Ende, J., Crijnen, A. A., Jaddoe, V. W., Moll, H. A., Mackenbach, J. P., Hofman, A., Hengeveld, M. W., Tiemeier, H., and Verhulst, F. C. 2009. Paternal depressive symptoms during pregnancy are related to excessive infant crying. *Pediatrics*, 124(1), e96–e103.

Veskrna, L. 2010. Peripartum depression – does it occur in fathers and does it matter? *Journal of Men's Health*, 7(4), 420–30.

Wee, K. Y., Skouteris, H., Pier, C., Richardson, B., and Milgrom, J. 2011. Correlates of ante- and postnatal depression in fathers: a systematic review. *Journal of Affective Disorders*, 130(3), 358–77.

WHO. 2011. *Depression* [online]. Available at: www.who.int/mental_health/management/depression/definition/en/ [Accessed 15 June 2012].

Chapter 14

Bipolar Affective Disorder in Men

Allan H. Young and Diego Hidalgo-Mazzei

Bipolar affective disorder (BD) is often a chronic and disabling illness that negatively impacts the quality life, functioning, and life expectancy of those affected (Whiteford et al., 2013). It mainly comprises recurrent pathological mood fluctuations ranging from manic to depressive episodes and the admixture of these, usually referred to as mixed states (Grande et al., 2016). Beyond these frank clinical episodes, many patients affected by BD are symptomatic, albeit subsyndromally, during almost half of their lifetime producing a high degree of functional and cognitive impairment (Martínez-Arán et al., 2004; Judd et al., 2002). As a consequence, the societal and economic burden of the disorder is highly challenging for any healthcare system due to high associated healthcare costs (Fajutrao et al., 2009).

Although current diagnostic criteria and treatment guidelines for BD don't provide separate and specific recommendations for women and men, there are nevertheless several gender-specific epidemiological, biological, clinical, and therapeutic differences that should be considered when approaching this disorder (Diflorio and Jones, 2010). Moreover, only a few publications report these differences and only a very few studies are designed or based on gender-specific BD characteristics (Flores-Ramos et al., 2017). In this new era of personalized medicine, it is certainly important that these differences are not taken for granted. Therefore, the main aim of this chapter is to provide a broad overview of BD as well as the updated general principles of its diagnosis and treatment, focusing especially on those aspects particularly relevant to men.

Epidemiology, Burden, and Costs

BD affects about 60 million people worldwide. It is estimated that the lifetime prevalence of BD is between 1% to 2% of the world population depending on the diagnostic criteria and region of the world considered (Merikangas et al., 2011; Ferrari et al., 2011). These prevalence rates are to some extent similar in most regions of the world, with slightly higher estimates in North Africa and the Middle East; however, in general, the BD diagnosis does not seem to be affected by ethnic origin or socioeconomic status (Clemente et al., 2015). The aggregated lifetime prevalence for BD type I has been estimated at 0.6%, 0.4% for type II and 1.4% for subthreshold BD. Although the overall BD 12-month and lifetime prevalence are similar for men and women according to most studies (Ferrari et al., 2011), some of them report relevant differences when this is analysed by subtypes of BD: there is some evidence suggesting that bipolar type I (BDI) might be more frequent in men in comparison to women, whereas females are more frequently diagnosed from bipolar type II (BDII) (Merikangas et al., 2011; Baldassano et al., 2005).

Due to the recurrent characteristics, persistent sub-threshold symptoms and associated cognitive as well as functional impairment, BD is now among the top five leading causes of disability for people of less than 25 years and the sixth ranked cause among working adults (Collins et al., 2011; Gore et al., 2011). The total Years Lived with Disability (YLD) attributed to BD in 2010 was 12,900, of which 45% pertained to men. It also accounted for 7% of disability-adjusted life years (DALYs) attributable to all mental disorders. Furthermore, it has been estimated that it is the second leading cause of days 'out of role' among all health conditions (Alonso et al., 2011). In spite of achieving medium and high education levels, in a large sample of nearly 3000 subjects diagnosed with bipolar disorder type I, 64% were unemployed (Kupfer et al., 2002), while in another study almost one-third were receiving a severe disablement benefit (Grande et al., 2013).

Consequently, the negative impact on the quality of life of people living with this disorder is substantial, even when they may be considered to be clinically euthymic (Bonnín et al., 2012; Michalak et al., 2006). This quality of life impairment is even more marked among BD men with co-morbid substance use (Adan et al., 2017). Even though most of the clinical assessments and follow-up evaluations undertaken by mental health professionals are focused on symptoms reduction and relapse prevention, it is of paramount importance also to assess functionality and cognition, as these are closely related to quality of life and overall clinical outcomes in BD (Bonnín et al., 2012). According to most studies, between 40 to 60% of all patients with BD have some degree of neurocognitive deficit during their lifetime and independently of acute episodes (Solé et al., 2017). There is a growing evidence that these cognitive deficits start even before illness onset (Martino et al., 2015). Those few studies that have explored gender-related differences in BD cognitive patterns have detected significant variations in several cognitive domains such as poorer scores in spatial working, and visual and immediate memory in men (Tournikioti et al., 2018; Suwalska and Łojko 2014). Hence, treatments seeking to remediate BD cognitive deficits should be tailored according to these differences (Solé et al., 2017).

In view of these data, it is not difficult to envision the immense healthcare costs associated with BD. In Europe, the total cost (direct, indirect and non-medical) of mental disorders has been recently estimated as €461 billion, one-third of which is related to direct healthcare costs. For BD, the total annual cost estimation is €21.4 billion and €111 billion (151 billion USD) in Europe and the USA, respectively. Indirect costs, such as early retirement, unemployment, time off work, and productivity lost, account for 75–86% of the total cost (Dilsaver 2011; Fajutrao et al., 2009).

Box 14.1   Epidemiology of BD

- Bipolar disorder (BD) is a highly prevalent, chronic illness afflicting between 1% and 2% of the world population
- The overall BD lifetime prevalence is similar for men and women, according to most studies
- The illness is now among the top five leading causes of disability among people of less than 25 years and the sixth highest among working adults
- BD is the second largest cause of days 'out of role' among all health conditions
- The disorder total annual cost is estimated to be of €21.4 billion in Europe

---

Aetiology and Pathophysiology

Despite extensive efforts to uncover the aetiology underlying the behavioural and cognitive dysfunctions in BD, the exact pathophysiologic mechanisms are still not fully understood. However, important advances and discoveries have been made during the last twenty years in the attempt to assemble this complex puzzle, allowing a tentative but better understanding of the disrupted genetic, biological, structural, and functional brain pathways affecting patients with BD (Maletic and Raison, 2014). What is clear is that, as many other illnesses, at least initially there is a strong interaction between genes and environment starting an early pathologic disruption at molecular, subcellular, and cellular levels with subsequent manifestations in neuroendocrine, autonomic, immune, and brain neuron regulation resulting in the final clinical manifestations.

The estimated heritability of BD is as high as 90%, with up to 70% concordance in monozygotic twins (Craddock and Sklar, 2013). However, the exact combination of genes underlying this heritability remains elusive, indicating a polygenetic multifunctional model. In this regard, in recent years a number of genes were identified that have been found to be associated with BD and related to intracellular or neurotransmission dysregulation such as the COMT, BDNF, NRG-1, MAOA, DAT, 5HTT, CACNA1C, GSK-3, and DISC-1. Some genes have been found to be gender-specific, such as the SEZ6L, RELN, or the DAT1 core promoter -67A/T polymorphism, conferring a specific risk only to males (Goes et al., 2010; Xu et al., 2013; Ohadi et al., 2007). Nonetheless, in vivo replication of these findings has delivered inconclusive results, and models predicting BD and correlations with neuroimaging findings are unsatisfactory (McCarthy et al., 2014). Moreover, there is a high degree of overlap of these genes with other severe mental disorders such as schizophrenia, making them too non-specific to associate directly with the phenotypic manifestation of BD (Maletic and Raison, 2014).

In parallel, advancements in structural and functional neuroimaging techniques have contributed to identifying those brain regions and circuits associated with BD. Among these, the frontal-subcortical, frontal-basal ganglia and prefrontal-limbic circuits seem to be the networks more frequently affected. There is also a growing body of evidence that repeated illness episodes impact brain structure and functionality, with impact on specific symptoms and deficits (Maletic and Raison, 2014). Likewise, studies have reported gender-specific differences in brain structure and function early in the course of BD, notably subcortical and cortical regions as well as hippocampus (Mitchell et al., 2018).

Several of the above-mentioned genes and brain regions, along with peripheral inflammatory blood molecules (e.g. interleukins (ILs), tumour-necrosis factors (TNFs), transforming growth factors (TGFs), interferons (INFs)), have been proposed as biomarkers for BD diagnosis, severity and prognosis (Carvalho et al., 2016). In addition, peripheral hormone levels have been implicated in the pathophysiology of BD and have been also proposed as potential biomarkers. Interestingly, in one of our studies, we found lower testosterone levels in depressed males with BD compared to male controls, whereas depressed women with BD had significantly higher testosterone levels than female controls. Although it could not be confirmed that this significant disturbance in BD was a causal, mediating, or moderating factor, it denotes some gender-specific neurobiological differences in BD (Wooderson et al., 2015). However, until now, the extensive research in the biomarkers field has not resulted in conclusive results which can be extrapolated to real-world clinical practice (Carvalho et al., 2016).

Box 14.2 Aetiology and neurobiology of BD

- The exact pathophysiologic mechanisms underlying BD are still not fully understood
- There is a strong interaction between genes and environment starting an early pathologic disruption at a molecular, subcellular, and cellular levels
- Many candidate genes have been associated with BD, implicating intracellular or neurotransmission dysregulation
- Structural and functional neuroimaging techniques have contributed to identifying brain areas and circuits associated with BD, such as the frontal-subcortical, frontal-basal ganglia and prefrontal-limbic circuits
- Despite these advances in generating putative biomarkers for BD diagnosis, severity, and prognosis, there are as yet no tests which could be extrapolated to real-world clinical practice

---

Symptoms, Diagnosis, Course, and Co-morbidities

Symptoms

Manic episodes are the hallmark of BD and comprise a persistently elevated, expansive, or irritable mood, lasting at least one week, and which are markedly different from the basal non-depressed mood (Belmaker and Bersudsky, 2004). Increased energy or activity is now seen as a core element, in DSM-5 (American Psychiatric Association, 2013). The syndrome includes sleep pattern disturbances, including a decreased need for sleep, inflated self-esteem as well as grandiose thoughts, racing thoughts with or without pressure of speech, decreased attention or focus, increased activity in terms of social or physical interaction, and augmented involvement in activities that suppose a high degree of pleasure but with a great risk to physical or psychological integrity. Additionally, psychotic features in the form of hallucinations or delusions can be present. Manic episodes are associated with a disturbance of social, educational, and occupational functioning that might require hospitalization to prevent the risk of harm to oneself or others. Some studies suggest that manic polarity in the initial episode, as well as psychotic symptoms, are more frequent and earlier in men than in women with BD (Kennedy et al., 2005; Kawa et al., 2005). Some studies suggest that behavioural and legal problems in manic episodes are more frequent in men than in women (Baldassano et al., 2005; Kawa et al., 2005).

Hypomanic episodes have almost all the same symptoms as manic episodes, but with lesser intensity of symptoms and a minimum duration of symptoms of at least 4 days. Psychotic symptoms are absent and the episodes are not severe enough to affect to a significant extent social or occupational functioning, or to require hospitalization.

In contrast, depressive episodes in BD are characterized by depressed mood and reduced motor activity that represents a change from the person's baseline mood pattern, lasting at least two weeks. The individual suffers from depressed mood or irritability most of the day, nearly every day as well as lack or decreased interests and the capacity to feel pleasure or joy. Moreover, a change in appetite and a consequent weight variation may be present. Sleep pattern changes, psychomotor retardation, loss of energy, guilt and worthlessness feelings, decreased concentration, and thoughts or plans of suicide can also manifest. Alongside these symptoms, psychotic symptoms can be present. Some studies suggesting that men suffer from comparatively fewer lifetime depressive episodes than women (Diflorio and Jones, 2010); however, this has not been confirmed by other studies (Baldassano et al., 2005).

Whilst 'textbook' characterization of BD is one of two illness 'poles', many people with BD experience states in which both manic and depressive symptoms overlap with each other; there have been denominated as the presence of mixed features – known as 'mixed states' in earlier editions of the DSM. To meet the DSM-5 specifier for mixed features, at least three manic/hypomanic symptoms that do not overlap with symptoms of major depression must be present in a depressed phase; and in the instance of mania or hypomania, the presence of at least three symptoms of depression jointly with the episode of mania/hypomania, are required.

Regarding symptom and episodes differences between men and women, there is some evidence that hypomanic and mixed symptoms are more common in women than in men (Diflorio and Jones 2010; Arnold 2003). Regardless of these differences, due to its diagnostic, prognostic, and treatment implications, both hypomanic and mixed symptoms should be meticulously and equally assessed in both genders.

Diagnosis and Types

The diagnosis of BD is based on clinical grounds from the symptoms and episodes reported by the individual and/or relatives. A careful longitudinal history review is required in order to identify the pattern of episodes. Such review is frequently conducted during clinical interviews in an unstructured manner, and it should be noted that there are structured interviews such as the Structured Clinical Interview for DSM Disorders (SCID)(First, 1995), which makes the systematic screening and diagnosis of BD as well as other frequent co-morbid mental disorders more reliable; they, are considered the gold standard diagnostic tools in clinical research but also informing daily clinical practice (Zimmerman, 2016). Furthermore, tools such as the 32-items Hypomanic Checklist (HCL-32), Mood Disorders Questionnaire (MDQ), and retrospective life-charts can also be useful, both to screen and characterize past episodes (Angst et al., 2005; Zimmerman et al., 2011). Even though the

above-mentioned tools can be helpful in supporting the diagnosis they have several limitations (Zimmerman et al., 2011) and ultimately it is the clinicians' judgement that is used to interpret them alongside other complementary and contextual information to reach a BD diagnosis.

Consistent with the most common diagnostic criteria used in clinical settings, the DSM-5, BD is formally diagnosed and further categorized into three types based mainly on the duration and severity of manic episodes. A diagnosis of BD Type I (BDI) requires at least one manic episode to make, even though this group of patients could also have had hypomanic and depressive episodes during the course of the disease. In contrast, a BD Type II (BDII) diagnosis requires the presence of at least one hypomanic episode and one depressive episode as well as the absence of a previous manic episode. Cyclothymic disorder is a diagnosis given to people who experience some hypomanic and depressive symptoms over at least two years, but without meeting all the required criteria to formally diagnose a depressive or hypomanic episode.

When hypomanic or manic symptoms manifest after the use of substances/medications or due to medical conditions, they are classified as substance/medication-induced bipolar and related disorder, and bipolar and related disorder due to another medical condition, respectively. However, if the manic/hypomanic episode persists after the physiological effect of the drug has abated the episode is considered to be mania (or hypomania). Finally, those cases in whom there are bipolar symptoms that do not fulfil all the criteria required to establish a bipolar type I, II, or cyclothymic disorders diagnosis, the category of Other Specified Bipolar and related Disorders is applicable (Figure 14.1; American Psychiatric Association, 2013).

Beyond the criteria mentioned above, the diagnosis of bipolar disorder can represent a complex challenge for any clinician and healthcare system, especially with the current lack of complementary objective measures. That is, bipolar symptoms have a wide array of presentations partially related to age as well as personal and cultural characteristics of the patient.

Most studies have reported a mean age of onset of BD under 25 years. According to some studies, males have an earlier disorder onset, detection, and treatment, probably due to the more frequent debut with

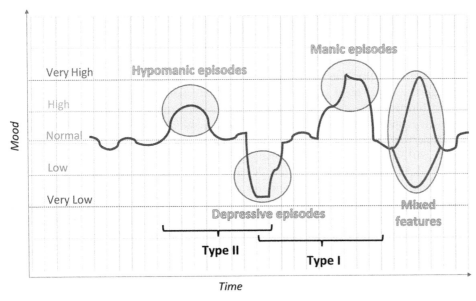

Figure 14.1 Scheme of the classifications of bipolar disorder type I, II, and mixed-features specifier based on the type of mood episodes according to the DSM-5

manic episodes with associated behavioural disturbances requiring more rapid medical attention (Kennedy et al., 2005). However, it is estimated that in developed countries it can take approximately eight to ten years since the first symptoms appear, until an appropriate diagnosis is made; the scenario in emergent economy countries could be much worse (Goldberg and Ernst, 2002). Furthermore, 40 to 50% of BD patients are initially misdiagnosed as having major depressive disorder (MDD) and 60% receive from one to four other different diagnoses over their lifetime (Scott and Leboyer, 2011). During this time they usually do not receive adequate treatments, or may be presented deleterious ones, resulting in higher rates of disability and mortality (Goldberg and Ernst, 2002). Consequently, newer cost-efficient, extended, and reliable screening and diagnostic methods that could integrate subjective information as well as emergent objective data are urgently needed to reach earlier diagnoses, inform appropriate treatments, and achieve better outcomes.

Course, Impairment, and Prognosis

A relapsing-recurring course of BD is the rule rather than the exception, despite treatment. For instance, the STEP-BD study followed 1469 BD patients receiving pharmacologic treatment for twenty-four months:

almost half of them experience a recurrence during this time, predominantly depressive ones. Recurrence and relapse rates are even higher without treatment or when there is irregular adherence to pharmacologic therapy (Perlis et al., 2006). If the frequency of these relapses increases to four or more mood episodes meeting criteria for mania, hypomania, or major depression within one year, the criteria for a rapid-cycling BD specifier is fulfilled. Rapid cycling is associated with a poorer prognosis, and thus potential causes (e.g. antidepressants, thyroid dysfunction, co-morbidities), as well as appropriate treatments, should be sought (Valentí et al., 2015). It is reportedly less common in women, but the reason for this is unclear (Diflorio and Jones, 2010).

Beyond mood episodes, many patients struggle with subsyndromal symptoms for almost half of their lifetime, predominantly depressive in nature. These sub-clinical symptoms, which often are not given sufficient clinical attention, are associated with impairment of quality of life, high rates of functional impairment, and disability (Bonnín et al., 2012).

One of the most important yet underestimated consequences of BD is the subtle and insidious cognitive deficits independently of the mood states and even persisting during periods of remission. It has been estimated that more than half of bipolar patients are affected by neurocognitive deficits (Solé et al.,

2012). The most impacted cognitive domains seem to be executive function and verbal memory (Martínez-Arán et al., 2004). Whether there is a progressive or accumulative cognitive decline after each episode is still a matter of debate (Martino et al., 2016). What is clear is that the resulting cognitive impairment can impair the quality of life and functionality of those affected, with very few recovery options available, albeit cognitive remediation interventions are showing some promise (Vieta et al., 2013).

The increased suicidal risk of patients with BD is one of the most concerning and worrisome symptoms, and which must have high priority during psychiatric risk evaluations. There is an eightfold increase of suicidal risk in male patients with BD in comparison to the general population, contributing to overall mortality rates (Crump et al., 2013). The most frequent general risk factors for attempted suicide include: recent mood episodes, hospitalizations or suicide attempts; and the presence of a co-morbid substance use disorder (SUD) in men (Tidemalm et al., 2014). Even though some studies reported higher suicide rates in men in comparison to women with BD, after controlling for several factors the risk seems to be equivalently high in both sexes (Diflorio and Jones, 2010).

Co-morbidities

BD frequently co-exist with other co-morbid psychiatric conditions such as anxiety disorders (40%), Borderline Personality Disorder (BPD) (20%), and

---

Box 14.3 Clinical manifestation and longitudinal course of BD

- BD subtypes are based on the type and intensity of episodes suffered by the patient
- The illness onset is most frequently before 25 years old
- The average diagnostic delay of BD is of about 8 to 10 years
- The relapsing-recurring course of the illness is the rule rather than the exception
- Beyond episodes, subsyndromal symptoms are present during almost half of BD patients' lifetime, contributing to impairment in functioning and quality of life
- More than half of all patients with BD will have some degree of neurocognitive deficit during their lifetime

---

SUDs (40–70%) (Baldassano et al., 2005). These co-morbidities, which are often not detected until late in the course of the illness, not only worsen the overall prognosis of the disorder but also make necessary a reconsideration of the diagnosis and treatment plan, which should be tailored or enhanced depending on each circumstance (Crump et al., 2013).

It is worth mentioning that the prevalence of some of these psychiatric co-morbidities is higher in men, notably SUDs, including alcohol, cannabis, and nicotine dependence (Frye et al., 2003; Kawa et al., 2005; Diflorio and Jones 2010). As mentioned above, the co-occurrence of these conditions affects the general health and functioning of male patients, having negative consequences for the long-term prognosis and functionality (Adan et al., 2017). Moreover, the summation effect of more than one of these increases the risk of the others (Hidalgo-Mazzei, Walsh, et al., 2015), and also increases the risk of suicide attempts (Zimmerman et al., 2014).

Co-morbidities are not limited to psychiatric disorders, extending also to medical conditions, the most prevalent conditions being migraine (23.7%), asthma (19.2%), dyslipidaemia (19.2%), hypertension (15%), thyroid disease (12.9%), and osteoarthritis (10.8%) (Forty et al., 2014). Dyslipidaemia seems to be particularly prevalent in men with BD, regardless of other sociodemographic or clinical factors, thus requiring regular lipid profile monitoring (Vemuri et al., 2011). Although thyroid dysfunction is more frequent in women on lithium treatment, it should be taken into account that the relative risk is also increased in men (Diflorio and Jones, 2010).

These high rates of medical co-morbidities contribute significantly to a worse course and prognosis of BD (number of episodes, psychiatric co-morbidities, rapid cycling, functional impairment) as well as with increased mortality (Forty et al., 2014; Crump et al., 2013). In fact, it has been estimated that men and women with bipolar disorder die nearly a decade earlier than the general population, with this increased risk attributable largely to medical causes (Crump et al., 2013). Thus, a comprehensive screening of potential medical co-morbidities must have high priority in the assessment, follow-up, and treatment of patients suffering from BD alongside those pertaining to their mental health. Additionally, prevention strategies through a balanced diet and regular exercise should be encouraged (Goodwin et al., 2016).

Box 14.4 Co-morbidities in BD

- Co-occurrence of BD with other psychiatric disorders is frequent
- Most frequent psychiatric co-morbidities are with anxiety disorders, Borderline Personality Disorder, and substance use disorders
- Co-morbid alcohol abuse or dependence is especially common in men with BD, thus a regular screening should be conducted and appropriate treatment offered
- Medical co-morbidities are also more prevalent in BD in comparison to the general population, contributing to the higher mortality in this group of patients
- Dyslipidaemia seems to be particularly prevalent in men with BD, requiring regular cardiovascular assessments and lipid profile monitoring
- Both medical and psychiatric co-morbidities significantly and negatively impact the course and prognosis of BD

Treatment

The treatment of BD depends on the illness phase: either acute treatments to address and resolve symptoms during episodes, or maintenance treatments to prevent them. In general terms, treatments can be classified into pharmacological, psychological, and non-pharmacological treatments. We provide a concise summary alongside an introduction to novel non-standard treatments. For more detailed information about specific treatment strategies in BD, the reader is referred to the most current and updated treatment guidelines (Goodwin et al., 2016; The National Institute for Health and Care Excellence, 2014; Yatham et al., 2018).

Pharmacological Treatments

The pharmacological treatment during subsyndromal or euthymic phases has shown to be effective in mitigating some symptoms of BD and decreasing the number of full-blown episodes (Vieta et al., 2013). The choice of the drug depends mainly on the current symptoms, as well as on the previous phases of the illness, tailored to the individual characteristics and preferences of the patient.

During euthymic or maintenance phases, there are a number of drugs, usually named mood-stabilizers, which have shown efficacy in preventing further episodes depending on the polarity of the previous ones (Popovic et al., 2012). The oldest of these is lithium, which has solid evidence for efficacy although the mechanism of action is still not fully understood. Lithium requires regular monitoring of plasma levels as well as other blood tests, including renal, thyroid, and para-thyroid function. Lithium has shown not only to reduce the risk of bipolar episodes, but also reduces suicidality (Goodwin et al., 2016; Severus et al., 2014). Nonetheless, among patients with BD there are about one-third of non-responders and partial responders to lithium, with no current reliable biomarker able to predict this (Licht et al., 2008). Moreover, lithium can have significant side effects in some patients such as tremors, diarrhoea, polyuria, weight gain, creatinine increase, and thyroid dysfunction. Hence, an early discontinuation is necessary in about half of patients. These discontinuation rates are similar in men and women, but men tend to discontinue more frequently without consulting with their psychiatrist (Öhlund et al., 2018).

Valproate is an anticonvulsant that has demonstrated efficacy in preventing manic episodes, as does – with less supporting evidence – carbamazepine. On the other hand, lamotrigine and quetiapine are among the other options available to reduce the risk of depressive relapses (Goodwin et al., 2016). It is worth mentioning that monotherapy with any one of these agents is preferable, but frequently this might not be sufficient to prevent further episodes, with many BD patients requiring a combination of two or more agents. Few studies have explored gender-specific efficacy among mood-stabilizers, and there is no consistent evidence that there are significant differences between the sexes in this regard (Flores-Ramos et al., 2017).

Regarding the treatment of acute episodes, pharmacological interventions can be effective in shortening the duration of the episodes alongside their behavioural, economic, and life-threating consequences. The choice of the drug depends upon the symptoms and personal characteristics of the patient. The medications recommended by evidence-based guidelines for the acute treatment of manic episodes are predominantly dopamine antagonists such as haloperidol, olanzapine, risperidone, and quetiapine. Partial dopamine agonist drugs such as aripiprazole are another potential option. The balance between efficacy and tolerability of each option should be considered on a case-by-case basis depending on episode characteristics, previous response, and co-morbidities. Again there are no specific gender effects in the management of acute mania, though males might require higher doses of antimanic agents than females.

The treatment of acute depressive episodes in BD is especially challenging. Quetiapine, olanzapine, olanzapine plus fluoxetine, and more recently lurasidone, all have established efficacy in bipolar depression. Even though antidepressants might still be considered an option in bipolar type II and for treatment-resistant cases, they are not generally considered as a first line option in the treatment of BD depression due to limited efficacy for evidence as well as potential deleterious short- and long-term consequences (switch to mania, rapid cycling, mixed states) (Pacchiarotti et al., 2013; Goodwin et al., 2016). In the presence of mixed features during either manic or depressive episodes, antidepressants should be discontinued and a mood-stabilizer initiated; olanzapine, aripiprazole, lurasidone, and ziprasidone could be considered (Verdolini et al., 2018).

During the last few years, promising new pharmacological treatment options have been explored and tested in BD. These compounds include the active glutamate NMDA-receptor antagonist ketamine, which has shown promising results in the treatment of bipolar depression, particularly in the setting of refractoriness and suicidality (Wilkinson et al., 2018). The main limitations of ketamine are related to its form of administration (intravenous being most common), short half-life (and therefore the need of repeated doses), and dissociative experiences that can be distressing for the patient. New clinical trials using esketamine (which can be administered intranasally), are starting to show preliminary encouraging results in the treatment of treatment-resistant unipolar depression (Canuso et al., 2018). Whilst these results require replication in bipolar depression, the fact that the original formulation has shown benefits in BD suggests esketamine might have a role as well. Other pharmacological add-on therapeutic pathways currently being explored – but with less consistent supporting evidence – include inositol, pramipexole, polyunsaturated fatty acids, n-acetylcysteine, anti-inflammatory agents, and probiotics (Vazquez et al., 2018).

It is important to note that the irregular or non-adherence is a problematic issue in BD, being associated with increased recurrences, greater morbidity, treatment nonresponse, and suicide (Baldessarini et al., 2008). It has been suggested that non-adherence is more frequent in men with BD (Vega et al., 2011; Kriegshauser et al., 2010). Hence, it is important to assess this situation in all patients, especially in males, and facilitate therapeutic strategies to increase medication adherence (Thase, 2012).

Despite its age and undeserved reputation, electroconvulsive therapy (ECT) continues to be a highly effective and relatively safe therapeutic option in severely ill patients in both depressive and poles of BD as well as in those with a rapid-cycling course or mixed states (Schoeyen et al., 2015).

Psychological Treatments

Adjunctive psychological interventions as an add-on to pharmacological treatment have been shown to improve long-term outcomes in BD. Those with rapidly growing evidence for efficacy are individual and group psychoeducation, family-focused interventions, cognitive behavioural therapy (CBT), interpersonal social rhythm therapy, and functional remediation. The third-generation therapies such as mindfulness-based approaches have been increasingly tested in this population, but with inconclusive results thus far (Reinares et al., 2014). Several barriers limit the broad implementation of these psychological treatments, the most important being the gap between availability and demand. There is a consensus in the literature that the shortcomings of traditional models of episodic care are suboptimal for improving chronic disease outcomes contributing to a high burden of chronic mental illness.

Many of the interventions afore-mentioned are offered exclusively through face-to-face individual or group meetings at few specialized clinics, unevenly geographically distributed and for a limited period. Adapting such interventions to individual characteristics in a cost-efficient way represents an important challenge (Reinares et al., 2014). There is an emerging interest in exploring new approaches to delivering these kinds of treatment, tailored to individual needs and in a continuous way (e.g., all year long) from any location, while maintaining their efficacy at a low cost through internet-based platforms (Hidalgo-Mazzei et al., 2015).

Other Therapeutic Approaches

Advances and progress have been made to improve the efficacy and safety of techniques such as light therapy with or without total sleep deprivation and repetitive transcranial magnetic stimulation (rTMS) in BD. These, when available, might have enough evidence to justify a role as an adjunctive therapy in BD (Yatham et al., 2018). Regarding more invasive options such as vagus nerve stimulation (VNS) and deep brain stimulation (DBS), considering that their evidence is limited and mostly extrapolated from unipolar depression cases, any use should be carefully and jointly evaluated by clinicians, specialists, and the patient after a case-by-case discussion of potential risk and benefits (Kisely et al., 2018).

Conclusions

BD is a chronic illness with often severe consequences for those suffering from it and for society as a whole. Considering the particular characteristics and course in men, early detection and timely treatment of the disorder are crucial to prevent relapses and increase the chances of a better prognosis. Optimal management requires regular and systematic lifetime follow-up by a multidisciplinary team of healthcare professionals as well as consistent commitment from the patient. There are several effective therapeutic options available which should be adapted to the patients' specific preferences and clinical circumstances. Promising advances in understanding and treating BD will hopefully provide a better understanding of the biologic mechanisms underlying the disorder, as well as more accurate, predictive, and diagnostic

biomarkers. In parallel, new technologies will be able to extend current treatments that could be tailored not only to gender but to personal and clinical characteristics.

Box 14.5 Principles of treatment in BD

- Long-term pharmacological treatment is the cornerstone of BD management, having shown to reduce relapses, mitigate symptoms, and improve the overall prognosis
- The choice of the drug depends mainly on the current symptoms as well as on the previous phases of the illness, tailored to the individual characteristics and preferences of the patient
- During euthymic phases, lithium has a solid evidence in prevention of relapse of both poles; valproate or dopamine antagonists for manic episodes, and lamotrigine for depressive episodes
- For acute episodes, dopamine antagonists demonstrated efficacy for manic episodes while olanzapine plus fluoxetine, quetiapine, and lurasidone are effective for depressive episodes
- The use of antidepressants during depressive phases should not generally be considered first choice due to potential short and long-term consequences
- Adjunctive psychological interventions as an add-on to pharmacological treatment have shown to improve long-term outcomes of BD

References

Adan, A., Marquez-Arrico, J. E., and Gilchrist, G. 2017. Comparison of health-related quality of life among men with different co-existing severe mental disorders in treatment for substance use. *Health and Quality of Life Outcomes*, 15(1), 209.

Alonso, J. et al. 2011. Days out of role due to common physical and mental conditions: results from the WHO World Mental Health surveys. *Molecular Psychiatry*, 16(12), 1234–46.

American Psychiatric Association. 2013. *Diagnostic and Statistical Manual of Mental Disorders, 5th Edition: DSM-5*. Arlington, VA: American Psychiatric Publishing.

Angst, J. et al. 2005. The HCL-32: towards a self-assessment tool for hypomanic symptoms in outpatients. *Journal of Affective Disorders*, 88(2), 217–33.

Arnold, L. M. 2003. Gender differences in bipolar disorder. *The Psychiatric Clinics of North America*, 26(3), 595–620.

Baldassano, C. F. et al. 2005. Gender differences in bipolar disorder: retrospective data from the first 500 STEP-BD participants. *Bipolar Disorders*, 7(5), 465–70.

Baldessarini, R. J., Perry, R., and Pike, J. 2008. Factors associated with treatment nonadherence among US bipolar disorder patients. *Human Psychopharmacology: Clinical and Experimental*, 23(2), 95–105.

Belmaker, R. H. and Bersudsky, Y. 2004. Bipolar disorder: mania and depression. *Discovery Medicine*, 4(23), 239–45.

Bonnín, C. M. et al. 2012. Subthreshold symptoms in bipolar disorder: impact on neurocognition, quality of life and disability. *Journal of Affective Disorders*, 136(3), 650–9.

Canuso, C. M. et al. 2018. Efficacy and Safety of Intranasal Esketamine for the Rapid Reduction of Symptoms of Depression and Suicidality in Patients at Imminent Risk for Suicide: Results of a Double-Blind, Randomized, Placebo-Controlled Study. *American Journal of Psychiatry*, 175(7), 620–30.

Carvalho, A. F. et al. 2016. Bias in emerging biomarkers for bipolar disorder. *Psychological Medicine*, 46(11), 2287–97.

Clemente, A. S. et al. 2015. Bipolar disorder prevalence: a systematic review and meta-analysis of the literature. *Revista Brasileira de Psiquiatria*, 37(2), 155–61.

Collins, P. Y. et al. 2011. Grand challenges in global mental health. *Nature*, 475(7354), 27–30.

Craddock, N. and Sklar, P. 2013. Genetics of bipolar disorder. *The Lancet*, 381(9878), 1654–62.

Crump, C. et al. 2013. Comorbidities and mortality in bipolar disorder. *JAMA Psychiatry*, 70(9), 931.

Diflorio, A. and Jones, I. 2010. Is sex important? Gender differences in bipolar disorder. *International Review of Psychiatry*, 22(5), 437–52.

Dilsaver, S. C. 2011. An estimate of the minimum economic burden of bipolar I and II disorders in the United States: 2009. *Journal of Affective Disorders*, 129(1–3), 79–83.

Fajutrao, L. et al. 2009. A systematic review of the evidence of the burden of bipolar disorder in Europe. *Clinical Practice and Epidemiology in Mental Health: CP and EMH*, 5, 3.

Ferrari, A. J., Baxter, A. J., and Whiteford, H. A. 2011. A systematic review of the global distribution and availability of prevalence data for bipolar disorder. *Journal of Affective Disorders*, 134(1–3), 1–13.

First, M. B. 1995. *Structured Clinical Interview for the DSM (SCID)*. Wiley Online Library.

Flores-Ramos, M. et al. 2017. Is it important to consider the sex of the patient when using lithium or valproate to treat the bipolar disorder? *Pharmacology Biochemistry and Behavior*, 152, 105–11.

Forty, L. et al. 2014. Comorbid medical illness in bipolar disorder. *The British Journal of Psychiatry: The Journal of Mental Science*, 205(6), 465–72.

Frye, M. A. et al. 2003. Gender differences in prevalence, risk, and clinical correlates of alcoholism comorbidity in bipolar disorder. *American Journal of Psychiatry*, 160(5), 883–9.

Goes, F. S. et al. 2010. Sex-specific association of the reelin gene with bipolar disorder. *American Journal of Medical Genetics Part B: Neuropsychiatric Genetics*, 153B(2), 549–53.

Goldberg, J. F. and Ernst, C. L. 2002. Features associated with the delayed initiation of mood stabilizers at illness onset in bipolar disorder. *The Journal of Clinical Psychiatry*, 63(11), 985–91.

Goodwin, G. M. et al. 2016. Evidence-based guidelines for treating bipolar disorder: revised third edition recommendations from the British Association for Psychopharmacology. *Journal of Psychopharmacology*, 30(6), 495–553.

Gore, F. M. et al. 2011. Global burden of disease in young people aged 10–24 years: a systematic analysis. *The Lancet*, 377(9783), 2093–2102.

Grande, I. et al. 2013. Occupational disability in bipolar disorder: analysis of predictors of being on severe disablement benefit (PREBIS study data). *Acta Psychiatrica Scandinavica*, 127(5), 403–11.

Grande, I. et al. 2016. Bipolar disorder. *The Lancet*, 387(10027), 1561–72.

Hidalgo-Mazzei, D., Mateu, A., et al. 2015. Internet-based psychological interventions for bipolar disorder: Review of the present and insights into the future. *Journal of Affective Disorders*, 188, 1–13.

Hidalgo-Mazzei, D., Walsh, E., et al. 2015. Comorbid bipolar disorder and borderline personality disorder and substance use disorder. *The Journal of Nervous and Mental Disease*, 203(1), 54–7.

Judd, L. L. et al. 2002. The long-term natural history of the weekly symptomatic status of bipolar

I disorder. *Archives of General Psychiatry*, 59(6), 530–7.

Kawa, I. et al. 2005. Gender differences in bipolar disorder: age of onset, course, comorbidity, and symptom presentation. *Bipolar Disorders*, 7(2), 119–25.

Kennedy, N. et al. 2005. Gender differences in incidence and age at onset of mania and bipolar disorder over a 35-year period in Camberwell, England. *American Journal of Psychiatry*, 162(2), 257–62.

Kisely, S. et al. 2018. A systematic review and meta-analysis of deep brain stimulation for depression. *Depression and Anxiety*, 35(5), 468–80.

Kriegshauser, K. et al. 2010. Gender differences in subjective experience and treatment of bipolar disorder. *The Journal of Nervous and Mental Disease*, 198(5), 370–2.

Kupfer, D. J. et al. 2002. Demographic and clinical characteristics of individuals in a bipolar disorder case registry. *The Journal of Clinical Psychiatry*, 63(2), 120–5.

Licht, R. W., Vestergaard, P., and Brodersen, A. 2008. Long-term outcome of patients with bipolar disorder commenced on lithium prophylaxis during hospitalization: a complete 15-year register-based follow-up. *Bipolar Disorders*, 10(1), 79–86.

Maletic, V. and Raison, C. 2014. Integrated neurobiology of bipolar disorder. *Frontiers in Psychiatry*, 5, 98.

Martínez-Arán, A. et al. 2004. Cognitive function across manic or hypomanic, depressed, and euthymic states in bipolar disorder. *The American Journal of Psychiatry*, 161(2), 262–70.

Martino, D. J. et al. 2015. Neurocognitive functioning in the premorbid stage and in the first episode of bipolar disorder: a systematic review. *Psychiatry Research*, 226(1), 23–30.

Martino, D. J. et al. 2016. A critical overview of the clinical evidence supporting the concept of neuroprogression in bipolar disorder. *Psychiatry Research*, 235, 1–6.

McCarthy, M. J. et al. 2014. Whole brain expression of bipolar disorder associated genes: structural and genetic analyses. *PloS One*, 9(6), e100204.

Merikangas, K. R. et al. 2011. Prevalence and correlates of bipolar spectrum disorder in the world mental health survey initiative. *Archives of General Psychiatry*, 68(3), 241–51.

Michalak, E. E. et al. 2006. Bipolar disorder and quality of life: a patient-centered perspective. *Quality of Life Research: An International Journal of Quality of Life Aspects of Treatment, Care and Rehabilitation*, 15(1), 25–37.

Mitchell, R. H. et al. 2018. Sex differences in brain structure among adolescents with bipolar disorder. *Bipolar Disorders*, 20(5), 448–58.

The National Institute for Health and Care Excellence. 2014. Bipolar disorder: assessment and management. NICE Clinical Guideline, 185 (February 2016).

Ohadi, M. et al. 2007. Gender dimorphism in the DAT1-67 T-allele homozygosity and predisposition to bipolar disorder. *Brain Research*, 1144, 142–5.

Öhlund, L. et al. 2018. Reasons for lithium discontinuation in men and women with bipolar disorder: a retrospective cohort study. *BMC Psychiatry*, 18(1), 37.

Pacchiarotti, I. et al. 2013. The International Society for Bipolar Disorders (ISBD) task force report on antidepressant use in bipolar disorders. *The American Journal of Psychiatry*, 170(11), 1249–62.

Perlis, R. H. et al. 2006. Predictors of recurrence in bipolar disorder: primary outcomes from the Systematic Treatment Enhancement Program for Bipolar Disorder (STEP-BD). *The American Journal of Psychiatry*, 163(2), 217–24.

Popovic, D. et al. 2012. Polarity index of pharmacological agents used for maintenance treatment of bipolar disorder. *European Neuropsychopharmacology*, 22(5), 339–46.

Reinares, M., Sánchez-Moreno, J., and Fountoulakis, K. N. 2014. Psychosocial interventions in bipolar disorder: what, for whom, and when. *Journal of Affective Disorders*, 156, 46–55.

Schoeyen, H. K. et al. 2015. Treatment-resistant bipolar depression: a randomized controlled trial of electroconvulsive therapy versus algorithm-based pharmacological treatment. *American Journal of Psychiatry*, 172(1), 41–51.

Scott, J. and Leboyer, M. 2011. Consequences of delayed diagnosis of bipolar disorders. *L'Encéphale*, 37, S173–S175.

Severus, E. et al. 2014. Lithium for prevention of mood episodes in bipolar disorders: systematic review and meta-analysis. *International Journal of Bipolar Disorders*, 2, 15.

Solé, B. et al. 2012. Neurocognitive impairment across the bipolar spectrum. *CNS Neuroscience and Therapeutics*, 18(3), 194–200.

Solé, B. et al. 2017. Cognitive impairment in bipolar disorder: treatment and prevention strategies. *The International Journal of Neuropsychopharmacology*, 20(8), 670–80.

Suwalska, A. and Łojko, D. 2014. Sex dependence of cognitive functions in bipolar disorder. *The Scientific World Journal*, 2014, article ID: 418432, 10pp., doi: 10.1155/2014/418432.

Thase, M. E. 2012. Strategies for increasing treatment adherence in bipolar disorder. *The Journal of Clinical Psychiatry*, 73(02), e08.

Tidemalm, D. et al. 2014. Attempted suicide in bipolar disorder: risk factors in a cohort of 6086 patients. K. Hashimoto, ed. *PLoS One*, 9(4), e94097.

Tournikioti, K. et al. 2018. Sex-related variation of neurocognitive functioning in bipolar disorder: focus on visual memory and associative learning. *Psychiatry Research*, 267, 499–505.

Valentí, M. et al. 2015. Risk factors for rapid cycling in bipolar disorder. *Bipolar Disorders*, 17(5), 549–59.

Vazquez, G. H. et al. 2018. Potential novel treatments for bipolar depression: ketamine, fatty acids, anti-inflammatory agents, and probiotics. *CNS and Neurological Disorders – Drug Targets*, 16(8), 858–69.

Vega, P. et al. 2011. Bipolar disorder differences between genders: special considerations for women. *Women's Health*, 7(6), 663–76.

Vemuri, M. et al. 2011. Gender-specific lipid profiles in patients with bipolar disorder. *Journal of Psychiatric Research*, 45(8), 1036–41.

Verdolini, N. et al. 2018. Mixed states in bipolar and major depressive disorders: systematic review and quality appraisal of guidelines. *Acta Psychiatrica Scandinavica*, 138(3), 196–222.

Vieta, E. et al. 2013. Clinical management and burden of bipolar disorder: results from a multinational longitudinal study (WAVE-bd). *The International Journal of Neuropsychopharmacology / Official Scientific Journal of the Collegium Internationale Neuropsychopharmacologicum (CINP)*, 16(8), 1719–32.

Vieta, E. et al. 2013. The clinical implications of cognitive impairment and allostatic load in bipolar disorder. *European Psychiatry: The Journal of the Association of European Psychiatrists*, 28(1), 21–9.

Whiteford, H. A. et al. 2013. Global burden of disease attributable to mental and substance use disorders: findings from the Global Burden of Disease Study 2010. *The Lancet*, 382 (9904), 1575–86.

Wilkinson, S. T. et al. 2018. The effect of a single dose of intravenous ketamine on suicidal ideation: a systematic review and individual participant data meta-analysis. *American Journal of Psychiatry*, 175 (2), 150–8.

Wooderson, S. C. et al. 2015. An exploration of testosterone levels in patients with bipolar disorder. *BJPsych Open*, 1(2), 136–8.

Xu, C. et al. 2013. Polymorphisms in seizure 6-like gene are associated with bipolar disorder I: Evidence of gene×gender interaction. *Journal of Affective Disorders*, 145(1), 95–9.

Yatham, L. N. et al. 2018. Canadian Network for Mood and Anxiety Treatments (CANMAT) and International Society for Bipolar Disorders (ISBD) 2018 guidelines for the management of patients with bipolar disorder. *Bipolar Disorders*, 20(2), 97–170.

Zimmerman, M. 2016. A review of 20 years of research on overdiagnosis and underdiagnosis in the Rhode Island Methods to Improve Diagnostic Assessment and Services (MIDAS) project. *Canadian Journal of Psychiatry / Revue canadienne de psychiatrie*, 61 (2), 71–9.

Zimmerman, M. et al. 2011. Are screening scales for bipolar disorder good enough to be used in clinical practice? *Comprehensive Psychiatry*, 52(6), 600–6.

Zimmerman, M. et al. 2014. Comorbid bipolar disorder and borderline personality disorder and history of suicide attempts. *Journal of Personality Disorders*, 28(3), 358–64.

Zimmerman, M. and Morgan, T. A. 2013. Problematic boundaries in the diagnosis of bipolar disorder: the interface with borderline personality disorder. *Current Psychiatry Reports*, 15(12), 422.

Chapter

15

The Mental Health of Men Who Offend

Daria Korobanova and Kimberlie Dean

The overwhelming majority of those who come into contact with the criminal justice system (CJS) as offenders are male; this is true even when considered across the spectrum of offence types (with specific exceptions), across jurisdictions and across time. Much of the research focused on the mental health of those in contact with the CJS has consequently been about male, rather than female, offenders.

What Are the Rates of Offending amongst Men?

According to the United Nations Crime Trend Survey (UN-CTS), men continue to make up the majority of persons suspected of crime (84%), convicted of crime (86%), and imprisoned (94%), worldwide (based on the 'most recent year data' provided by each country included in the survey for the period 2009–13; Heiskanen and Lietonen, 2017). Globally, the number of men and women imprisoned has risen steadily but the overall male-to-female ratio has remained much the same. Imprisonment patterns do, however, vary across jurisdictions, with some countries witnessing a recent decrease in male imprisonment rates (e.g., of 4.2% from 2006 to 2016 in the USA) (Carson, 2018). In addition, some countries have seen an emerging reduction in the gender gap for imprisonment. In Australia, for example, the growth of imprisonment (total number and imprisonment rate) for men has been slower than it has for women during the period 2007 to 2017 (Australian Bureau of Statistics, 2017b).

What Explains the Gender Gap amongst Offenders?

The dramatic over-representation of men in samples of offenders has been the focus of much investigation. Differences in the seriousness of offending behaviour and the consequent length of custodial sentences received are likely to explain at least some of the very wide gender gaps seen in incarcerated populations. For example, the gender gap in the Australian prison population for offences that involve physical violence towards another person (e.g., sexual assault; abduction and harassment; robbery and extortion; acts intended to cause injury; homicide) is greater than for non-violent offences (e.g., illicit drug offences, theft and related offences; and fraud, deception and related offences; Australian Bureau of Statistics, 2017b). Another factor likely to contribute to the wide gender gap in incarcerated populations relates to the possibility of biases operating in the CJS (i.e., the differential rates, by gender, of being suspected of crime, of conviction and of being given a prison sentence following conviction, for a particular offence). In the UN-CTS study highlighted earlier, 13% of men suspected of a crime were subsequently convicted, compared to 5% of women (i.e., almost three times higher; Heiskanen and Lietonen, 2017), while 25% of convicted men compared to 10% of convicted women were sentenced to imprisonment (i.e., almost two and a half times more likely; Heiskanen and Lietonen, 2017). Thus, in addition to the consequences of more serious offending, it is argued that courts are more likely to find men guilty of an offence, compared to women charged with the same offence; and that following conviction, they are more likely to imprison men and sentence them to longer periods of incarceration (see also Heidensohn and Silverstri, 2012; Rodriguez et al., 2006; Starr, 2014). It has also been demonstrated that men with mental illness may be less likely than women to be diverted from the CJS into mental health treatment (Box 15.1; Soon et al., 2018).

Beyond the nature of offences committed and the potential for gender biases to operate in the CJS, a wide range of factors and theories have been proposed to explain the large gender gap still seen when relative rates of offending behaviour – particularly violent and aggressive behaviour – are considered. These include both biological (e.g., genes, hormonal differences, neurobiological differences) and environmental factors (e.g., societal expectations/reinforcement of gender roles and behaviour), as well as a consideration of the potential for interaction between factors (Staniloiu and Markowitsch, 2012). Intermediate between such potential causal factors and the gender gap seen in offending behaviour, men have been shown to demonstrate behaviour strongly associated with offending, such as higher levels of trait impulsivity and lower levels of self-control (Strüber et al., 2008). Rebellon et al. (2016) provide a review of many of the psychosocial theories that attempt to explain the gender gap, including learning theory (e.g., Akers, 1990, 2009), control theories (e.g., Gottfredson and Hirschi, 1990; Hagan et al., 1990; Hagan et al., 1987), and strain theory (e.g., Broidy and Agnew, 1997). The authors also explore the role of anticipated guilt in explaining gender differences in rates of delinquency; while Bennett et al. (2005) consider the role of differences in the development of socio-cognitive skills between men and women. Overall, the picture of factors underpinning the gender gap in offending behaviour, and in the rates of contact with the CJS, is a complex one.

What Are the Characteristics of Men Who Offend?

As suggested by the identified factors and postulated theories arising from an examination of the gender gap amongst offenders, some differences in the characteristics of male and female offenders have been found, including in terms of both socio-demographic and offending profiles. Table 15.1 presents data from several Australian sources, including from the state of New South Wales (NSW), to provide a profile of male and female prisoners, where the latest figures indicate that men make up 92.0% of the prison population (Australian Bureau of Statistics, 2018). Male prisoners in NSW were found to have better pre-custody employment histories than women, but the prevalence of being single and living alone prior to imprisonment did not appear to differ greatly by gender. Men in Australian prisons were, on average, serving longer sentences than women, and women were slightly more likely to be held on remand (Corben, 2016). For both men and women, the three most common offences (with the exception of sexual offences for men) were illicit drug offences, acts intended to cause injury, and unlawful entry with intent; this group of offences accounted for approximately 50% of the most serious offences for both men and women. Sexual assault and related offences were, however, more common amongst male prisoners (12.5%) than female prisoners (1.6%), while a higher proportion of women had illicit drug offences (21.4%), theft and related offences (7.7%), and fraud, deception, and related offences (8.5%) recorded as their most serious offence, compared to men (14.4%, 3.6%, and 1.8%, respectively). Finally, men were more likely to have been imprisoned previously (57.4% vs 45.6% in women), a finding that may reflect differences in the life-course patterns of offending between men and women.

It should also be noted that men of indigenous and other ethnic minority backgrounds are often over-represented in prison populations, although in Australian prisons the extent of over-representation of individuals with an Aboriginal and/or Torres Strait Islander background is even greater for women than it is for men (36.8% for men and 50.6% for women compared to 2.8% for both sexes in the general population; Australian Bureau of Statistics, 2017a). Elevated incarceration rates for Indigenous peoples have also been reported in New Zealand, where 50% of the prison population identify as Maori (New Zealand Department of Corrections, 2015), compared to 14.9% in the general population.

Table 15.1 Key characteristics of men and women in custody in Australia, including specifically in the state of New South Wales (NSW)

Characteristics	Men	Women
Demographic Characteristics		
Aboriginal and/or Torres Strait Islander[1] (Australia)	36.8%	50.6%
Age group[2] (Australia):		
18–29 years	33.8%	34.7%
30–39 years	33.2%	34.3%
40 + years	33.0%	31.0%
Single/never married[3] (NSW)	55.8%	54.9%
Employed prior to prison[3] (NSW)	48.2%	26.1%
Lived alone prior to prison[3] (NSW)	19.0%	18.5%
Offending Characteristics		
Most serious offence/charge[2] in current episode (Australia):		
Assault, abduction, harassment, and other offences against the person	24.5%	20.9%
Illicit drug offences	14.4%	21.4%
Sexual assault and related offences	12.5%	1.6%
Unlawful entry with intent	10.5%	9.5%
Other offences	8.3%	8.5%
Robbery, extortion, and related offences	7.6%	5.8%
Homicide and related offences	7.5%	8.0%
Theft, fraud, deception, and related offences	5.4%	16.2%
Property damage, public order, traffic, and miscellaneous offences	3.9%	4.2%
Dangerous or negligent acts endangering persons	3.8%	3.4%
Prohibited and regulated weapons and explosives offences	1.6%	0.6%
Length of aggregate sentence[4] (NSW):		
Not under sentence (i.e., on remand)	32.1%	42.4%
< 6 months	3.5%	6.1%
≥ 6 months to < 1 year	8.4%	11.0%
1 year to < 5 years	29.6%	25.7%
5 years to < 10 years	13.6%	8.1%
10 years to < 20 years	7.5%	3.1%
20 years or more	3.8%	3.2%
Life	0.8%	0.3%
Forensic patient[5]	0.7%	0.2%
Prior imprisonment[2] (Australia)	57.4%	45.6%

[1] Australian Bureau of Statistics (2018), *Corrective Services, Australia, March Quarter 2018*. Canberra: Australian Bureau of Statistics, retrieved from www.abs.gov.au/ausstats/abs@.nsf/mf/4512.0
[2] Australian Bureau of Statistics (2017), *Prisoners in Australia, 2017*. Canberra: Australian Bureau of Statistics retrieved from www.abs.gov.au/ausstats/abs@.nsf/mf/4517.0
[3] Justice Health and Forensic Mental Health Network (2017), 2015 Network Patient Health Survey Report. Sydney, Australia: Justice Health and Forensic Mental Health Network.
[4] Corben, 2016. NSW Inmate Census 2016: Summary of characteristics, NSW: Department of Corrective Services.
[5] In NSW, Australia, either found Not Guilty by Reason of Mental Illness (NHMI) or found unfit to plead and ordered to be detained.

Mental Health of Men in Contact with the CJS

Severe Mental Illness

It is well recognized that both men and women in contact with the CJS, particularly those incarcerated, experience high rates of mental illness compared to the general population (Butler et al., 2006). In a systematic review and meta-analysis, Fazel and Seewald (2012) reported a pooled prevalence of 3.6% for psychosis and 10.2% for major depression for imprisoned men. In the United Kingdom, one recent study found that 14.2% of men in custody met the diagnostic criteria for psychosis and 20.3% met the criteria for a depressive episode (Bebbington et al., 2017). A similar rate of psychosis (14%) was reported in an earlier New Zealand study and an even higher prevalence of depression (47%) was found (Brinded et al., 2001). The prevalence of psychiatric morbidity varies considerably between jurisdictions, likely due to differences in case ascertainment methodology (e.g., self-report vs diagnostic interviews), sampling (e.g., violent vs non-violent offenders), and differences in legal provisions intended to reduce the burden of mental illness amongst prisoners (e.g., legal support for diversion of the mentally ill at court; Fazel et al., 2016). One of the more consistent findings is that men on remand experience higher levels of psychiatric morbidity than men who are sentenced (Brinded et al., 2001; Butler et al., 2005). Related to this finding, it appears that cross-sectional surveys are likely to underestimate the true level of mental health need amongst prisoners, since studies focused specifically on prison entrants have reported even higher rates of illness (Butler et al., 2005; Dirkzwager and Nieuwbeerta, 2018). The burden of mental illness amongst incarcerated males is also seen in samples of young men in juvenile detention. A systematic review of twenty-five surveys of young people in custody reported that 3.3% of adolescent boys experienced psychotic illness, 10.6% were diagnosed with depression, and 11.7% had ADHD (Fazel et al., 2008).

Whilst not all studies include both male and female prisoners – or if they do the numbers of women may be too small to enable rigorous comparison – it does appear that the prevalence of mental illness is higher amongst female compared to male prisoners (Andersen et al., 1996; Brinded et al., 2001; Bronson and Berzofsky, 2017; James and Glaze,

2006). This is consistent with the finding that the gender gap seen in the general population with regard to risk of offending is considerably narrowed amongst those with serious mental illness. Although the difference was not found to be statistically significant, one meta-analysis of the association between psychosis and violence found the relative risk to be doubled in women (pooled OR 7.9; 95% CI 4.0–15.4) compared to men (pooled OR 4.0; 95% CI 3.0–5.3; Fazel et al., 2009). Interestingly, the gender gap for victims of crime and violence in the general population mirrors that for offenders and is similarly narrowed (or even reversed) amongst those with serious mental illnesses (Khalifeh and Dean, 2010).

Research focused on mental illness amongst prisoners has been dominated by cross-sectional studies, but in a recent longitudinal sample of men entering custody in the Netherlands, prospective follow-up to determine the course of mental health symptoms was undertaken over 18 months (Dirkzwager and Nieuwbeerta, 2018). The level of mental health symptoms declined during the period of imprisonment, although even at the end of follow-up, men in custody in this sample continued to experience mental health symptoms that were significantly higher than men in the community. The finding of levels of mental health symptoms or psychological distress peaking at entry into custody is consistent with other longitudinal prison studies with shorter follow-up periods (Hassan et al., 2011).

Fewer studies of mental illness in samples of male offenders have been conducted outside custodial settings. In an Australian cross-sectional study of police detainees (Baksheev et al., 2010), male detainees were approximately ten times more likely to have a mood disorder and fifteen times more likely to have a diagnosis of a psychotic disorder than men in the community. In a UK police-contact study, those individuals detained in police cells overnight presented with significantly higher rates of psychiatric diagnoses at a magistrates court than those who were attending court from the community (Shaw et al., 1999). It is likely that those with more serious mental disorders are detained overnight due to disorganized and other behaviours associated with the presence of severe mental illness.

From a life-course perspective, the majority of men who offend as adults are likely to have had their first conviction when much younger (McGee and Farrington, 2010), but the impact of mental illness on life-course patterns of offending is not well established. There is some evidence to indicate that the presence of a severe mental illness such as schizophrenia or bipolar disorder may be associated with a higher risk of recidivism (Baillargeon et al., 2009; Fazel and Yu, 2011). Beyond risk of reoffending, ex-prisoners with a history of mental disorder are at increased risk of a range of adverse outcomes, including higher rates of substance use, unemployment, psychological distress, self-harm, and the need for ongoing contact with mental health and primary care services (Cutcher et al., 2014).

Substance Use Disorders

Substance use problems are overall more common in males than females (see Chapter 18). Substance use is highly prevalent amongst those in contact with the CJS, and the level of substance use problems co-morbid with mental illness is also high (Butler et al., 2011; Fazel and Seewald, 2012). In a systematic review of prison-based studies, the overall prevalence of alcohol use disorders was found to range from 17.7% to 30.0%, and prevalence of drug use disorders was estimated to be between 10.0% and 48.0%, with prevalence rates found to be higher in male prison entrants than in cross-sectional prison samples (Fazel et al., 2006). Among Dutch male prison entrants, for example, 39.2% reported heavy drinking and 43.3% reported heavy drug use in the twelve months prior to imprisonment (Dirkzwager and Nieuwbeerta, 2018). The presence of substance use disorders, particularly when co-morbid with severe mental illness, is associated with a number of adverse outcomes for male prisoners, including a higher risk of self-harm and suicide (Baillargeon, Penn, et al., 2009). Following release from prison, substance use problems are also associated with an increased risk of mortality (Chang et al., 2015), due to accidental overdose as well as from suicide.

Self-Harm and Suicide

Prisoners are at elevated risk of self-harm and suicide, as are those in contact with the CJS more generally. One national-register study in Denmark found that more than a third of all adult male suicides in the general population had a history of some contact with the CJS (Webb et al., 2011). In a large international study of prison suicide, rates amongst men in prison were found to be much higher than in the general population, with rate ratios ranging from 1.6 (95% CI 1.4–1.8) in the USA to 10.2 (95% CI 4.6–22.7) in Norway (Fazel et al., 2017). In the UK National Confidential Inquiry into Suicide and Homicide by People with Mental Illness, investigators found that one-third of all suicides in custody (both sexes; sample included 92% men) occurred within one week of imprisonment (Shaw et al., 2004). Those who completed suicide exhibited high rates of mental health problems prior to death and one-third had been in contact with community mental health services prior to imprisonment. This finding regarding the possibility of early imprisonment being a high-risk period is supported by the results of the longitudinal prison studies described earlier (Dean and Korobanova, 2018; Dirkzwager and Nieuwbeerta, 2018; Hassan et al., 2011). Historical factors, such as previous suicide attempts, having been diagnosed with a mental illness, and having been prescribed psychotropic medications, have been identified as predictors of suicide in one prison sample (comprising 97% men; Fruehwald et al., 2004).

Surveys of prisoners also find high rates of reported self-harm, both in custody, prior to prison entry, and following release. In Australia, 20% of non-Indigenous and 10% of Indigenous men entering prison reported a history of self-harm (Australian Institute of Health and Welfare, 2015), and in a large cross-sectional prison health survey conducted in the Australian state of New South Wales (NSW), 22.8% of men reported having self-harmed during the current period of imprisonment (Justice Health and Forensic Mental Health Network, 2017). In the UK, the annual rate of self-harm amongst men in custody was found to be 5% during the period between 2004 and 2009 (Hawton et al., 2014), with an average rate of two events per year. Risk factors for self-harm amongst prisoners in this study are shown in Box 15.2. In the UK, the mean annual rate of suicide amongst male inmates who self-harmed has been estimated to be 334 per 100,000; (the comparable rate amongst those

---

Box 15.2 Risk factors for self-harm amongst prisoners in the UK (Hawton et al., 2014)

- Being on remand
- Serving a life sentence
- Young age
- Being of white ethnicity
- Being in a high-security environment

without a history of self-harm being 79 per 100,000 in male inmates (Hawton et al., 2014).

Interventions for Men in Contact with the CJS

Mental health interventions and models of service delivery have been developed to address the needs of men at all stages of CJS contact (see Box 15.3) , but they have developed largely in the absence of a rigorous evidence base. Most mental health interventions and service models have been borrowed from other non-criminal justice settings, with adaptations that have been little tested, even after implementation.

Court Diversion

In the context of a need to address the burden of mental illness amongst those in contact with the CJS, particularly in prisons, mental health courts, court liaison, and court diversion services have been established in many jurisdictions internationally. These services aim to identify offenders with mental health needs at an early stage in the criminal justice process and divert them into mental health treatment. Internationally, the models adopted vary from the establishment of mental health courts with a problem-solving approach, as in many US states (Richardson and McSherry, 2010), to court-based mental health diversion and liaison services, common in the UK (James, 2010), and in many Australian states (Davidson et al., 2016). Limited information is available on court diversion approaches internationally and, in particular, with regard to the pathways and outcomes for individuals who come into contact with such services, although emerging research indicates that the impact of diversion may be positive. In the US, for example, a number of studies have found positive outcomes, including reduced recidivism rates, decreased incarceration time, improved mental health service access, and improved psycho-social functioning, at least in the short term (Broner et al., 2004; Richardson and McSherry, 2010; Steadman et al., 1999). The extent to which outcomes following court diversion might differ by sex is, however, unclear. As mentioned earlier, in one NSW cohort of individuals found eligible for diversion at local court, the majority of whom were male (75.9%), the odds of being diverted by the magistrate were lower for men compared to women (OR for women compared to men 1.40; 95% CI 1.30–1.64; Soon et al., 2018).

Box 15.3 Interventions for men in contact with the CJS

- Mental health courts
- Court liaison
- Court diversion
- Mental health service provision in prisons

  ○ Mental health screening
  ○ In-reach assessment and case management
  ○ 'prison hospital wings'

- Pre-release planning
- Post-release continuum of care

Custodial-Based Interventions and Services Models

Interventions and service models for male prisoners with mental illness have been developed largely on the basis of attempting to replicate community provision, supported by the widely accepted, but not fully enacted, principle of care equivalence that has been enshrined in policy documents at the level of the Office of the High Commission for Human Rights within the United Nations (United Nations, 1990). Mental health service provision in prisons, at least in those of sufficient size and in Western jurisdictions, typically consists of the following: universal brief screening for mental health problems amongst those entering custody; in-reach assessment and case management provided to those in the general prison population; and designated 'prison hospital wings' intended to house those inmates with the most serious mental health problems (see also Chapter 16 for a detailed discussion of mental illness in imprisoned men).

Screening for health problems, including mental illness, at prison entry is a unique element of the typical health service model seen in custodial settings and is without an obvious comparator in a non-custodial environment. Universal screening of individuals entering prison thus represents a potential opportunity to identify those with unaddressed mental health needs from amongst a group known to have high levels of morbidity but low levels of successful help-seeking in the community (Australian Institute of Health and Welfare, 2015; Howerton et al., 2007). Until recently, however, bespoke approaches to such screening had not been well developed or tested (Martin et al., 2013), and few prison studies have followed screened prisoners up over time. The extent to which screening approaches should differ for male and female prisoners, if at all, is unclear. In one UK study of prison screening that included both male and female prisoners, the prevalence of severe mental illness determined on the basis of a structured diagnostic tool was 23%, while only one-quarter of this group were identified by routine prison screening and referred to mental health services for assessment (Senior et al., 2013); 13% were taken on by in-reach services for case management. Interestingly, while the results of this study were not stratified by the sex of the prisoner, the authors did find that male gender was an independent and positive predictor of the likelihood of being taken on for case management.

In-reach services and hospital wings – together forming the key elements of most post-screening models of mental health care provision in prisons – have also been largely unevaluated, apart from simple descriptions of the models employed and the characteristics of prisoners seen by clinicians (Levy, 2005). The extent to which treatment for mental health problems in prison is effective, in terms both of mental health and other potentially related outcomes such as reoffending, is untested, as is the possibility of any differential impact by the sex of the inmate. The National Evaluation of Prison Mental Health In-Reach report (Shaw et al., 2009), a survey of in-reach services in the UK, found that while in-reach team leaders supported the idea of such services, they also thought that these services were poorly resourced and implemented. In New Zealand, a new model of care for male prisoners with serious mental illness has been trialled, with a positive impact on prison numbers seen across screening, referral, treatment, and engagement phases (Pillai et al., 2016). The new model of care in this study focused on a broadening of triggers for referral to mental health services and the addition of a triaging stage following referral.

One of the key areas of prison mental health service provision that remains to be developed and adopted is pre-release planning and post-release support. The vast majority of prisoners will return to the community, many after a relatively short period, and the disruption to mental healthcare relationships caused by incarceration can be difficult to repair on release. The post-release period is a high-risk time for prisoners, with research indicating that the early post-release period is associated with an increased risk of self-harm and suicide (Borschmann et al., 2017; Kariminia et al., 2007), among other adverse health and related outcomes. One study of over 85,000 released prisoners in

NSW, Australia, found that men had a higher post-release suicide rate than women, and that the same was true for the rate of suicides in custody (Kariminia et al., 2007). A number of research groups have begun developing and testing interventions designed to improve the continuity of mental health care during the prison-to-community transition in order to address the vulnerability of prisoners during the initial post-release period. These so-called critical-time interventions are modelled on approaches taken to mitigate risk of a return to homelessness following hospital admission and have so far demonstrated promising results (Jarrett et al., 2012; Kinner et al., 2016). Developments in interventions and models of service provision for the prison-to-community transition period are in their infancy and the extent to which benefits seen to date are replicated in both male and female prisoners is yet to be established.

Forensic Patients

In most Western jurisdictions, legal provision is made to accommodate circumstances in which an individual charged with an offence, typically a serious violent offence, is deemed to be so mentally unwell at the time of committing the offence that they are regarded as being unable, fully or partially, to be held responsible for their actions. Others may be so mentally unwell or cognitively impaired that they are unable to plead to the charges against them and/or are unfit to stand trial. While terminology and definitions, legal processes and practices, as well as models of mental health service response, vary considerably between jurisdictions, a great deal of research has been undertaken for the purpose of describing this group of mentally disordered offenders and, in particular, their risks of reoffending following release from secure care or incarceration (Fazel et al., 2016). In keeping with the evidence demonstrating a reduced gender gap for offending behaviour amongst those with severe mental illness, samples of such forensic patients tend to be dominated by men (but to a reduced extent). In a systematic review of outcomes following release from secure care, male forensic patients made up 75% of the pooled sample, with data taken from 35 individual studies (Fazel et al., 2016). Whilst overall reoffending rates were found to be low compared to those reported for comparative groups, including released prisoners, findings were not stratified by sex. In one Australian study, 85.3% of the forensic patient sample were male;

reoffending rates were relatively low for the sample as a whole and male gender was not found to predict either general or violent offending post-conditional release (Hayes, Kemp, Large, and Nielssen, 2014).

Conclusions

Men are much more likely than women to have contact with the CJS as offenders and, although both male and female offenders are known to have high rates of mental illness, the burden appears to be somewhat lower for men. There are many factors thought to explain the large 'gender gap' in offending seen in the general population and the narrowing of this gap seen in samples of individuals with mental illness, including consideration of gender differences in type/severity of offending behaviour, possible biases operating in the CJS, and gender differences in a variety of biological and environmental factors. Amongst those men in contact with the CJS, the key mental health problems that need to be identified and addressed include severe mental illnesses such as schizophrenia, co-occuring substance use disorders and risk of self-harm/suicide. Interventions and service models intended to address the mental health burden of men in contact with the CJS include court diversion, screening at prison entry, prison in-reach, and special prison wings; and, most recently, the development of interventions to improve outcomes following release from custody. Forensic patients are a group of offenders with severe mental illness who have typically committed serious violent offences and are diverted into specialized and secure forensic mental health services. The majority of forensic patients are male, although men dominate forensic patient samples to a reduced extent, and their reoffending rates post-release appear to be relatively low.

References

Akers, R. L. 1990. Rational choice, deterrence, and social learning theory in criminology: the path not taken. *J. Crim. L. and Criminology*, 81, 653.

Akers, R. L. 2009. *Social Learning and Social Structure: A General Theory of Crime and Deviance.* Piscataway, NJ: Transaction Publishers.

Andersen, H. S., Sestoft, D., Lillebæk, T., Gabrielsen, G., and Kramp, P. 1996. Prevalence of ICD-10 psychiatric morbidity in random samples of prisoners on remand. *International Journal of Law and Psychiatry*, 19(1), 61–74. doi: 10.1016/0160-2527(95)00025-9

Australian Bureau of Statistics. 2017a. *Census of Population and Housing: Reflecting Australia – Stories from the Census, 2016 – Aboriginal and Torres Strait Islander Population.* Canberra: Australian Bureau of Statistics. Retrieved from www.abs.gov.au/AUSSTATS/ abs@.nsf/Lookup/2071.0Main +Features1132016?OpenDocument.

Australian Bureau of Statistics. 2017b. *Prisoners in Australia, 2017.* Canberra: Australian Bureau of Statistics. Retrieved from www.abs .gov.au/ausstats/abs@.nsf/mf/4517.0.

Australian Bureau of Statistics. 2018. *Corrective Services, Australia, March quarter 2018.* Canberra: Australian Bureau of Statistics. Retrieved from www.abs.gov.au/ausstats/abs@.nsf/ mf/4512.0.

Australian Institute of Health and Welfare. 2015. *The Health of Australia's Prisoners 2015.* Canberra: AIHW.

Baillargeon, J., Binswanger, I. A., Penn, J. V., Williams, B. A., and Murray, O. J. 2009. Psychiatric disorders and repeat incarcerations: the revolving prison door. *American Journal of Psychiatry*, 166(1), 103–9.

Baillargeon, J., Penn, J. V., Thomas, C. R., Temple, J. R., Baillargeon, G., and Murray, O. J. 2009. Psychiatric disorders and suicide in the nation's largest state prison system. *Journal of the American Academy of Psychiatry and the Law*, 37(2), 188.

Baksheev, G. N., Thomas, S. D. M., and Ogloff, J. R. P. 2010. Psychiatric disorders and unmet needs in Australian police cells. *Australian and New Zealand Journal of Psychiatry*, 44(11), 1043–51.

Bebbington, P., Jakobowitz, S., McKenzie, N., Killaspy, H., Iveson, R., Duffield, G., and Kerr, M. 2017. Assessing needs for psychiatric treatment in prisoners: 1. Prevalence of disorder. *Soc Psychiatry Psychiatr Epidemiol*, 52(2), 221–9.

Bennett, S., Farrington, D. P., and Huesmann, L. R. 2005. Explaining gender differences in crime and violence: the importance of social cognitive skills. *Aggression and Violent Behavior*, 10(3), 263–88.

Borschmann, R., Thomas, E., Moran, P., Carroll, M., Heffernan, E., Spittal, M. J., . . . and Kinner, S. A. 2017. Self-harm following release from prison: a prospective data linkage study. *Australian and New Zealand Journal of Psychiatry*, 51(3), 250–9.

Brinded, P. M. J., Simpson, A. I. F., Laidlaw, T. M., Fairley, N., and Malcolm, F. 2001. Prevalence of psychiatric disorders in New Zealand prisons: a national study. *Australian and New Zealand Journal of Psychiatry*, 35(2), 166–73.

Broidy, L. and Agnew, R. 1997. Gender and crime: a general strain theory perspective. *Journal of Research in Crime and Delinquency*, 34(3), 275–306.

Broner, N., Lattimore, P. K., Cowell, A. J., and Schlenger, W. E. 2004. Effects of diversion on adults with co-occurring mental illness and substance use: outcomes from a national multi-site study. *Behav Sci Law*, 22(4), 519–41.

Bronson, J. and Berzofsky, M. 2017. *Indicators of Mental Health Problems Reported by Prisoners and Jail*

Inmates, 2011–12. Washington, DC: Bureau of Justice Statistics, pp. 1–16.

Butler, T., Allnutt, S., Cain, D., Owens, D., and Muller, C. 2005. Mental disorder in the New South Wales prisoner population. *Australian and New Zealand Journal of Psychiatry*, 39(5), 407–13.

Butler, T., Andrews, G., Allnutt, S., Sakashita, C., Smith, N. E., and Basson, J. 2006. Mental disorders in Australian prisoners: a comparison with a community sample. *Australian and New Zealand Journal of Psychiatry*, 40(3), 272–6.

Butler, T., Indig, D., Allnutt, S., and Mamoon, H. 2011. Co-occurring mental illness and substance use disorder among Australian prisoners. *Drug and Alcohol Review*, 30(2), 188–94.

Carson, E. A. 2018. *Prisoners in 2016*. Washington, DC: Bureau of Justice Statistics.

Chang, Z., Lichtenstein, P., Larsson, H., and Fazel, S. 2015. Substance use disorders, psychiatric disorders, and mortality after release from prison: a nationwide longitudinal cohort study. *The Lancet Psychiatry*, 2(5), 422–30.

Corben, S. 2016. *NSW Inmate Census 2016: Summary of Characteristics*. NSW: Department of Corrective Services.

Cutcher, Z., Degenhardt, L., Alati, R., and Kinner, S. A. 2014. Poor health and social outcomes for ex-prisoners with a history of mental disorder: a longitudinal study. *Australian and New Zealand Journal of Public Health*, 38(5), 424–9.

Davidson, F., Heffernan, E., Greenberg, D., Butler, T., and Burgess, P. 2016. A critical review of mental health court liaison services in Australia: a first national survey. *Psychiatry, Psychology and Law*, 23(6), 908–21.

Dean, K. and Korobanova, D. 2018. Brief mental health screening of prison entrants: psychiatric history versus symptom screening for the prediction of in-prison outcomes. *The Journal of Forensic Psychiatry and Psychology*, 29(3), 455–66.

Dirkzwager, A. and Nieuwbeerta, P. 2018. Mental health symptoms during imprisonment: a longitudinal study. *Acta Psychiatrica Scandinavica*, 138(4), 300–11.

Fazel, S., Bains, P., and Doll, H. 2006. Substance abuse and dependence in prisoners: a systematic review. *Addiction*, 101(2), 181–91.

Fazel, S., Doll, H., and Långström, N. 2008. Mental disorders among adolescents in juvenile detention and correctional facilities: a systematic review and metaregression analysis of 25 surveys. *Journal of the American Academy of Child and Adolescent Psychiatry*, 47(9), 1010–19.

Fazel, S., Fimińska, Z., Cocks, C., and Coid, J. 2016. Patient outcomes following discharge from secure psychiatric hospitals: systematic review and meta-analysis. *The British Journal of Psychiatry*, 208(1), 17–25.

Fazel, S., Gulati, G., Linsell, L., Geddes, J. R., and Grann, M. 2009. Schizophrenia and violence: systematic review and meta-analysis. *PLoS Med*, 6(8), e1000120.

Fazel, S., Hayes, A. J., Bartellas, K., Clerici, M., and Trestman, R. 2016. Mental health of prisoners: prevalence, adverse outcomes, and interventions. *The Lancet Psychiatry*, 3(9), 871–81.

Fazel, S., Ramesh, T., and Hawton, K. 2017. Suicide in prisons: an international study of prevalence and contributory factors. *The Lancet Psychiatry*, 4(12), 946–52.

Fazel, S. and Seewald, K. 2012. Severe mental illness in 33 588 prisoners worldwide: systematic review and meta-regression analysis. *The British Journal of Psychiatry*, 200(5), 364–73.

Fazel, S. and Yu, R. 2011. Psychotic disorders and repeat offending: systematic review and meta-analysis. *Schizophr Bull*, 37(4), 800–10.

Fruehwald, S., Matschnig, T., Koenig, F., Bauer, P., and Frottier, P. 2004. Suicide in custody: case–control study. *The British Journal of Psychiatry*, 185(6), 494–8.

Gottfredson, M. R. and Hirschi, T. 1990. *A General Theory of Crime*. Stanford, CA: Stanford University Press.

Hagan, J., Gillis, A. R., and Simpson, J. 1990. Clarifying and extending power-control theory. *American Journal of Sociology*, 95(4), 1024–37.

Hagan, J., Simpson, J., and Gillis, A. R. 1987. Class in the household: a power-control theory of gender and delinquency. *American Journal of Sociology*, 92(4), 788–816.

Hassan, L., Birmingham, L., Harty, M. A., Jarrett, M., Jones, P., King, C., . . . and Senior, J. 2011. Prospective cohort study of mental health during imprisonment. *The British Journal of Psychiatry*, 198(1), 37–42.

Hawton, K., Linsell, L., Adeniji, T., Sariaslan, A., and Fazel, S. 2014. Self-harm in prisons in England and Wales: an epidemiological study of prevalence, risk factors, clustering, and subsequent suicide. *The Lancet*, 383(9923), 1147–54.

Hayes, H., Kemp, R. I., Large, M. M., and Nielssen, O. B. 2014. A 21-year retrospective outcome study of New South Wales forensic patients granted conditional and unconditional release. *Australian and New Zealand Journal of Psychiatry*, 48(3), 259–82.

Heidensohn, F. and Silverstri, M. 2012. Gender and crime. In M. Maguire, R. Morgan, and R. Reiner (eds) The Oxford Handbook of Criminology, vol. 5. Oxford: Oxford University Press.

Heiskanen, M. and Lietonen, A. 2017. *Crime and Gender: A Study on How Men and Women Are Represented in International Crime Statistics*. Helsinki: HEUNI.

Howerton, A., Byng, R., Campbell, J., Hess, D., Owens, C., and Aitken, P. 2007. Understanding help seeking behaviour among male offenders: qualitative interview study. *BMJ*, 334(7588), 303.

James, D. J. and Glaze, L. E. 2006. *Bureau of Justice Statistics Special Report: Mental Health Problems of Prison and Jail Inmates*.

Washington, DC: US Department of Justice, Office of Justice Programs.

James, D. V. 2010. Diversion of mentally disordered people from the criminal justice system in England and Wales: an overview. *International Journal of Law and Psychiatry*, 33(4), 241–8.

Jarrett, M., Thornicroft, G., Forrester, A., Harty, M., Senior, J., King, C., . . . and Shaw, J. 2012. Continuity of care for recently released prisoners with mental illness: a pilot randomised controlled trial testing the feasibility of a Critical Time Intervention. *Epidemiology and Psychiatric Sciences*, 21(02), 187–93.

Justice Health and Forensic Mental Health Network. 2017. *2015 Network Patient Health Survey Report.* Sydney, Australia: Justice Health and Forensic Mental Health Network. Retrieved from www .justicehealth.nsw.gov.au/ publications/2015_NHPS_ FINALREPORT.pdf.

Kariminia, A., Law, M., Butler, T., Levy, M., Corben, S., Kaldor, J., and Grant, L. 2007. Suicide risk among recently released prisoners in New South Wales, Australia. *Medical Journal of Australia*, 187(7), 387.

Khalifeh, H. and Dean, K. 2010. Gender and violence against people with severe mental illness. *Int Rev Psychiatry*, 22(5), 535–46.

Kinner, S. A., Alati, R., Longo, M., Spittal, M. J., Boyle, F. M., Williams, G. M., and Lennox, N. G. 2016. Low-intensity case management increases contact with primary care in recently released prisoners: a single-blinded, multisite, randomised controlled trial. *J Epidemiol Community Health*, 70 (7), 683–8.

Levy, M. 2005. Prisoner health care provision: Reflections from Australia. *International Journal of Prisoner Health*, 1(1), 65–73.

Martin, M., Colman, I., Simpson, A., and McKenzie, K. 2013. Mental

health screening tools in correctional institutions: a systematic review. *BMC Psychiatry*, 13(1), 275.

McGee, T. R. and Farrington, D. P. 2010. Are there any true adult-onset offenders? *The British Journal of Criminology*, 50(3), 530–49.

New Zealand Department of Corrections. 2015. *Trends in the Offender Population 2014/15.* Online report. Retrieved from www .corrections.govt.nz/resources/ research_and_statistics/corrections-volumes-report/trends_in_the_ offender_population_201415.

Pillai, K., Rouse, P., McKenna, B., Skipworth, J., Cavney, J., Tapsell, R., . . . and Madell, D. 2016. From positive screen to engagement in treatment: a preliminary study of the impact of a new model of care for prisoners with serious mental illness. *BMC Psychiatry*, 16(1), 9.

Rebellon, C. J., Manasse, M. E., Agnew, R., Van Gundy, K. T., and Cohn, E. S. 2016. The relationship between gender and delinquency: assessing the mediating role of anticipated guilt. *Journal of Criminal Justice*, 44, 77–88.

Richardson, E. and McSherry, B. 2010. Diversion down under – Programs for offenders with mental illnesses in Australia. *International Journal of Law and Psychiatry*, 33(4), 249–57.

Rodriguez, F. S., Curry, T. R., and Lee, G. 2006. Gender differences in criminal sentencing: do effects vary across violent, property, and drug offenses? *Social Science Quarterly*, 87(2), 318–39.

Senior, J., Birmingham, L., Harty, M. A., Hassan, L., Hayes, A. J., Kendall, K., . . . and Shaw, J. 2013. Identification and management of prisoners with severe psychiatric illness by specialist mental health services. *Psychol Med*, 43(07), 1511–20.

Shaw, J., Baker, D., Hunt, I. M., Moloney, A., and Appleby, L. 2004. Suicide by prisoners: national clinical survey. *The British Journal of Psychiatry*, 184(3), 263–7.

Shaw, J., Creed, F., Price, J., Huxley, P., and Tomenson, B. 1999. Prevalence and detection of serious psychiatric disorder in defendants attending court. *The Lancet*, 353(9158), 1053–6.

Shaw, J., Senior, J., Lowthian, C., Foster, K., Clayton, R., Coxon, N., and Hassan, L. 2009. *A national evaluation of prison mental health in-reach services. Offender Health Research Network.* Retrieved from www.ohrn.nhs.uk/resource/ Research/Inreach.pdf.

Soon, Y.-L., Rae, N., Korobanova, D., Smith, C., Gaskin, C., Dixon, C., . . . and Dean, K. 2018. Mentally ill offenders eligible for diversion at local court in New South Wales (NSW), Australia: factors associated with initially successful diversion. *The Journal of Forensic Psychiatry and Psychology*, 29(5), 705–16.

Staniloiu, A. and Markowitsch, H. 2012. Gender differences in violence and aggression – a neurobiological perspective. *Procedia-Social and Behavioral Sciences*, 33, 1032–6.

Starr, S. B. 2014. Estimating gender disparities in federal criminal cases. *American Law and Economics Review*, 17(1), 127–59.

Steadman, H. J., Cocozza, J. J., and Veysey, B. M. 1999. Comparing outcomes for diverted and nondiverted jail detainees with mental illnesses. *Law Hum Behav*, 23(6), 615–27.

Strüber, D., Lück, M., and Roth, G. 2008. Sex, aggression and impulse control: an integrative account. *Neurocase*, 14(1), 93–121.

United Nations. 1990. *Basic principles for the treatment of prisoners.* Retrieved from www.ohchr.org/EN/ ProfessionalInterest/Pages/ BasicPrinciplesTreatmentOf Prisoners.aspx.

Webb, R. T., Qin, P., Stevens, H., Mortensen, P. B., Appleby, L., and Shaw, J. 2011. National study of suicide in all people with a criminal justice history. *Arch Gen Psychiatry*, 68(6), 591–9.

Chapter 16

The 'Mad and the Bad' behind Bars
Men's Mental Illness in Prisons

Joel Peter Eigen

If an eighteenth-century social reformer were to find himself suddenly in the late twentieth century and surveyed the characteristics of inmates in prison, he could be forgiven for thinking that nothing had happened regarding criminal justice policy in the intervening two-and-a-half centuries. The initial Western practice of housing the criminal and the mentally infirm under the same roof seems to have come full circle; before the 1750s, 'Houses of Correction' served to aggregate all manner of inconvenient folk: debtors, street-walkers, the mentally ill, criminal offenders. Since that time, an array of professions and academic disciplines – psychiatry, criminology, penology – parcelled out 'the mad and the bad' into separate populations, the better for study and treatment.

Accordingly, the nineteenth century witnessed the parallel construction of asylums and prisons (including juvenile institutions), fuelled by the abiding conviction that the newly envisioned buildings and the isolation from society's pressures they provided would create the optimal setting to reform a host of deviant activities and patterns of thought (Rothman, 1971). With the closure of many stand-alone psychiatric hospitals in the 1960s and 1970s, however, and with the building of 600 prisons in the USA since 1980 alone, it should come as little surprise that among the burgeoning population of Americans behind bars, the prevalence of serious mental derangement has grown to crisis proportions (Kupers, 1999).

Men's Mental Health in Prisons

Jails and prisons have of course always served as warehouses for the mentally deranged; indeed, the co-morbidity of insanity and criminality has been recognized since antiquity (Walker, 1985). The question of *how* to treat the criminal lunatic, though, has been approached in a host of ways, rarely yielding satisfactory or enduring policy (see also Chapter 5). Perhaps

the reason is that persons both deranged and criminal engage two of our most passionate social sentiments: that the sick and the infirm deserve society's solicitous care, and that the morally transgressive deserve censure and punishment. The common law's acknowledgement that violence and madness might exist in the same offender has been manifested most clearly in the Insanity Defence, formalized in the nineteenth century, although common-law acquittals on the basis of mental unsoundness can be traced to 1505 (Walker, 1968). The common law's acknowledgement of the legal significance of mental debility dates to the Middle Ages, when the element of malicious intention was required to accompany the physical doing of an act in order for criminal culpability to attach to the behaviour (Eigen, 1995).

As dramatic and vivid as historic (and contemporary) insanity trials continue to be, the plea of insanity is raised in a fraction of the criminal court's caseload: only one percent of criminal trials yearly. The Defence garners an acquittal in approximately one trial in four (Steadman et al., 1993). Focusing upon the infrequency of the formal defence, however, obscures the staggering number of mentally ill prisoners in jails and state or federal US prisons. With current estimates of 40 to 50% of inmates in need of psychiatric care and with 90% of inmates being male, the enduring and largely unmet need for medical treatment constitutes an urgent topic for any consideration of men's health (Kupers, 2005).

This chapter examines men's psychological needs in prison in the following manner. First, the elusive connection between emptying mental hospitals and the massive escalation in the size of the prison population in the USA is explored. The possible shift in populations from the state hospital to the state penitentiary – a process referred to as *transinstitutionalization* – will be the focus here. Next, the chapter takes up the challenges to mental health that prisons and jails pose to inmates, challenges that could easily

---

Box 16.1 Mass incarceration and mental illness

- Mass incarceration is the result of aggressive criminal justice policies
- Released mental patients make up only 4–7% of current prison population
- Mentally ill persons are at major disadvantage in negotiating bail, plea, and parole
- Prisoners found Incompetent to Stand Trial make up half of all patients in state hospitals

---

generate mental derangement among men with no prior history of medical diagnosis or treatment at all.

How incarceration threatens the psychological resources of those with a history of mental problems can be captured by examining the prison culture awaiting men upon admission, and why it presents such obstacles to treatment, particularly for those most in need of counselling. Whether the mentally deranged receive medical attention and the manner in which it is carried out is examined through the administrators' need to strike a balance between the institutional prerogatives to ensure security with the inmates' needs for counselling. The chapter concludes with a possible solution to prison overcrowding that threatens both the life of the mentally ill prisoner as well as the availability of care to attend to his psychological needs. The reader is also referred to Chapter 15 for a broader discussion of criminality and mental illness in men. This chapter focusses on the US prison context.

The Sociocultural Political Context

It has become commonplace to look to the shutting down of state hospitals as a powerful contributory element to the burgeoning population of prison inmates several decades later. The reasons traditionally given for the closing of state asylums include the introduction of powerful psychotropic drugs, the attractive argument that community mental health centres were by far the preferred setting to restore mental and emotional equanimity, and the federal government's decision to divert public expenditure from psychiatric hospitals to the oft-envisioned decentralized mental health centres to be located in residential communities (Scull, 1977; Harcourt, 2011a; Issac and Armat, 1990).

Were patients who would have made up the state hospital population caught up in the process eventually known as mass incarceration? The effort to account for what *might have happened* to patients

released from hospital – as well as speculating where subsequent patients would now be housed – is a daunting task that has not discouraged researchers. Indeed, the change of address for the mentally ill from asylum to prison has received much scholarly work, with most attention focused on the titanic growth in prison population *after* 1980. Yet those historians and social scientists who maintain a connection between decarceration and mass incarceration can point to only a modest, indeed *very* modest, share in the newly grown prison population: somewhere between 4 to 7% (Raphael and Stoll, 2013: 187). But had these *soi-disant* hospital patients been swept up en masse by the policies that contributed to mass incarceration, one would expect a late twentieth-century prison population of predominantly white, elderly females. Given that today's US prisons house a disproportionate number of poor African American and Hispanic young men, it is difficult to see decarceration as a significant element in the monumental rise in the number of Americans in prison (Kupers, 2005).

Regarding the gender and class composition of the inmate population, is it possible to find a more subtle connection between the last century's fundamental changes in housing the mentally ill offender? Today's students of criminal justice policy agree that mass incarceration – which significantly engaged issues of gender, race, and social class – was much more the result of modifications in criminal sentencing, aggressive policing, and increasingly punitive prosecutors routinely opting to aim for the most severe criminal charges upon conviction (Roth, 2018; Katzen, 2011). This is not to suggest, however, that aggressive police and prosecutorial efforts had little impact on the newly discharged mental patients (and for those who likely would have been candidates for hospitalization).

The result of closing state hospitals fell most directly on the poor, for whom the hospital was likely their one opportunity to obtain medical treatment. Tens of thousands of former patients suddenly faced a world without familial, occupational, medical resources. It is not difficult to imagine that zero-tolerance policing swept the vagrant, the homeless, the mentally ill sleeping rough on the streets into the maw of the criminal justice system (Kupers, 1999). After taking crime suspects – and those *not* suspected of an offence, merely annoying and obtrusive – into custody, the police have immense discretion regarding the disposition of disruptive and annoying persons: to the Emergency Room of a general hospital, to the admitting desk of a state hospital ward, or to the county jail. Once in jail, disorderly, acting-out behaviour can become a matter of further detention and eventual incarceration if the individual reacts with anger and strikes out violently.

The critical piece in the downward spiral of the indigent mentally ill is the crippling disadvantage they face when encountering a justice system ambitious in its indictment and draconian in its sentencing. How, for example, do the mentally deranged negotiate bail, navigate plea bargaining, or learn how to comport themselves at a parole hearing (Roth, 2018)? This is a justice system not only weighted on the side of the state but more than ever employed to extract the lengthiest sentence possible. In the USA, if the accused appears not just bewildered, but clueless regarding the proceedings against him, the court may opt to find him Incompetent to Stand Trial (IST) and commit him to a state hospital until such time that he recovers a sufficient level of coherence to understand the proceedings against him and to aid in his own defence (Roth, 2018).

The court's decision to interrupt the prosecution is not rare: fully half of all beds in the remaining state hospitals are occupied by these 'forensic patients'. The current estimate is that some 50,000 to 60,000 defendants are held for psychiatric evaluation each year; almost a quarter eventually deemed IST and remain in jail indefinitely (Roth, 2018: 184). There is no term limit to the disposition; the accused offender will remain in confinement until he understands enough of a trial's proceedings to satisfy the common law's requirement that he be able to provide assistance to his legal counsel. The most the Supreme Court has intruded into this process is to rule that detention before trial should take only a 'reasonable length of time'. Of course, the meaning of *reasonable* is hardly self-evident, nor is the definition of *deliberate*, in terms of the trial proceeding 'with all deliberate speed'.

Box 16.2   Mental illness, prison, and 'toxic masculinity'

- Inmate subculture consists of hyper-male traits of aggression and domination
- Physical and sexual assault are ubiquitous, constant threats
- Mentally ill prisoners are victimized by both fellow inmates and correctional guards
- 'Cell therapy' is limited; prisons opt for widespread use of powerful psychotropic drugs

---

The Impact of Imprisonment on the Mental Health of Men

Mentally ill defendants who do not escape conviction with an insanity defence (or commitment as a forensic patient, awaiting a finding of competency) encounter a criminal justice system fraught with peril, all the more tricky to navigate because of their derangement. Many mentally ill defendants enter the court system with a history of personal trauma, leaving them brittle and suspicious of what they're being told. Gender plays not only a critical role in their interactions with the police but often in the aetiology of their distress. Boys who suffered childhood abuse – physical or sexual – respond in one of two ways: either by withdrawing into social isolation or by striking out with violence (Kupers, 1999). Years later, upon encountering the apparatus of the state, they can fall back to familiar patterns. A determined effort to *remove* themselves from their immediate social setting leaves them looking uncooperative and sullen; a ready resort to violence, on the other hand, leaves them vulnerable to harsh treatment in the form of lock-up in a segregated, maximum security unit. Given the estimates quoted earlier, the correctional system is tasked with the management of mentally disturbed inmates numbering in the hundreds of thousands. One wonders, then, how these disturbed prisoners adjust to their new environment.

Ever since the publication of Gresham Sykes's pioneering study, *Society of Captives*, criminologists and mental health professionals have examined the lives of prisoners through the lens of the author's proposed 'Pains of Imprisonment' (Sykes, 1958). The assaults on one's self were framed as a series of deprivations: the denial of liberty, of goods, and services, of heterosexual relations, of autonomy. Perhaps the most searing among these is the deprivation of security. It cannot give one a tremendous sense of comfort to learn that his cell-mate is a convicted murderer (or rapist). The inmate soon learns that physical and sexual assaults are ubiquitous and frequent in prisons and jails, constituting a perpetual nightmare for prisoners, whether mentally stable or perfectly coherent (Kupers, 1996).

One of the inmates' few resources for self-protection is to subscribe conspicuously to the inmate code, complete with its own normative guidelines and differentiated role hierarchy.

Reading the social landscape of the prison ward and incorporating the demands of an unfamiliar and frankly frightening social world require the newly imprisoned to be a quick study, able to grasp where lies the power to brutalize and to victimize. He then must learn to strike strategic alliances to avoid being assaulted. In sum, he must grasp the essentials of 'toxic masculinity': a web of hyper-male traits of domination and wonton violence (Kupers, 2005). Any weakness, any vulnerability, will be quickly seized upon, marking the raw inmate as an easy target. Indeed, any display of emotion at all is an invitation for trouble; he must learn to suffer in silence, keeping any assault to himself because reporting an attack to a guard is the most unforgiven of transgressions: snitching.

Finding oneself in such an unfamiliar and confronting human environment, the mentally ill offender is ripe for victimization by both fellow inmates and correctional guards. A disproportionate share of the mentally unwell are subject to sexual assault; there are picked on precisely because they are widely perceived as 'weak in the head' (Kupers, 2005). They are also over-represented among those inmates selected for punitive segregation (Kupers, 1999). Once transported to these solitary security units, prisoners are prey to a host of psychological torments that attend sensory deprivation: hallucinations, perceptual distortions, illusions, vivid and frightening fantasies (Grassian and Friedman, 1986). Forced segregation and solitary confinement generate their own unique type of derangement, 'Stress Response Syndrome', characterized by persecutory ideation, necessarily augmenting whatever delusions the prisoner first presented on admission (Kupers, 1996). Episodes of violent verbal and behavioural histrionics are likely to be interpreted by correctional personnel as wilful infractions of discipline rather than as signs of a more thoroughgoing psychosis. Preyed upon therefore by both his fellow inmates and mishandled by the correctional guards, the psychological toll taken on these male inmates' health cannot be overestimated.

Risks of victimization are not uniform across the population of mentally ill prisoners. Some researchers have found that prisoners with bouts of depression, paranoia, and hallucinations experienced the highest rates of victimization by other inmates (Drapalski et al., 2009). These findings should be examined with caution, however; intake interviews are most likely conducted by nonmedical professionals – often social workers – who do their best to contour the patents' reported symptoms to familiar diagnostic categories. There is no way of assessing the reliability of these disease designations.

In consequence, further attempts to parcel out the generic category of 'mentally ill offender' into discrete diagnoses have employed a more systematic survey of symptoms. Asking inmates a range of questions about mood, previous diagnoses, and their experiences with the predatory prison culture suggests that inmates with Depressive Personality Disorder suffer the highest rates of assault; those diagnosed with Psychotic Disorder suffer the least, presumably because they routinely confine themselves (or *are* confined) to their cells. Inmates labelled as paranoid were most likely to initiate physical and verbal assaults, while those classified as suffering Borderline Personality Disorder, exhibiting impulsive, reckless behaviours, were believed to 'respond violently to perceived threats with aggression of their own' (Daquin and Daigle, 2008).

There remains, however, the disquieting sense that one really cannot determine the validity of the diagnosis in the first place. Systematic screening upon admission is more apparent than real; interviews are often a rushed affair, given increasing demands on the intake officer due to overcrowding. There is also the attitude of the classifier to take into consideration: prisoners reporting psychological torment are often greeted with barely concealed suspicion. Even the medically qualified observer may readily assume he is being manipulated for a variety of reasons, not least the desire for a change in cell assignment or an easier work detail (Kupers, 1999). There is also the protean nature of mental derangement itself, challenging even the most perspicacious of medical professionals to grasp the defining nature of the inmate's illness given the abbreviated experience he has with the inmate. Ultimately, grasping the dynamics that result in a formal diagnosis is thwarted by the Department of Corrections at the state level, restricting access to prison files and observation of the medical interaction. Regardless of the precise disease category, it is nonetheless true that the mentally ill *across* diagnoses face a disproportionate risk of physical and sexual assault, and suspicion among the correctional personnel to whom they must report any such attack.

Also standard across all prisons is the inmates' reluctance to ask for counselling or indeed even to admit not being tough enough to survive in a culture where only silent strength and the capacity to endure suffering are prized. For those prisoners who receive psychological counselling of some kind, the challenges are formidable. Because of the added correctional personnel required to transport an inmate from his cell to a private room, most prisoners are forced to engage in 'cell therapy', where they are examined and counselled *through* the bars. This of course undermines any sense of privacy or any belief that the content of his anxiety or fears will be kept confidential. Even the admission that one is willing to admit he needs help flies in the face of the masculine ideal, so the mere appearance of the therapist in the cell block marks off the inmate as vulnerable and easy prey.

Treatment, of course, is not limited to one-to-one counselling; indeed, the frequency of psychotherapy pales in comparison with the use of powerful psychotropic medication. Chlorpromazine – later, Thorazine – had been introduced in state hospitals beginning in 1954 as a way to quiet unruly patients, to 'slow them down' whilst in a manic episode (Roth, 2018: 89). Psychopharmacology has of course undergone qualitative refinement since the mid-twentieth century, but the use of psychotropic drugs remains integral to the institution's functioning as much a means of ensuring the ordered management of prisoners as the possible relief of prisoner's symptoms. The balancing of the inmates' psychological needs with the institution's overall exigency for security is likely weighted in the interests of the latter.

A prison, after all, is a 'total institution' in the words of Erving Goffman: a defining characteristic is bureaucratic efficiency (Goffman, 1961). Even the phenomenal growth in prison construction beginning in the 1980s could not keep pace with the escalating population of the newly convicted, sentenced to harsh and lengthy terms. New prison capacity was immediately constrained: a cell built for one prisoner had to accommodate two; gyms and dayrooms needed for relaxation and tension release were filled into dormitory-style bunk beds (Kupers, 1999; 2005). The crippling effects of overcrowding taxed the security and medical resources of each prison, adding still further to the pressure-cooker environment behind bars. Individual states soon discovered that the exorbitant costs of prison construction had drained the treasury, precluding increases in medical staff and rehabilitative efforts. In consequence, psychologically distressed inmates would be

> **Box 16.3 Assessing men's health in prison: any way forward?**
> - After initial separation, the deranged and the criminal are now incarcerated together
> - Given the closing of state hospitals, prisons and jails have become asylums by default
> - Community treatment, so enthusiastically proffered, has not materialized
> - A remedy for the dire state of mental illness in prison begins with criminal sentencing reform

fortunate to see a medical specialist for a few minutes at a time, and that only on a monthly basis. Medication proves to be the treatment of first resort, therefore, especially given the premium placed on a docile inmate population, required for the management of any *total* institution.

These features together – toxic masculinity, prison overcrowding, woefully underfunded medical resources – have made prisons a particularly pernicious setting for men's physical and psychological health. Suicide – nine times that of the general public – accounts for half of all deaths in custody (Kupers, 1999). Other mortality risks include head trauma (often the result of a brutal arrest), drug overdose, heart attack, and diabetes crisis (Katzen, 2011). Regarding psychological peril, mentally ill offenders are likely the least able to tolerate the pressures they encounter inside the prison. Inmates suffering some form of post-traumatic stress disorder, for example, often becoming highly distressed as early as their admission. They are then moved to a secure ward where social isolation only invites repeated flashbacks and panic attacks.

Drug therapy of course is available (and plentiful), but the accommodation period required for the body's chemistry to adapt to the newly ingested chemicals can require weeks, while the barely tolerable behavioural and mood side effects are immediate. Given the tremors, the confusion, the drooling, and slurred speech that often accompany the drug's consequences, a distressed, perhaps paranoid inmate could easily be excused for thinking the medication to be poison, to be avoided at all costs. Of course, he may have no choice in the matter: he is hardly a voluntary agent given the coercion of prison discipline. Physical restraints applied during an episode of behavioural disturbance will not be removed unless the pill is swallowed. Similarly, a recommendation for parole may only be made if the prisoner takes the medication and effects a pacific and compliant demeanour in front of his assessors. Upon release, there is no guarantee that former prisoners will continue the medication; indeed, there is reason to believe quite the otherwise. The return to prison following discharge is highest among inmates with serious mental debility, leading one to suspect that the drug is more an institutional than a therapeutic fix.

Potential Solutions

Is there any way to intrude upon criminal justice policies that have put so many men at risk to their mental health? The most obvious remedy is to radically decrease the size of the inmate population – most responsible for overcrowding – which limits the time any medical professional can devote to any one inmate, resulting in the cursory screening of inmates during the intake interview. As it happens, reducing mass incarceration is currently on the US political agenda: prison reform – taking aim specifically at mandatory sentencing and 'three strikes' policies – has resulted in a joint effort by unlikely bedfellows. Conservative, right-wing legislators are finally balking at the astronomical costs required to build and maintain one new prison after another; left-wing activists see a population suffering from overcrowding, with fewer recreational opportunities to relieve stress, and the near disappearance of programmes that embraced rehabilitation and education. Further, both sides are increasingly anxious about the effects of mass incarceration on the community left behind: families suffering hardship as one bread winner is removed for an increasingly long period of time, a social network bereft of older adult males that can provide guidance to young boys. For any number of reasons, mass incarceration has been a monumental financial drain on state and federal budgets, a sociological crisis for inner-city culture, and a medical nightmare for those men who enter the prison with a history of mental distress. And for those who enter prison with no history of mental derangement, the need to confront and absorb a frightening new world of toxic masculinity can amount to a daily encounter with unbridled fear.

That the mentally unwell and the criminal felon now share the same institution is of interest not only to the eighteenth-century time traveller we met at the beginning, but to historians of psychiatry, social scientists, and legislators trying to construct a more economical as well as, one hopes, more humane treatment of both populations. The nineteenth century witnessed an embrace of the 'rehabilitative ideal' – a conception of human personality as endlessly malleable – and of the penitentiary as the optimal setting for reconstructing the criminal's personality (Allen, 1964; Ignatieff, 1968). In parallel fashion, the brutal warehousing of the mentally infirm witnessed the enthusiastic proffering of another carceral setting – the 'well-ordered asylum' – that would curb pernicious family and community indulgence, surrounding the patient with proper discipline and *moral* treatment.

The ideology of personal and social reform was eagerly advanced by the new professions of psychiatry and criminology, each claiming sovereignty in rehabilitating 'the bad and the mad'. Not surprisingly, parallel dilemmas faced both innovative settings. However different they appeared on paper, the penitentiary and the asylum faced the exigency of running an institution of social control: maintaining safety, order, and discipline, while simultaneously attempting to minister to the developmental and psychological needs of persons deemed too dangerous to in society. Was this an intractable dilemma?

Forced separation of the mentally ill from their community is a relatively modern phenomenon; the family and the parish had traditionally been the locus of care and treatment. As migration from rural to urban centres accompanied other social dislocations following industrialization, however, the sheer volume of disturbed persons and the waning of family and community ties compelled the state to assume a greater share of the supervisory responsibility, manifest in public asylums, which grew in number and size from the early 1800s. Their sorry history – overcrowding, filth, and descent into simply warehousing the mad – left the state hospital system ripe for criticism and, in time, eventual abandonment. But the much-heralded community mental health centres failed to emerge: the former would-be mental patients drifted into homeless shelters or slept rough on the streets. Although there are scarce data to suggest that the population of mental patients simply changed institutions, it is nonetheless true that today's prisons and jails have become society's default psychiatric institution (Roth, 2018).

Rather that conclude from the above that the state is simply ill-equipped to assume the role that family and parish once performed, it would be wise to consider how the state's criminal justice system – from apprehension, to conviction, to sentencing – might ameliorate what has become a nightmare scenario, even for those entering with no history of mental distraction. If current political trends continue, mass incarceration numbers will be lowered appreciably simply by restrictions on mandatory minimum sentencing, to be reserved largely in future for those committing violent crimes. Given that three in four federal prisoners have been convicted in non-violent drug offences, this should lessen the overcrowding considerably. If states choose to consider these drug offences as better disposed through drug courts as some jurisdictions are doing, all the better still.

There seems to be little appetite for community mental health centres, however, leaving correctional institutions as the likely default for mentally-ill offenders. With the resources saved by admitting fewer prisoners, the administration would be in a position to concentrate on better and more extensive screening of inmates' needs upon admission, and more sustained one-to-one counselling, perhaps *not* carried on through prison bars. The conflict between security and treatment, however, will remain, regardless of the size of the institution. Caught in a system ill-prepared to address long-standing mental torment – and distracted states generated by overcrowding and toxic male codes themselves – the mentally ill find themselves prisoners to political policies that loom much larger than their own medical needs.

References

Alexander, R. and Meshelemiah, J. C. A. 2010. Gender identity disorders in prison: what are the legal implications for prison mental health professionals and administrators? *Prison J*, 90(3), 269–87.

Allen, F. 1964. *The Borderlands of Criminal Justice: Essays in Law and Criminology*. Chicago: University of Chicago Press.

Creese, R., Bynum, W. F., and Bearn, J. 1995. *The Health of Prisoners: Historical Essays*. Amsterdam: Editions Rodopi.

Daquin, J. and Daigle, L. 2008. Mental disorder and victimization in prison, examining the role of mental health treatment. *Crim Behav and Men Hlth*, 28, 141–51.

Drapalski, A. L., Youman, K., Stuewig, J., and Tangney, J. 2009. Gender differences in jail inmates' symptoms of mental illness, treatment history, and treatment seeking. *Criml Behav and Men Hlth*, 19, 193–206.

Eigen, J. P. 1995. *Witnessing Insanity: Madness and Mad-Doctors in the English Court*. New Haven, CT: Yale University Press.

Goffman, E. 1961. *Asylums: Essays on the Social Situation of Mental Patients and Other Inmates*. New York: Random House.

Gonzalez, J. and Connell, N. M. 2014. Mental health of prisoners: identifying barriers to mental health treatment and medication continuity. *Amer Public Hlth Assoc*, 1–4(12), 2328–33.

Grassian, S. and Friedman, N. 1986. Effects of sensory deprivation in psychiatric seclusion and solitary confinement. *Int J Law and Psych*, 8, 49–65.

Harcourt, B. E. 2011a. Reducing mass incarceration: lessons from the deinstitutionalization of mental hospitals in the 1960s. *Ohio St J Crim Law*, 9, 53–88.

Harcourt, B. E. 2011b. An institutionalization effect: the impact of mental hospitalization and imprisonment on homicide in the United States, 1934–2001. *J Leg Stud*, 40, 38–83.

Ignatieff, M. 1968. *A Just Measure of Pain: The Penitentiary in the Industrial Revolution, l750–1850*. New York: Pantheon Books.

Isaac, R. J. and Armat, V. C. 1990. *Madness in the Streets: How Psychiatry and the Law Abandoned the Mentally Ill*. New York: The Free Press.

Katzen, A. L. 2011. African American men's health and incarceration: access to care upon reentry and eliminating invisible punishments. *Berk J Gend, Law and Just*. 26. 221 52.

Kupers, T. 1996. Trauma and its sequelea in male prisoners: effects of confinement, overcrowding, and diminished services. *Am J Orthopsychi*, 66, 189–96.

Kupers, T. 1999. *Prison Madness: The Mental Health Crisis behind Bars and What We Must Do about It*. San Francisco: Jossey-Bass.

Kupers, T. 2005. Toxic masculinity as a barrier to mental health treatment in prison. *J Clin Psych*, 61, 713–24.

Raphael, S. and Stoll, M. 2013. Assessing the contribution of the de-institutionalization of the mentally ill to growth in U.S. incarceration rates. *J of Leg Stud*, 42, 187–221.

Roth, A. 2018. *Insane: America's Criminal Treatment of Mental Illness*. New York: Basic Books.

Rothman, D. 1971. *Discovery of the asylum: social order and disorder in the new republic*. Boston: Little, Brown and Company.

Rothman, D. 1980. *Conscience and Convenience: The Asylum and Its Alternatives in Progressive America*. Boston: Little, Brown and Company.

Sabo, D., Kupers, T. A., and London, W., eds. 2001. *Prison Masculinities.* Philadelphia: Temple University Press.

Scull, A. T. 1977. *Decarceration: Community Treatment and the Deviant – A Radical View.* New York: Prentice Hall.

Scull, A. T. 1979. *Museums of Madness: The Social Organization of Insanity* *in 19th Century England.* London: Allen Lane.

Steadman, H., McGreevy, M. A., Morrisey, J., Callahan, L., Robbins, P. C., and Cirincione, C. 1993. *Before and After Hinckley: Evaluating Insanity Defense Reform.* London: The Guilford Press.

Sykes, G. 1958. *The Society of Captives: A Study of a Maximum Security* *Prison.* Princeton, NJ: Princeton University Press.

Walker, N. D. 1968. *Crime and Insanity in England, Vol 1: The Historical Part.* Edinburgh: Edinburgh University Press.

Walker, N. D. 1985. The insanity defense before 1800. *Ann Am Acad Pol and Soc Sci,* 477, 25–30.

Domestic Violence and Men's Mental Health

Anna F. Taylor, Deirdre MacManus, and Louise M. Howard

This chapter focuses on the link between domestic violence and men's mental health and outlines recommendations for identifying men experiencing or perpetrating domestic violence, as well as interventions and strategies for recovery.

Domestic violence and abuse (DVA) is defined by the UK Government as an incident, or pattern of incidents, of controlling, coercive, threatening behaviours, violence, or abuse between people who are aged 16 or over, who are or have been intimate partners or family members, regardless of gender or sexuality (Home Office, 2012). It includes psychological, physical, sexual, financial, and emotional abuse. It also includes 'honour'-based violence and forced marriage. Other definitions used (e.g., in Australia) use broader definitions to include the impact on the whole family (e.g., children witnessing the abuse). However defined, it is recognized as a major public health and clinical problem for individuals, families, communities, and society (WHO, 2013). For example, DVA has been estimated to cost the UK almost £16 billion per annum (Walby, 2009).

Intimate partner violence (IPV), another term frequently used in the literature, refers to a more specific form of violence occurring between intimate partners, defined by the World Health Organization as behaviour by a current or ex-partner that causes physical, sexual, or psychological harm, including controlling behaviours (WHO, 2013). IPV is often conceptualized into distinct typologies; 'situational or common couple violence' and 'intimate terrorism'. Situational violence is defined as mutual, less severe violence, whereas intimate terrorism includes a strong element of coercive control and physical violence (Johnson et al., 2014).

Although it is recognized that both sexes can be either victims and perpetrators of domestic violence, the phenomenon is regularly viewed from the perspective of male-to-female violence, with an extensive body of research on female victimization. It is widely recognized within the literature that men can be perpetrators of domestic violence. However, consistent evidence now shows that a substantial number of men are victims of domestic violence, and yet the impacts of this are far less understood. Research suggests it has far-reaching and serious consequences for both physical and mental health in men (Hines and Douglas, 2015).

DVA Victimization in Men

Despite lower prevalence of victimization in men than women, the rates of incidents are still very high. In 2017, the Crime Survey for England and Wales estimated that 713,000 men and 1.2 million women aged 16–59 years experienced DVA. In the prior year 4.3% of men and 7.5% of women in England and Wales reported that they were victims of domestic violence (Office for National Statistics, 2017). It is estimated that 2.4 million men (15%) and 4.4 million women (26%) aged 16–59 have experienced some form of DVA. In the USA, the National Intimate Partner and Sexual Violence Survey (2011) found that one in nine men and one in four women were victims of severe intimate partner violence (i.e., sexual violence physical violence and/or stalking), with one in six men and one in three women experiencing some form of sexual violence during their lifetime. However, data on incidents of violence have been criticized by many, as they do not measure impact, and mask the extent of repeated, severe violent incidents (and domestic homicides), which are more likely to be experienced by women than men (Walby et al., 2017; Trevillion et al., 2012).

Less research has been conducted on same-sex relationships, but some studies suggest men in male-to-male relationships may be more likely to be victims than men in heterosexual relationships (Greenwood et al., 2002). In male-to-male couples, self-reported lifetime experience of IPV has been found to vary between 15.4% and 51% (Nowinski and Bowen, 2012; Stanley et al., 2006; Goldberg and Meyer, 2013) with variability in estimates in part due to differences in study methodologies (Nowinski and Bowen, 2012; Finneran and Stephenson, 2013). Studies of same-sex relationships have shown the prevalence of physical abuse reported is similar in men and women, with 35.5% of men and 40.1% of women reporting physical abuse from a same-sex partner (Rollè et al., 2018; Stiles-Shields and Carroll, 2015); the rates are markedly higher than in heterosexual couples. US research suggests that men who have sex with men report higher rates of victimization than heterosexual men, with 34% reporting psychological, 22% physical, and 5% sexual violence (Greenwood et al., 2002); in heterosexual men, studies have found the prevalence of sexual and physical assault to be 7.5% (Burke and Follingstad, 1999; Tjaden et al., 1999; Zierler et al., 2000).

Risk factors for being a victim of DVA, in men and women, include witnessing DVA in childhood, a history of childhood abuse, substance misuse, and poverty (Capaldi et al., 2012; Office for National Statistics, 2017). However, due to the limited number of studies on male victimization, research has not yet been able to identify distinct risk factors for male victims. The WHO highlights, in its ecological framework, that violence and abuse are also influenced by societal (e.g., attitudes to abuse) and community factors (e.g., neighbourhood violence), (Heise, 1998) and this is as much the case for men as it is for women.

DVA Perpetration and Men

Internationally, it is estimated that over 75% of violence against women is perpetrated by their male intimate partners (Garcia-Moreno et al., 2005). A systematic review reported that more than one in four women (28.3%) and one in five men (21.6%) report perpetrating physical violence in an intimate relationship (Desmarais et al., 2012)

In men, key risk factors for IPV perpetration include childhood experience of, or exposure to, violence (e.g., physical or sexual abuse) and having permissive attitudes regarding violence against women (whilst believing in gender equality has been found to be protective against perpetration; Jewkes, 2002; Jewkes et al., 2011; Abramsky et al., 2011; Fleming et al., 2015). Mental disorders and substance abuse

(Oram et al., 2014b) are also key risk factors for IPV perpetration in men. Co-occurrence of depression, post-traumatic stress disorder symptoms, and substance abuse have been found to be associated with IPV (Kiene et al., 2017; Machisa et al., 2016; Rhodes et al., 2009). Research has also shown a relationship between poverty and education and perpetration of IPV, as well as a history of physical abuse perpetration (Schumacher et al., 2001). When examining domestic homicides in the UK perpetrated by people with mental disorders with a history of contact with psychiatric services, 82% were male (Oram et al., 2014b; see Box 17.1).

Exposure to DVA in childhood has been found to have a range of adverse impacts, specifically on mental health problems (e.g., depression and anxiety), under-developed emotional regulation skills, and a tendency towards aggression (Card et al., 2008; Malinosky-Rummell and Hansen, 1993; Ruddle et al., 2017). It has been suggested that this is due to poor formation of attachments with parents (Dutton and White, 2012) and learning negative behaviours from peers (Dodge et al., 1995). Experience of violence or abuse may affect children differently, depending on gender (Costa et al., 2015). A study of men who had been victims of childhood abuse reported that 34–56% were likely to become DVA perpetrators (Margolin and Gordis, 2004), suggesting that exposure to DVA in childhood may increase the likelihood of engaging in these types of behaviours in the future. Further research on how this contributes to adult perpetration of violence is needed, as it could highlight areas where interventions could be used to prevent future violence (Fazel et al., 2018).

Box 17.1 Risk factors for IPV men

- Childhood experience of abuse
- Childhood exposure to domestic violence
- Poor early attachments
- Peer attitudes and behaviours
- Permissive attitudes to violence against women
- Mental health problems, including:

  o Depression
  o Post-traumatic stress disorder
  o Personality disorder (antisocial, borderline)

- Substance use and abuse
- Poverty
- Lower educational levels

Measurement Issues in the Literature

It is important to acknowledge that studies of DVA may present an unclear picture of the prevalence and impact of DVA, as the methods of measurement vary greatly from study to study. Research studies often find similar rates of self-reported violence perpetration in males and females (Archer, 2002; Holtzworth-Munroe, 2005) and occasionally even higher rates of violence perpetrated by women than men (Carney et al., 2007). However, in studies that consider severity of violence, severe violence is more likely to be perpetrated by men (Holtzworth-Munroe, 2005). Similarly, studies that have measured the impact of physical aggression find that men were more likely to have injured their partners than women (Archer, 2000; Graham-Kevan, 2007; Palmetto et al., 2013). The bidirectional nature of violence also needs to be considered when interpreting prevalence rates (e.g., when a victim retaliates to the perpetrator), as this is not captured in some measures used in the research (Capaldi and Owen, 2001).

Issues of reporting bias also need to be considered. A large international systematic review of studies of the prevalence of DVA concluded that underreporting within population surveys may be a problem, with the number of people willing to disclose being lower than the actual rates of DVA (Alhabib et al., 2010). For men, underreporting of victimization and the lack of recognition of psychological abuse as a crime may be a particular issue. A study on the arrest and prosecution rate for spousal assault suggests that male victims of IPV were reluctant to report the abuse and police were unwilling to arrest women accused of perpetrating violence where there were no physical injuries, leading to only 2% of suspected female perpetrators being arrested compared to 53.4% of men (Brown, 2004). These issues within the literature mean that the research to date may not accurately reflect the true prevalence or impact of IPV on both men and women.

DVA Victimization and Mental Disorder

Research on DVA has consistently found a link between IPV victimization and mental disorders in the general population. For men and women, research has found links between IPV and a wide spectrum of disorders, including depression, PTSD, anxiety disorders, and substance misuse (Bundock et al., 2013; Campbell, 2002; Coker et al., 2002; Oram et al., 2013b; Kamperman et al., 2014; Trevillion et al., 2014). Research suggests there may be a causal association between IPV and mental disorders, as IPV can lead to mental disorders and can also make an individual more vulnerable to experiencing IPV (Howard et al., 2010).

In the case of men, this may be an important area to consider. Preliminary evidence has in fact suggested that men with mental disorders are at particularly increased risk of victimization (Goodman et al., 2001; Teplin et al., 2005). In psychiatric populations the gender difference in prevalence of male and female victims is attenuated, though a recent systematic review highlights that women with severe mental illness are still at increased risk of being victims of DVA than men (Khalifeh et al., 2016). Several studies report higher prevalence rates of victimization in men with severe mental health issues compared to the general population. A study found that in men with mental illness, particularly those with severe mental illness (SMI), the risk for victimization is increased compared to the general population (Khalifeh et al., 2015). It was reported that 13% of men with SMI had experience of recent domestic violence (past year) vs 5% of control men (Khalifeh et al., 2015). Another study estimated that 18% of male patients in psychiatric settings had experienced physical violence and 4% sexual violence by a partner (Chang et al., 2011). Across mixed psychiatric settings 31.6% of male patients reported lifetime partner violence (Oram et al., 2013b), a considerably higher rate compared to the general population. Studies have also shown that men with severe mental illness are more likely to be a victim of DVA than a perpetrator (Ehrensaft et al., 2006). This suggests that men with severe mental illnesses may be particularly vulnerable to being victims of IPV. Men are also less likely to seek help for IPV victimization (Brown, 2004), which may have implications for their recovery.

DVA Perpetration and Mental Disorder

A smaller but growing body of research supports an association between DVA perpetration and a broad range of mental disorders, including depression, anxiety disorders, PTSD, ADHD, personality disorders, and substance misuse (Oram et al., 2014a; Hahn et al., 2015; Okuda et al., 2015; Buitelaar et al., 2020).

A systematic review found that psychiatric disorders are associated with a high prevalence of ever having perpetrated domestic violence in both men and women (Oram et al., 2014a). Moreover, in men diagnosed with common mental disorders (depression, generalized anxiety disorder, and panic disorder) there were increased odds of them having ever been physically violent against a partner (Oram et al., 2014a). This association was also found in women with common mental disorders.

Some research in the USA and emerging data from the UK have suggested that within military populations the prevalence and severity of partner violence (victimization and perpetration) is higher than in civilian populations (Heyman and Neidig, 1999; Griffin and Morgan, 1988; MacManus et al., under review).

Researchers have begun to explore the causal links between mental health and DVA perpetration. A systematic review of ADHD reported that cohort studies identified hyperactive, impulsive, and inattention symptoms as risk factors for adult IPV; conduct disorder and antisocial personality disorder were regarded as mediators in three studies; other research suggests that when ADHD is associated with alcohol misuse there is an increased likelihood of male–female IPV (Wymbs et al., 2017; Buitelaar et al., 2020). Some researchers have hypothesized that the link between ADHD and IPV may be explained by co-morbid traits of antisocial personality disorder (APD), which are shown to predict IPV perpetration (Holtzworth-Munroe and Stuart, 1994; Walther et al., 2017). Other studies highlight the role of co-morbid alcohol consumption in those with ADHD (Molina et al., 2007; Wymbs et al., 2017), given its strong link to IPV perpetration in both males and females (Capaldi et al., 2012).

Research has frequently shown that borderline and antisocial personality features (Costa and Babcock, 2008) are key risk factors for IPV perpetration and that men with these traits are likely to commit more serious violence and cause more injuries to their partners (Ehrensaft et al., 2006; Ross and Babcock, 2009). Recent research found that among young men the pathway from early trauma to IPV can be mediated by personality disorder (González et al., 2016). In borderline personality disorder (BPD) multiple longitudinal studies show emotional dysregulation and interpersonal dysfunction (features that characterize the disorder) mediate the link between BPD and IPV (Jackson et al., 2015; Newhill et al., 2012; Stepp et al., 2012). It has been hypothesized that

individuals with BPD features will perpetrate IPV in response to real or imagined threats of abandonment, to try to prevent their partners from leaving them (Ross and Babcock, 2009). However, in antisocial personality disorder, it has been suggested IPV perpetration is due to deficiencies in empathy, rather than fear of abandonment (Bovasso et al., 2002) and they may use violence as way to resolve conflict or maintain power and control in the relationships (Babcock et al., 2000). Substance misuse has also been suggested as a potential mediator between personality disorder and IPV. In one study, men who had substance abuse issues (drugs or alcohol) had more borderline personality features and committed more severe IPV than those who did not use drugs or alcohol (Thomas et al., 2013).

Research has also consistently found a direct link between higher rates of IPV perpetration and substance misuse (O'Farrell et al., 2004; El-Bassel et al., 2007; Yu et al., 2019; Gilchrist et al., 2015). Studies have found that men receiving treatment for substance abuse (O'Farrell et al., 2004; El-Bassel et al., 2007; Gilchrist et al., 2015) report higher rates of IPV perpetration (34–60% in past year) than men in the general population (Fleming et al., 2015; O'Farrell et al., 2003). Studies have suggested that men are eight to eleven times more likely to perpetrate IPV on a day when they have been drinking (Fals-Stewart, 2003) and physical harm is more likely and more severe (Wupperman et al., 2009; Testa et al., 2003; Shorey et al., 2014). In those arrested for perpetration, men were also significantly more likely than women (73% vs 53%) to have used alcohol or drugs prior to the event (Friend et al., 2011).

Psychosis may also play a role in DVA perpetration (Coid et al., 2016). Of homicides committed by people with mental illness, 14% of intimate partner homicide perpetrators and 23% of adult family homicide perpetrators had been in recent contact with a mental health service. Psychosis was more prevalent in family homicides (Oram et al., 2013a). Although the association between psychosis and violence is generally modest (Coid et al., 2006; Douglas et al., 2009) and most people with psychosis are not violent (Fazel et al., 2009), when compared to the general population they are more likely to perpetrate acts of violence, including homicide (Fazel et al., 2009; Nielssen and Large, 2010). The link between psychosis and DVA could be due in part to paranoid ideation (Coid et al., 2016). Previous victimization may also play an important role, as research has found that people suffering from schizophrenia are approximately fourteen times more likely to be victims of violence than to commit violence toward others (Brekke et al., 2001).

Identification and Interventions of DVA in Men with Mental Health Issues

Mental health professionals have an important role in responding to DVA (Chapman and Monk, 2015) and it has been health policy in England and some parts of the USA and New Zealand for many years to carry out routine enquiry into domestic violence in all mental health assessments (Read and Fraser, 1998; Department of Health, 2020). However, DVA remains under-detected in mental health settings with only 10–30% of cases being identified by mental health professionals (Howard et al., 2010).

Research on responding to DVA has focused largely on women, due to its greater prevalence and impacts. This has meant that what is known about the identification and interventions is often based on female samples, particularly for victimization, with very few men included. For mental health service users, there is a growing body of evidence on the identification of DVA and interventions that may be effective, but again studies mostly focus on female samples, with very few men (Trevillion et al., 2016).

Identifying Service Users with DVA

Enquiry about DVA is low in mental health services (Howard et al., 2010; Trevillion et al., 2016), which impacts negatively on the disclosure of DVA by service users and its identification. A UK study found that amongst 131 psychiatrists and psychiatric nurses only 15% reported routinely enquiring about DVA (Nyame et al., 2013). A study in a US emergency department found that service users with substance use disorders were less likely to be asked about DVA, whilst for other mental health disorders, no differences were found (Choo et al., 2010). This may be particularly detrimental for the identification of male perpetrators, as studies have shown that men being treated for substance abuse are more likely to have been perpetrators of IPV, with around four in ten having been physically or sexually violent and seven in ten having been psychologically violent to their intimate partner in the previous twelve months,

which is far higher than in the general population (O'Farrell et al., 2004; El-Bassel et al., 2007).

Studies from service user's perspectives reflect that there is a general lack of enquiry about DVA in mental health settings. A US survey highlighted that only 27% (43 out of 158) of male service users reported being screened for DVA compared to the female service users, where over half (55%) reported being screened for DVA (Chang et al., 2011). In that survey, a fifth of male service users (18%) reported lifetime DVA and 6% past year DVA. The results suggest that professionals are not enquiring about DVA, particularly with male service users.

Identification/Enquiry

As previously mentioned, charities working with male victims (RESPECT – a UK charity that offers helpline support for male and female perpetrators of domestic violence and abuse) have highlighted issues in misdiagnosing men as victims, when they are in fact perpetrators (especially if their partner has used violent resistance) or in unhappy relationships without any abuse.

RESPECT have developed a toolkit on identification of IPV in men. Due to the complexity of a relationship they suggested specific questions to help identify whether the man is a perpetrator or victim (see Box 17.2). In addition, a toolkit on identification and response to domestic violence in psychiatric patients has been developed by our group and is free to download here: www.kcl.ac.uk/psychology-systems-sciences/research/lara-vp-download-form

RESPECT also suggests that male victims will have many common experiences that may help to identify them. For example, they will all have experienced incidents of violence or abuse from a partner, they may have been injured or require medical attention due to their partners behaviour, they will be in fear of violence to themselves or children, they have

---

Box 17.2 Questions to understand IPV

- 'If violence took place, who ended it? (As opposed to started it)'
- 'Who suffered most physical injury? (Consistently over time)'
- 'Which person is in fear of the other? (Often for their lives)'

experienced controlling behaviour from their partner, they are fearful of violence at separation, they are able to give authentic descriptions of the abuse, and they typically do not speak badly of their partner.

Identification of DVA Perpetration

There is a lack of research on the detection of DVA perpetration in mental health services (Trevillion et al., 2016). However, a UK survey of service users attending community mental health teams found that one in ten disclosed lifetime perpetration of DVA (Khalifeh, 2015). Several reports from third sector organisations and national confidential enquiries have highlighted the failure of mental health services to assess risk of DVA perpetration (https://static1 .squarespace.com/static/5ee0be2588f1e349401c832c/t/ 5efb6ce1d305a44006cb5ab9/1593535715616/STADV_ DHR_Report_Final.pdf; The National Confidential Inquiry into Suicide and Homicide by People with Mental Illness, 2017). Moreover, within perpetrator programmes in the UK, very few referrals come from mental health services (Kelly and Westmarland, 2015), highlighting the lack of identification and awareness of referral pathways amongst mental health professionals.

UK charities and research have highlighted that, given that the majority of perpetrators are male and may manipulate or minimize their actions, those assessing for DVA should be aware that some men who present as victims are in fact perpetrators (RESPECT; Bancroft, 2002; Bala, 2000). Evidence from the Men's Advice Line suggests this, as a significant number of men calling who initially identify as victims later change their own identification or provide information that suggests they are a perpetrator. Research on male perpetrators has suggested that they routinely deny their abusive behaviour, minimize the severity and the impacts of the abuse, and blame it on others (Scott and King, 2007; Bancroft, 2002). Accurate identification is therefore key in order to provide the correct interventions and advice and to prevent situations becoming dangerous for the partners of men who identify as victims but are actually perpetrators.

Studies with mental health service users have highlighted that direct enquiry helps to facilitate disclosure of DVA (Eckhardt et al., 2008; Khalifeh, 2015) and is necessary with those who perpetrate DVA as they are unlikely to identify themselves as

perpetrators or seek help without encouragement (Chapman and Monk, 2015; Eckhardt et al., 2008).

Research also suggests incidents of DVA are inadequately documented by mental health services (Cobo et al., 2010); however, these studies include predominantly females (Cobo et al., 2010). A recent review highlighted that mental health professionals may be unsure of how to respond to service user's reporting DVA. A UK survey of mental health professionals showed that only 27% reported providing information to service users after disclosure of abuse (Nyame et al., 2013).

Barriers to Identifying and Responding to DVA

Mental health professionals identify several barriers to enquiring about DVA. As summarized in Box 17.3 it not being a part of their role; their not being trained in enquiry or interventions for DVA; and lacking confidence in undertaking these tasks (Rose et al., 2011). Professionals also report concerns about assessment in people with psychosis and the veracity of their reports or causing offence by asking intrusive questions (Rose et al., 2011). Other reasons include a perceived lack of expertise (Salyers et al., 2004), lack of rapport or strong therapeutic relationship with the service user (Currier et al., 1996), lack of time or competing demands (Phelan et al., 2005), the presence of the partners during appointments or fear of offending or re-traumatizing service users (Trevillion et al., 2014). One study suggested that male clinicians may be less likely to enquire about DVA than female clinicians (Nyame et al., 2013).

Research suggests that female service users find routine enquiry acceptable but less is known about male service-user's attitudes (Feder et al., 2006). Seeking help may be more difficult for men; one study

---

Box 17.3 Perceived barriers to enquiring about PIV amongst mental health professionals

- Not seen as part of role
- Not trained
- Not sure how to ask
- Not sure how to respond
- Fear of causing offence
- Fear of undermining therapeutic relationship
- Presence of partners during interview
- Lack of time/competing demands

suggested that men may face prejudice from healthcare professionals. Counsellors who worked with male victims of DVA reported surprise at the occurrence of male abuse, as well as with the severity of the abuse (Hogan et al., 2012). Moreover, mental health service users may find it even harder to disclose DVA as they are likely to have experienced discrimination due to their mental illness, which may make them reluctant to seek help (Du Mont and Forte, 2014; Trevillion et al., 2016). It is therefore important that professionals in mental health service undergo training and education in the identification and response to DVA in men (Tsui et al., 2010).

Research has suggested that despite having knowledge on DVA, professionals lack confidence in assessing and responding to it. A survey in the UK of 131 psychiatrists and psychiatric nurses found that despite psychiatrists reporting significantly greater knowledge about DVA than nurses, they did not feel as ready to use it to assess or respond to service users (Nyame et al., 2013). Another qualitative study found that staff lacked confidence in when and how to tell other relevant professionals and new partners about service users who had perpetrated DVA (Oram et al., 2016). A substantial training gap was similarly identified in a survey of Australian psychiatrists and trainees (Forsdike et al., 2019). However, training interventions may be effective in improving professional responses. A study found that after GPs and nurses completed a training intervention on the identification, documentation, and referral of male patients experiencing of perpetrating DVA, their self-reported preparedness to meet the needs of male patients significantly increased and there was a small increase in the numbers of male patients identified in the records (Williamson et al., 2015).

Interventions for Victims of DVA

Much of the healthcare literature on interventions focuses on female victims of IPV (Salber and Taliaferro, 2006) and research on interventions with male victims is quite limited, particularly in mental health populations. A recent systematic review reports that tailored mental health interventions such as cognitive behavioural therapy (CBT) and empowerment-based advocacy are effective for female victims of DVA when they include development of cognitive and emotional skills and are targeted at problem solving, focusing on strengths and attention to

ongoing safety risks (Trabold et al., 2018). However, these studies did not include men. Research into interventions with male victims of domestic violence with mental health issues are sorely needed.

Of the guidance that is available, NICE (PH50) highlights the need for training on DVA for all mental health professionals to deliver effective interventions. Staff (some of whom may be affected by DVA) should also be given support for their personal experiences through their Mental Health Trust. For victims of IPV, NICE recommends psychological therapy (for example, trauma-focused cognitive behavioural therapy), medication, and support. Risk assessment should also be an ongoing process to ensure the victim's safety, as well as safety planning with the person and referral to other DVA support services if relevant (depending on the person's individual preference and whether the abuse is current or historic).

NICE advises that clinicians should be careful when considering couples interventions as they can prevent the victim from being empowered and allow the perpetrator's abuse to continue. If this is the chosen intervention, the victim should have several sessions separately as well.

Interventions for Perpetrators of DVA

Currently interventions for IPV perpetration include holding the perpetrator legally and practically accountable for their actions, helping them understand how their behaviour is unacceptable and promoting equitable gender attitudes through perpetrator programmes (Bancroft, 2002). There is limited research that has considered interventions for mental health service users who have perpetrated DVA. Systematic reviews of IPV perpetrator programmes based on CBT, which aim to prevent reoffending suggest small to no effects (Feder et al., 2008; Smedslund et al., 2007). Some researchers suggest this is due to the rigid criteria for what counts as an improvement in IPV, as many studies use a complete absence of reoffending post-intervention as their desired outcome. The current results suggest some improvements in attitudes towards women, but no consistent improvements in recidivism of the violence. However, these programmes often exclude men with significant mental disorders (Feder et al., 2008; Smedslund et al., 2007), therefore further research in mental health populations on prevention strategies is needed.

Interventions that address specific modifiable risk factors for perpetration in men may be effective in reducing DVA; examples include: evidence-based treatments for PTSD, substance misuse, paranoid ideation in psychosis and personality disorders (O'Farrell et al., 2004; El-Bassel et al., 2007; Radcliffe and Gilchrist, 2016). A randomized control trial (RCT) of an integrated CBT intervention for men with alcohol dependence found that participants in the CBT intervention group reported significantly lower DVA perpetration, and their wives scored significantly lower on depression, anxiety, and stress levels at a three-month follow-up (Satyanarayana et al., 2016). A systematic review of interventions targeting men's alcohol use and family relationships in low- and middle-income countries found six studies documenting modest improvements in drinking and couple or family outcomes after interventions. These included CBT techniques, communication skills training, narrative therapy, and participatory learning. The study found that gender-transformative approaches were associated with a reduction in IPV. Motivational interviewing and behavioural approaches reduced men's alcohol use (Giusto and Puffer, 2018). More research is needed in this area but addressing specific risk factors such as trauma or alcohol misuse could reduce DVA perpetration in men.

Conclusions

Domestic violence is an issue that men with mental health issues face. However, research on how to detect and address this is very limited and as a result, current guidelines on DVA do not include much research with males. Further research on interventions for DVA in males is needed to understand what is effective. From what is known, all mental health services need to receive training in identifying and responding DVA and clear referral pathways need to be developed to work with other DVA agencies.

References

Abramsky, T., Watts, C. H., Garcia-Moreno, C., Devries, K., Kiss, L., Ellsberg, M., Jansen, H. A. and Heise, L. 2011. What factors are associated with recent intimate partner violence? Findings from the WHO multi-country study on women's health and domestic violence. *BMC Public Health*, *11*(1), 109.

Alhabib, S., Nur, U., and Jones, R. 2010. Domestic violence against women: systematic review of prevalence studies. *Journal of Family Violence*, *25*(4), 369–82.

Archer, J. 2000. Sex differences in aggression between heterosexual partners: a meta-analytic review. *Psychological Bulletin*, *126*(5), 651.

Archer, J. 2002. Sex differences in physically aggressive acts between heterosexual partners: a meta-analytic review. *Aggression and Violent Behavior*, *7*(4), 313–51.

Babcock, J. C., Jacobson, N. S., Gottman, J. M., and Yerington, T. P. 2000. Attachment, emotional regulation, and the function of marital violence: differences between secure, preoccupied, and dismissing violent and nonviolent husbands. *Journal of Family Violence*, *15*(4), 391–409.

Bala, N. 2000. A differentiated legal approach to the effects of spousal abuse on children: a Canadian context. In: R. Geffner, P. Jaffe, and M. Sudermann (eds) *Children Exposed to Domestic Violence: Current Issues in Research, Intervention, Prevention, and Policy Development*. New York: The Haworth Trauma and Maltreatment Press, 301–28.

Bancroft, L. 2002. *Why Does He Do That? Inside the Minds of Angry and Controlling Men*. New York: The Berkley Publishing Group.

Bovasso, G. B., Alterman, A. I., Cacciola, J. S., and Rutherford, M. J. 2002. The prediction of violent and nonviolent criminal behavior in a methadone maintenance population. *Journal of Personality Disorders*, *16*(4), 360–73.

Brekke, J. S., Prindle, C., Bae, S. W., and Long, J. D. 2001. Risks for individuals with schizophrenia who are living in the community. *Psychiatric Services*, *52*(10), 1358–66.

Brown, G. A. 2004. Gender as a factor in the response of the law-enforcement system to violence against partners. *Sexuality and Culture*, *8*(3–4), 3–139.

Buitelaar, N. J., Posthumus, J. A., and Buitelaar, J. K. 2020. ADHD in childhood and/or adulthood as a risk factor for domestic violence or intimate partner violence: a systematic review. *Journal of Attention Disorders*, *24*(9), 1203–14.

Bundock, L., Howard, L. M., Trevillion, K., Malcolm, E., Feder, G., and Oram, S. 2013. Prevalence and risk of experiences of intimate partner violence among people with eating disorders: a systematic review. *Journal of Psychiatric Research*, *47*(9), 1134–42.

Burke, L. K. and Follingstad, D. R. 1999. Violence in lesbian and gay relationships: theory, prevalence, and correlational factors. *Clinical Psychology Review*, *19*(5), 487–512.

Campbell, J. C. 2002. Health consequences of intimate partner violence. *The Lancet*, 359(9314), 1331–6.

Capaldi, D. M. and Owen, L. D. 2001. Physical aggression in a community sample of at-risk young couples: gender comparisons for high frequency, injury, and fear. *Journal of Family Psychology*, 15(3), 425.

Capaldi, D. M., Knoble, N. B., Shortt, J. W., and Kim, H. K. 2012. A systematic review of risk factors for intimate partner violence. *Partner Abuse*, 3(2), 231–80.

Card, N. A., Stucky, B. D., Sawalani, G. M., and Little, T. D. 2008. Direct and indirect aggression during childhood and adolescence: a meta-analytic review of gender differences, intercorrelations, and relations to maladjustment. *Child Development*, 79(5), 1185–1229.

Carney, M., Buttell, F., and Dutton, D. 2007. Women who perpetrate intimate partner violence: a review of the literature with recommendations for treatment. *Aggression and Violent Behavior*, 12(1), 108–15.

Chang, J. C., Cluss, P. A., Burke, J. G., Hawker, L., Dado, D., Goldstrohm, S., and Scholle, S. H. 2011. Partner violence screening in mental health. *General Hospital Psychiatry*, 33(1), 58–65.

Chapman, A. and Monk, C. 2015. Domestic violence awareness. *American Journal of Psychiatry*, 172(10), 944–5.

Choo, E. K., Nicolaidis, C., Jenkinson, R. H., Cox, J. M., and John Mcconnell, K. 2010. Failure of intimate partner violence screening among patients with substance use disorders. *Academic Emergency Medicine*, 17(8), 886–9.

Cobo, J., Muñoz, R., Martos, A., Carmona, M., Pérez, M., Cirici, R., and García-Parés, G. 2010. Violence against women in mental health departments: is it relevant for mental health professionals? *Revista de Psiquiatría y Salud Mental (English Edition)*, 3(2), 61–7.

Coid, J. W., Ullrich, S., Bebbington, P., Fazel, S., and Keers, R. 2016. Paranoid ideation and violence: meta-analysis of individual subject data of 7 population surveys. *Schizophrenia Bulletin*, 42(4), 907–15.

Coid, J., Yang, M., Roberts, A., Ullrich, S., Moran, P., Bebbington, P., Brugha, T., Jenkins, R., Farrell, M., Lewis, G., and Singleton, N. 2006. Violence and psychiatric morbidity in the national household population of Britain: public health implications. *The British Journal of Psychiatry*, 189(1), 12–19.

Coker, A. L., Davis, K. E., Arias, I., Desai, S., Sanderson, M., Brandt, H. M., and Smith, P. H. 2002. Physical and mental health effects of intimate partner violence for men and women. *American Journal of Preventive Medicine*, 23(4), 260–8.

Costa, B. M., Kaestle, C. E., Walker, A., Curtis, A., Day, A., Toumbourou, J. W., and Miller, P. 2015. Longitudinal predictors of domestic violence perpetration and victimization: a systematic review. *Aggression and Violent Behavior*, 24, 261–72.

Costa, D. M. and Babcock, J. C. 2008. Articulated thoughts of intimate partner abusive men during anger arousal: correlates with personality disorder features. *Journal of Family Violence*, 23(6), 395.

Currier, G. W., Barthauer, L. M., Begier, E. and Bruce, M. L. 1996. Training and experience of psychiatric residents in identifying domestic violence. *Psychiatric Services*, 47(5), 529–30.

Department of Health. 2020 March. Refocusing the Care Programme Approach Policy and Positive Practice Guidance. Available from https:// webarchive.nationalarchives.gov.uk/ 20130124042407/http://www.dh.gov .uk/prod_consum_dh/groups/dh_ digitalassets/@dh/@en/documents/ digitalasset/dh_083649.pdf

Desmarais, S. L., Reeves, K. A., Nicholls, T. L., Telford, R. P., and

Fiebert, M. S. 2012. Prevalence of physical violence in intimate relationships, part 2: rates of male and female perpetration. *Partner Abuse*, 3(2), 170–98.

Dodge, K. A., Pettit, G. S., Bates, J. E., and Valente, E. 1995. Social information-processing patterns partially mediate the effect of early physical abuse on later conduct problems. *Journal of Abnormal Psychology*, 104(4), 632.

Douglas, K. S., Guy, L. S., and Hart, S. D. 2009. Psychosis as a risk factor for violence to others: a meta-analysis. *Psychological Bulletin*, 135(5), 679.

Du Mont, J. and Forte, T. 2014. Intimate partner violence among women with mental health-related activity limitations: a Canadian population based study. *BMC Public Health*, 14(1), 51.

Dutton, D. G. and White, K. R. 2012. Attachment insecurity and intimate partner violence. *Aggression and Violent Behavior*, 17(5), 475–81.

Eckhardt, C. I., Samper, R. E., and Murphy, C. M. 2008. Anger disturbances among perpetrators of intimate partner violence: clinical characteristics and outcomes of court-mandated treatment. *Journal of Interpersonal Violence*, 23(11), 1600–17.

Ehrensaft, M. K., Cohen, P., and Johnson, J. G. 2006. Development of personality disorder symptoms and the risk for partner violence. *Journal of Abnormal Psychology*, 115(3), 474.

Ehrensaft, M. K., Moffitt, T. E., and Caspi, A. 2006. Is domestic violence followed by an increased risk of psychiatric disorders among women but not among men? A longitudinal cohort study. *American Journal of Psychiatry*, 163(5), 885–92.

El-Bassel, N., Gilbert, L., Wu, E., Chang, M., and Fontdevila, J. 2007. Perpetration of intimate partner violence among men in methadone treatment programs in New York City. *American Journal of Public Health*, 97(7), 1230–2.

El-Bassel, N., Gilbert, L., Wu, E., Chang, M., Gomes, C., Vinocur, D., and Spevack, T. 2007. Intimate partner violence prevalence and HIV risks among women receiving care in emergency departments: implications for IPV and HIV screening. *Emergency Medicine Journal*, 24(4), 255–9.

Fals-Stewart, W. 2003. The occurrence of partner physical aggression on days of alcohol consumption: a longitudinal diary study. *Journal of Consulting and Clinical Psychology*, 71(1), 41.

Fazel, S., Långström, N., Hjern, A., Grann, M., and Lichtenstein, P. 2009. Schizophrenia, substance abuse, and violent crime. *Jama*, 301(19), 2016–23.

Fazel, S., Smith, E. N., Chang, Z., and Geddes, J. R. 2018. Risk factors for interpersonal violence: an umbrella review of meta-analyses. *The British Journal of Psychiatry*, 213(4), 609–14.

Feder, G. S., Hutson, M., Ramsay, J., and Taket, A. R. 2006. Women exposed to intimate partner violence: expectations and experiences when they encounter health care professionals: a meta-analysis of qualitative studies. *Archives of Internal Medicine*, 166(1), 22–37.

Feder, L., Wilson, D. B., and Austin, S. 2008. Court-mandated interventions for individuals convicted of domestic violence. *Campbell Systematic Reviews*, 12(4), 1–46.

Finneran, C. and Stephenson, R. (2013) Intimate partner violence among men who have sex with men. A systematic review. Trauma Violence Abuse, 14, 168–85.

Fleming, P. J., McCleary-Sills, J., Morton, M., Levtov, R., Heilman, B., and Barker, G. 2015. Risk factors for men's lifetime perpetration of physical violence against intimate partners: results from the international men and gender equality survey (IMAGES) in eight

countries. *PloS One*, 10(3), e0118639.

Forsdike, K., O'Connor, M., Castle, D., and Hegarty, K. 2019. Exploring Australian psychiatrists' and psychiatric trainees' knowledge, attitudes and preparedness in responding to adults experiencing domestic violence. *Australasia Psychiatry*, 27(1), 64–8. doi:10.1177/1039856218789778

Friend, J., Langhinrichsen-Rohling, J., and Eichold, B. H. 2011. Same-day substance use in men and women charged with felony domestic violence offenses. *Criminal Justice and Behavior*, 38(6), 619–33.

Frye, V., Latka, M. H., Wu, Y., Valverde, E. E., Knowlton, A. R., Knight, K. R., Arnsten, J. H., O'leary, A., and INSPIRE Study Team. 2007. Intimate partner violence perpetration against main female partners among HIV-positive male injection drug users. *JAIDS Journal of Acquired Immune Deficiency Syndromes*, 46, S101–S109.

García-Moreno, C., Jansen, H. A., Ellsberg, M., Heise, L., and Watts, C. 2005. *WHO Multi-Country Study on Women's Health and Domestic Violence against Women: Initial Results on Prevalence, Health Outcomes and Women's Responses*. Switzerland: World Health Organization.

Gilchrist, G., Blazquez, A., Segura, L., Geldschläger, H., Valls, E., Colom, J., and Torrens, M. 2015. Factors associated with physical or sexual intimate partner violence perpetration by men attending substance misuse treatment in Catalunya: a mixed methods study. *Criminal Behaviour and Mental Health*, 25(4), 239–57.

Giusto, A. and Puffer, E. 2018. A systematic review of interventions targeting men's alcohol use and family relationships in low- and middle-income countries. *Global Mental Health (Cambridge Core)*, 5, e10. doi:10.1017/gmh.2017.32

Goldberg, N. G. and Meyer, I. H. 2013. Sexual orientation disparities in history of intimate partner violence: Results from the California Health Interview Survey. *Journal of Interpersonal Violence*, 28(5), 1109–18.

González, R. A., Kallis, C., Ullrich, S., Barnicot, K., Keers, R., and Coid, J. W. 2016. Childhood maltreatment and violence: mediation through psychiatric morbidity. *Child Abuse and Neglect*, 52, 70–84.

Goodman, L. A., Salyers, M. P., Mueser, K. T., Rosenberg, S. D., Swartz, M., Essock, S. M., Osher, F. C., Butterfield, M. I., and Swanson, J. 2001. Recent victimization in women and men with severe mental illness: prevalence and correlates. *Journal of Traumatic Stress*, 14(4), 615–32.

Graham-Kevan, N. 2007. Domestic violence: Research and implications for batterer programmes in Europe. *European Journal on Criminal Policy and Research*, 13(3–4), 213–25.

Greenwood, G. L., Relf, M. V., Huang, B., Pollack, L. M., Canchola, J. A., and Catania, J. A. 2002. Battering victimization among a probability-based sample of men who have sex with men. *American Journal of Public Health*, 92(12), 1964–9.

Griffin, W. A. and Morgan, A. R. 1988. Conflict in maritally distressed military couples. *American Journal of Family Therapy*, 16(1), 14–22.

Hahn, J. W., Aldarondo, E., Silverman, J. G., McCormick, M. C., and Koenen, K. C. 2015. Examining the association between posttraumatic stress disorder and intimate partner violence perpetration. *Journal of Family Violence*, 30(6), 743–52.

Heise, L. L. 1998. Violence against women: an integrated, ecological framework. *Violence against Women*, 4(3), 262–90.

Henderson, L. 2003. Prevalence of domestic violence among lesbians and gay men. Data report to Flame

TV. https://sigmaresearch.org.uk/reports/item/report2003

Heyman, R. E. and Neidig, P. H. 1999. A comparison of spousal aggression prevalence rates in US Army and civilian representative samples. *Journal of Consulting and Clinical Psychology*, 67(2), 239.

Hines, D. A. and Douglas, E. M. 2015. Health problems of partner violence victims: comparing help-seeking men to a population-based sample. *American Journal of Preventive Medicine*, 48(2), 136–44.

Hogan, K. F., Hegarty, J. R., Ward, T., and Dodd, L. J. 2012. Counsellors' experiences of working with male victims of female-perpetrated domestic abuse. *Counselling and Psychotherapy Research*, 12(1), 44–52.

Holtzworth-Munroe, A. and Stuart, G. L. 1994. Typologies of male batterers: three subtypes and the differences among them. *Psychological Bulletin*, 116(3), 476.

Holtzworth-Munroe, A. 2005. Male versus female intimate partner violence: putting controversial findings into context. *Journal of Marriage and Family*, 67(5), 1120–5.

Home Office. 2012. www.gov.uk/government/news/new-definition-of-domestic-violence

Howard, L. M., Oram, S., Galley, H., Trevillion, K., and Feder, G. 2013. Domestic violence and perinatal mental disorders: a systematic review and meta-analysis. *PLoS Medicine*, 10(5), e1001452.

Howard, L. M., Trevillion, K., Khalifeh, H., Woodall, A., Agnew-Davies, R., and Feder, G. 2010. Domestic violence and severe psychiatric disorders: prevalence and interventions. *Psychological Medicine*, 40(6), 881–93.

Jackson, M. A., Sippel, L. M., Mota, N., Whalen, D., and Schumacher, J. A. 2015. Borderline personality disorder and related constructs as risk factors for intimate partner violence perpetration. *Aggression and Violent Behavior*, 24, 95–106.

Jewkes, R. 2002. Intimate partner violence: causes and prevention. *The Lancet*, 359(9315), 1423–9.

Jewkes, R., Sikweyiya, Y., Morrell, R., and Dunkle, K. 2011. Gender inequitable masculinity and sexual entitlement in rape perpetration South Africa: findings of a cross-sectional study. *PloS One*, 6(12), e29590.

Johnson, M. P., Leone, J. M., and Xu, Y. 2014. Intimate terrorism and situational couple violence in general surveys: ex-spouses required. *Violence against Women*, 20(2), 186–207.

Kamperman, A. M., Henrichs, J., Bogaerts, S., Lesaffre, E. M., Wierdsma, A. I., Ghauharali, R. R., Swildens, W., Nijssen, Y., Van Der Gaag, M., Theunissen, J. R., and Delespaul, P. A. 2014. Criminal victimisation in people with severe mental illness: a multi-site prevalence and incidence survey in the Netherlands. *PLoS One*, 9(3), e91029.

Kelly, L. and Westmarland, N. 2015. Domestic violence perpetrator programmes: Steps towards change. Project Mirabal final report. www.nr-foundation.org.uk/downloads/Project_Mirabal-Final_report.pdf

Khalifeh, H. 2015. Violent and non-violent crime against people with severe mental illness. Doctoral thesis, University College London.

Khalifeh, H., Moran, P., Borschmann, R., Dean, K., Hart, C., Hogg, J., Osborn, D., Johnson, S., and Howard, L. M. 2015. Domestic and sexual violence against patients with severe mental illness. *Psychological Medicine*, 45(4), 875–6.

Khalifeh, H., Oram, S., Osborn, D., Howard, L. M., and Johnson, S. 2016. Recent physical and sexual violence against adults with severe mental illness: a systematic review and meta-analysis. *International Review of Psychiatry*, 28(5), 433–51.

Kiene, S. M., Lule, H., Sileo, K. M., Silmi, K. P., and Wanyenze, R. K. 2017. Depression, alcohol use, and intimate partner violence among outpatients in rural Uganda: vulnerabilities for HIV, STIs and high risk sexual behavior. *BMC Infectious Diseases*, 17(1), 88.

Machisa, M. T., Christofides, N., and Jewkes, R. 2016. Structural pathways between child abuse, poor mental health outcomes and male-perpetrated intimate partner violence (IPV). *PloS One*, 11(3), e0150986.

Malinosky-Rummell, R. and Hansen, D. J. 1993. Long-term consequences of childhood physical abuse. *Psychological Bulletin*, 114(1), 68.

Margolin, G. and Gordis, E. B. 2004. Children's exposure to violence in the family and community. *Current Directions in Psychological Science*, 13(4), 152–5.

Mary Beth Phelan, M. D. 2004. *Domestic Violence Screening and Intervention in Medical and Mental Healthcare Settings*. New York: Springer Publishing Company.

Molina, B. S., Pelham, W. E., Gnagy, E. M., Thompson, A. L., and Marshal, M. P. 2007. Attention-deficit/hyperactivity disorder risk for heavy drinking and alcohol use disorder is age specific. *Alcoholism: Clinical and Experimental Research*, 31(4), 643–54.

Newhill, C. E., Eack, S. M., and Mulvey, E. P. 2012. A growth curve analysis of emotion dysregulation as a mediator for violence in individuals with and without borderline personality disorder. *Journal of Personality Disorders*, 26(3), 452–67.

NICE. 2016. Domestic violence and abuse. Quality standard [QS116]. www.nice.org.uk/guidance/qs116/resources/domestic-violence-and-abuse-pdf-75545301469381

Nielssen, O. and Large, M. M. 2010. Rates of homicide during the first episode of psychosis and after treatment: a systematic review and meta-analysis. *Schizophrenia Bulletin*, 36(4), 702–12. doi:10.1093/schbul/sbn144

Nowinski, S. N. and Bowen, E. 2012. Partner violence against heterosexual and gay men: prevalence and correlates. *Aggression and Violent Behavior*, 17(1), 36–52.

Nyame, S., Howard, L. M., Feder, G., and Trevillion, K. 2013. A survey of mental health professionals' knowledge, attitudes and preparedness to respond to domestic violence. *Journal of Mental Health*, 22(6), 536–43.

O'Farrell, T. J., Fals-Stewart, W., Murphy, M., and Murphy, C. M. 2003. Partner violence before and after individually based alcoholism treatment for male alcoholic patients. *Journal of Consulting and Clinical Psychology*, 71(1), 92.

O'farrell, T. J., Murphy, C. M., Stephan, S. H., Fals-Stewart, W., and Murphy, M. 2004. Partner violence before and after couples-based alcoholism treatment for male alcoholic patients: the role of treatment involvement and abstinence. *Journal of Consulting and Clinical Psychology*, 72(2), 202.

Office for National Statistics. 2017. Domestic abuse in England and Wales: year ending March 2018. www.ons.gov.uk/peoplepopulationandcommunity/crimeandjustice/bulletins/domesticabuseinenglandandwales/yearendingmarch2018.

Okuda, M., Olfson, M., Wang, S., Rubio, J. M., Xu, Y., and Blanco, C. 2015. Correlates of intimate partner violence perpetration: results from a National Epidemiologic Survey. *Journal of Traumatic Stress*, 28(1), 49–56.

Oram, S., Capron, L., and Trevillion, K. 2016. Promoting recovery in mental health: evaluation report. www.kcl.ac.uk/ioppn/depts/hspr/research/CEPH/wmh/projects/A-Z/antidepressant-pregnancy/PRIMH-Evaluation-Report-FINAL.pdf.

Oram, S., Flynn, S., Shaw, J., Appleby, L., and Howard, L. M. 2013a. Mental illness and domestic homicide: a population-based descriptive study. *Psychiatric Services*, 64(10), 1006–11. doi:10.1176/appi.ps.201200484

Oram, S., Khalifeh, H., Trevillion, K., Feder, G., and Howard, L. M. 2014a. Perpetration of intimate partner violence by people with mental illness. *European Journal of Public Health*, 24(suppl. 2).

Oram, S., Trevillion, K., Feder, G., and Howard, L. M. 2013b. Prevalence of experiences of domestic violence among psychiatric patients: systematic review. *British Journal of Psychiatry*, 202, 94–9. doi:10.1192/bjp.bp.112.109934

Oram, S., Trevillion, K., Khalifeh, H., Feder, G., and Howard, L. M. 2014b. Systematic review and meta-analysis of psychiatric disorder and the perpetration of partner violence. *Epidemiology and Psychiatric Sciences*, 23(4), 361–76.

Palmetto, N., Davidson, L. L., Breitbart, V., and Rickert, V. I. 2013. Predictors of physical intimate partner violence in the lives of young women: victimization, perpetration, and bidirectional violence. *Violence and Victims*, 28 (1), 103–21.

Phelan, M. B., Hamberger, L. K., Guse, C. E., Edwards, S., Walczak, S., and Zosel, A. 2005. Domestic violence among male and female patients seeking emergency medical services. *Violence and Victims*, 20(2), 187–206.

Radcliffe, P. and Gilchrist, G. 2016. 'You can never work with addictions in isolation': addressing intimate partner violence perpetration by men in substance misuse treatment. *International Journal of Drug Policy*, 36, 130–40.

Read, J. and Fraser, A. 1998. Staff response to abuse histories of psychiatric inpatients. *Australian and New Zealand Journal of Psychiatry*, 32, 206–13.

Read, J., Sampson, M., and Critchley, C. 2016. Are mental health services getting better at responding to abuse, assault and neglect? *Acta Psychiatrica Scandinavica*, 134(4), 287–94.

Rhodes, K. V., Houry, D., Cerulli, C., Straus, H., Kaslow, N. J., and McNutt, L. A. 2009. Intimate partner violence and comorbid mental health conditions among urban male patients. *The Annals of Family Medicine*, 7(1), 47–55.

Rollè, L., Giardina, G., Caldarera, A. M., Gerino, E., and Brustia, P. 2018. When intimate partner violence meets same sex couples: a review of same sex intimate partner violence. *Frontiers in Psychology*, 9, article 1506, 1–13. doi:10.3389/fpsyg.2018.01506 [published correction appears in *Frontiers in Psychology* 2019 July 19; 10, article 1706].

Rose, D., Trevillion, K., Woodall, A., Morgan, C., Feder, G., and Howard, L. 2011. Barriers and facilitators of disclosures of domestic violence by mental health service users: qualitative study. *The British Journal of Psychiatry*, 198(3), 189–94.

Ross, J. M. and Babcock, J. C. 2009. Proactive and reactive violence among intimate partner violent men diagnosed with antisocial and borderline personality disorder. *Journal of Family Violence*, 24(8), 607–17.

Ruddle, A., Pina, A., and Vasquez, E. 2017. Domestic violence offending behaviors: a review of the literature examining childhood exposure, implicit theories, trait aggression and anger rumination as predictive factors. *Aggression and Violent Behavior*, 34, 154–65.

Salber, P. R. and Taliaferro, E. 2006. *The Physician's Guide to Violence against Women and Abuse. A Reference for All Health Care Professionals*. Volcano, CA: Volcano Press.

Salyers, M. P., Evans, L. J., Bond, G. R., and Meyer, P. S. 2004. Barriers to assessment and treatment of posttraumatic stress disorder and other trauma-related problems in people with severe mental illness: clinician perspectives. *Community Mental Health Journal*, 40(1), 17–31.

Satyanarayana, V. A., Nattala, P., Selvam, S., Pradeep, J., Hebbani, S., Hegde, S., and Srinivasan, K. 2016. Integrated cognitive behavioral intervention reduces intimate partner violence among alcohol dependent men, and improves mental health outcomes in their spouses: a clinic based randomized controlled trial from South India. *Journal of Substance Abuse Treatment*, 64, 29–34.

Schumacher, J. A., Feldbau-Kohn, S., Slep, A. M. S., and Heyman, R. E. 2001. Risk factors for male-to-female partner physical abuse. *Aggression and Violent Behavior*, 6(2–3), 281–352.

Scott, K. and King, C. 2007. Resistance, reluctance, and readiness in perpetrators of abuse against women and children. *Trauma, Violence, and Abuse*, 8(4), 401–17.

Shorey, R. C., Stuart, G. L., McNulty, J. K., and Moore, T. M. 2014. Acute alcohol use temporally increases the odds of male perpetrated dating violence: a 90-day diary analysis. *Addictive Behaviors*, 39(1), 365–8.

Smedslund, G., Dalsbø, T. K., Steiro, A., Winsvold, A., and Clench-Aas, J. 2007. Cognitive behavioural therapy for men who physically abuse their female partner. *Cochrane Database of Systematic Reviews*, (3), CD006048. doi: 10.1002/14651858. CD006048.pub2.

Stanley, J. L., Bartholomew, K., Taylor, T., Oram, D., and Landolt, M. 2006. Intimate violence in male same-sex relationships. *Journal of Family Violence*, 21(1), 31–41.

Stepp, S. D., Smith, T. D., Morse, J. Q., Hallquist, M. N., and Pilkonis, P. A. 2012. Prospective associations among borderline personality

disorder symptoms, interpersonal problems, and aggressive behaviors. *Journal of Interpersonal Violence*, 27(1), 103–24.

Stiles-Shields, C. and Carroll, R. A. 2015. Same-sex domestic violence: prevalence, unique aspects, and clinical implications. *Journal of Sex and Marital Therapy*, 41(6), 636–48.

Teplin, L. A., McClelland, G. M., Abram, K. M., and Weiner, D. A. 2005. Crime victimization in adults with severe mental illness: comparison with the National Crime Victimization Survey. *Archives of General Psychiatry*, 62(8), 911–21. doi:10.1001/ archpsyc.62.8.911

Testa, M., Quigley, B. M., and Leonard, K. E. 2003. Does alcohol make a difference? Within-participants comparison of incidents of partner violence. *Journal of Interpersonal Violence*, 18(7), 735–43.

The National Confidential Inquiry into Suicide and Homicide by People with Mental Illness. Annual Report: England, Northern Ireland, Scotland and Wales. October 2017. University of Manchester, http:// documents.manchester.ac.uk/ display.aspx?DocID=37591.

Thomas, M. D., Bennett, L. W., and Stoops, C. 2013. The treatment needs of substance abusing batterers: a comparison of men who batter their female partners. *Journal of Family Violence*, 28(2), 121–9.

Tjaden, P., Thoennes, N., and Allison, C. J. 1999. Comparing violence over the life span in samples of same-sex and opposite-sex cohabitants. *Violence and Victims*, 14(4), 413.

Trabold, N., McMahon, J., Alsobrooks, S., Whitney, S., and Mittal, M. 2018. A systematic review of intimate partner violence interventions: state of the field and implications for practitioners. *Trauma, Violence, and Abuse*, 21(2), 1–15.

Trevillion, K., Byford, S., Cary, M., Rose, D., Oram, S., Feder, G., Agnew-Davies, R., and Howard, L.

M. 2014. Linking abuse and recovery through advocacy: an observational study. *Epidemiology and Psychiatric Sciences*, 23(1), 99–113.

Trevillion, K., Corker, E., Capron, L. E., and Oram, S. 2016. Improving mental health service responses to domestic violence and abuse. *International Review of Psychiatry*, 28(5), 423–32.

Trevillion, K., Oram, S., Feder, G., and Howard, L. 2012. Experiences of domestic violence and mental disorders: a systematic review and meta-analysis. *PLoS One*, 7(12), e51740. doi:10.1371/journal.pone .0051740

Tsui, V., Cheung, M., and Leung, P. 2010. Help-seeking among male victims of partner abuse: men's hard times. *Journal of Community Psychology*, 38(6), 769–80.

Walby, S. (2009). *The Cost of Domestic Violence*. Lancaster: Lancaster University Press.

Walby, S., Towers, J., Balderston, S., Corradi, C., Francis, B., Heiskanen, M., Helweg-Larsen, K., Mergaert, L., Olive, P., Palmer, E., and Stöckl, H. 2017. *The Concept and Measurement of Violence against Women and Men*. Bristol: Policy Press.

Weiner, D. A. 2005. Crime victimization in adults with severe mental illness: comparison with the National Crime Victimization Survey. *Archives of General Psychiatry*, 62(8), 911–21.

WHO. 2013. Responding to intimate partner violence and sexual violence against women: WHO clinical and policy guidelines. http://apps.who .int/iris/bitstream/10665/85240/1/ 9789241548595_eng.pdf

Williamson, E., Jones, S. K., Ferrari, G., Debbonaire, T., Feder, G., and Hester, M. 2015. Health professionals responding to men for safety (HERMES): feasibility of a general practice training intervention to improve the response to male patients who have experienced or perpetrated domestic violence and abuse. *Primary Health Care Research and Development, 16*(3), 281–8.

Wupperman, P., Amble, P., Devine, S., Zonana, H., Fals-Stewart, W., and Easton, C. 2009. Violence and substance use among female partners of men in treatment for intimate-partner violence. *Journal of the American Academy of Psychiatry and the Law Online, 37*(1), 75–81.

Wymbs, B. T., Walther, C. A., Cheong, J., Belendiuk, K. A., Pedersen, S. L., Gnagy, E. M., Pelham, Jr, W. E., and Molina, B. S. 2017. Childhood ADHD potentiates the association between problematic drinking and intimate partner violence. *Journal of Attention Disorders, 21*(12), 997–1008.

Yu, R., Nevado-Holgado, A. J., Molero, Y., D'Onfrio, B. M., Larsson, H., Howard, L. M., and Fazel, S. 2019. Mental disorders and intimate partner violence perpetrated by men towards women: a Swedish population-based longitudinal study. *PLoS Medicine, 16*(12), e1002995. doi:10.1371/journal.pmed.1002995

Zierler, S., Cunningham, W. E., Andersen, R., Shapiro, M. F., Nakazono, T., Morton, S., Crystal, S., Stein, M., Turner, B., St Clair, P., and Bozzette, S. A. 2000. Violence victimization after HIV infection in a US probability sample of adult patients in primary care. *American Journal of Public Health, 90*(2), 208.

Chapter

18

Alcohol and Substance Misuse in Men

Yvonne Bonomo and J. Buckley Lennox

There are considerable differences between men and women when it comes to substance use and misuse. In general, men commence alcohol and other substance use earlier than women (United Nations Office of Drugs and Crime [UNODC] 2015). The prevalence and the characteristics of alcohol and drug use also differ when comparing men to women. In addition, across the world, men still outnumber women with regard to alcohol and other drug treatment (UNODC, 2015). Box 18.1 summarizes substance use in males and the chapter then takes a lifespan approach to substance use substance use disorders in males.

Adolescent Males and Substance Use

As outlined in Chapter 4 of this book, adolescence is a key developmental period. It can be considered in three phases – early, middle, and late adolescence. Early adolescence typically covers the ages 11–14 years and the focus in this developmental stage is whether the changes that the young person is going through are 'normal'. Middle adolescence typically covers the age range 15–17 years and during this period, the focus of the individual is usually identity, including a sense of to which peer group does the young person belong. Late adolescence refers to the age of 18 years and older and in this developmental phase, the focus is often on what the individual will 'do' with their life, the establishment of intimate relationships, and planning for the future. These stages are a guide only, and it is important to be aware that sometimes the developmental stage of an individual may not quite be aligned with their chronological age. Some older adolescents are delayed in the capacities normally expected for their age, and vice versa.

The brain undergoes significant change during adolescence (Giedd et al., 1999; Gogtay et al., 2004). As the brain matures, substantial pruning of less 'useful' neural pathways occurs while at the same time myelination of other neural pathways is effected,

> **Box 18.1** **Alcohol and substance use in males**
> - Alcohol and substance use differs between men and women
> - Alcohol and substance use varies across the lifespan of the male
> - Psychosocial, psychological approaches, and pharmacotherapy should be considered in the approach to substance use problems
> - The approach to the male with problem alcohol or other substance use needs to take into consideration the life stage of the male
> - Whatever the life stage, improvements can be achieved in the majority of men with problem alcohol or substance use

enabling more efficient and more effective transmission of neuronal signals. The maturation process starts from the posterior of the brain and moves toward the prefrontal cortex. The latter is the last part of the brain to mature, and is responsible for executive function. Executive function includes the ability to determine the consequences of different actions, to suppress urges, and to discern between conflicting thoughts or concepts. These processes are in their early stages at the commencement of adolescence, and clinically, they can manifest as concrete thinking rather than abstract reasoning or logical deductive thinking in young adolescents.

Male teenagers who drink alcohol or use substances in early adolescence frequently make suboptimal decisions related to their substance use or other behaviour, in part because they have less capacity to fully comprehend potential negative consequences that might occur. By middle adolescence, young people are usually able to think in more abstract terms about their health and they are better at recognizing the impact of drinking alcohol or using drugs on their health and well-being and on that of others, albeit they are often inconsistent in their thoughts and behaviour. Peers are a very significant influence in middle adolescence, and it is generally accepted that peers play a crucial role in the initiation of substance use in adolescents.

Prevalence of Substance Use in Adolescent Males

Experimentation with potentially risky behaviours, including substance use, typically occurs in adolescence. Early adolescents most commonly experiment first with alcohol and tobacco. Some early adolescent males will experiment with other substances, such as inhalants, sometimes referred to as 'chroming' or 'sniffing' volatile hydrocarbons such as those in spray paints, glue, or petrol. This form of substance use most often occurs in certain subgroups of youth in whom the psychosocial risk factors greatly outweigh protective factors; these include Indigenous young people and disadvantaged groups (Swaim and Stanley, 2018; Zhu and Rieder, 2012). Health-risk behaviours usually emerge by middle adolescence, including experimentation with cannabis, which is the most commonly used illicit drug globally (UNODC, 2015). Experimentation also occurs with MDMA ('ecstasy') and new psychoactive substances (NPS) at this age, usually at music festivals and other similar contexts. Progression to methamphetamine, heroin, or other opioids and injecting drug use generally occurs in the minority of young people who tend to have a number of vulnerabilities.

Characteristics of Substance Use in Adolescent Males

Longitudinal studies have consistently shown that young males who experiment heavily with substances typically have a greater number of 'risk factors' than 'protective factors' in their psychosocial profile. Risk factors are those factors in a young person's life that make it more likely that they will engage in behaviours that lead to negative outcomes in health and well-being (Hawkins et al., 1992; Resnick et al., 1997). Risk and protective factors may occur in a number of domains including social (e.g., socioeconomic class), family (e.g., family relations, parenting style, parental use of substances or mental illness), peers and social skills, academic ability and school adjustment, personality and behaviours (e.g., externalizing or internalizing, other behaviours). Examples of risk factors

Box 18.2 Factors impacting substance use in young adolescent males

- Social class
- Economic family burden
- Family conflict
- Parenting style
- Parental substance use
- Peer pressure
- Academic ability
- Bullying
- Personality problems

include lack of engagement with school, being bullied, and familial conflict. Protective factors are those factors that reduce the likelihood that the risks adolescents, take will result in harm. Some examples of protective factors are strong parental guidance, good peer relationships, and participation in sporting or in creative activities(Box 18.2; Hawkins et al., 1992; Resnick et al., 1997).

Alcohol remains the most commonly used and misused substance in young people and its prevalence far exceeds other substance use, including illicit substance use. Tobacco smoking is often associated with heavy drinking in young people. By and large, alcohol and tobacco smoking in young people are driven by behavioural and social factors. Physiological dependence on substances is rare in adolescence, tending to occur later in life, at the earliest in late adolescence but more commonly in young adulthood or later. A minority of smoking youth have, however, been described as having an early onset of nicotine dependence that appears to be driven by biological factors. These young people report similar symptoms to nicotine-dependent adults to maintain a steady state of nicotine, including smoking soon after waking or continuing to smoke even when unwell (Adelman, 2004). In these young people, quitting is particularly difficult and nicotine cessation pharmacotherapies to date have not yielded high rates of success (Karpinski et al., 2010).

Interventions for Male Adolescent Substance Use

Interventions for substance use vary depending on the context and on the individual. Most importantly, the developmental stage of the adolescent must be taken into account as the approach should be tailored to that stage. A holistic approach, rather than one focusing mainly on the substance use, and multidisciplinary input is required with a focus on behavioural strategies and interventions for mental health and well-being. Most young people do not engage with health professionals who appear to be more interested in the substance use than in a more holistic approach to the individual. Increasing access to interventions for adolescents is of paramount importance because young people are less likely than adults to proactively follow up health care. Hence, outreach, opportunistic health care, and assistance with transition from adolescent to adult services at the appropriate time, are all key aspects of the approach to adolescent substance use.

Prevention Approaches in Adolescent Males

Prevention of substance use problems in adolescents can occur on a systemic level or an individual level.

At a systemic level, public health approaches such as regulation of advertising and product placement for alcohol are important. Local government strategies such as sporting club policies also have an important role to play, such as the Good Sports programme in Australia (Duff et al., 2007).

On an individual level, promoting resilience is a key approach to prevention of substance use problems in adolescents. One way in which to promote resilience is to strengthen protective factors that help the adolescent feel connected to family, school, peers, or other social contexts such as sporting or religious groups. Parents also have an important role to play in prevention. Harsh parenting, poor parent–child communication, and parental alcohol use have been associated with male alcohol use into emerging adulthood (Diggs et al., 2017). Communication and approaches to parenting that focus on a warm relationship and positive regard are protective factors against substance use. Health professionals should advise parents not to supply their sons and daughters with alcohol, or facilitate their access to, and consumption of, alcohol. Parental supply of alcohol has generally been associated with increased rates of drinking (Kaynak et al., 2014; Mattick et al., 2017). Longitudinal data indicates that the later the onset of alcohol use in the young person, the less likelihood there is of alcohol-related problems later (Liang and Chikritzhs, 2015).

Young Adult Males and AOD Use

Young adulthood typically refers to ages 18 to 24 years. Young adult males, when compared to adolescents, generally have a better understanding of the broader implications of their substance use, and misuse. From a bio-psycho-social perspective, young adults tend to be more focused on their future and often have greater motivation to address education and employment, mental health, and substance use. Intimate relationships are frequently an important driver of behaviours at this stage of life.

Prevalence of Substance Use in Young Adult Males

General population surveys globally show that more than half of young adults report drinking alcohol (Australian Institute of Health and Welfare [AIHW], 2017; Office for National Statistics, 2018; Substance Abuse and Mental Health Services Administration, 2016). The prevalence of other substance use and dependence (e.g., cannabis, opioids, amphetamines) often peaks in this age group and the decade after (Degenhardt et al., 2013).

Characteristics of Substance Use in Young Adult Males

Longitudinal studies have consistently shown that the majority of young adult males who drink, smoke, or use illicit drugs transition out of regular or heavy use as the responsibilities and commitments to study, gain employment, and develop intimate relationships grow. A subgroup of young adult males persist with their substance use and are at increased risk of problem use and substance dependence. In these young men, there may be a history of trauma such as childhood sexual abuse (Fergusson et al., 2013), antisocial personality disorder (Mattick et al., 2017), or a genetic predisposition to substance use problems. Indicators of an individual predisposition to developing problems include how the young male responds to alcohol. Alcohol-related blackouts, for example, have been shown to be a predictor of problem alcohol use (Hingson et al., 2016; Marino and Fromme, 2018). Loss of control in drinking during adolescence and young adulthood may also be a marker of vulnerability to ongoing problem drinking (Olsson et al., 2016). A strong family history of alcohol or other substance use problems may also be a marker of inherent vulnerability, and these individuals are best advised to delay onset of, or ideally abstain from, alcohol or drug use.

Interventions for Young Adult Substance Use Problems

Most young adult males can address their substance use themselves and benefit from health information and advice about risks of harm and potential treatment options if they are having difficulty. However, there is an important subgroup of young adult males who need a much more intensive approach. Some of these individuals have been linked with services as an adolescent, and in these cases, assistance with the transition from youth to adult services may be needed. Adult services differ from adolescent services in that they expect the individual to have more autonomy and self-efficacy and there is therefore a greater onus on the young adult to drive their own healthcare. This may need to be explained to the individual, who may not appreciate the difference in approaches between adolescent and adult services and may be surprised or even distressed at the change in paradigm that they experience. Typically, adult treatment services are less able to accommodate opportunistic healthcare, or provide outreach services and they are generally speaking less flexible in coordinating appointments.

Other young adults may not have accessed adolescent services, their problems presenting for the first time in young adulthood. Underlying mental health concerns such as depression, anxiety, or other mental health disorders may be present and the substance use may be a form of 'self-medication'. The approach to treatment therefore needs to address these underlying mental health conditions.

Some young adult males may have already progressed to substance dependence, and in these individuals, behavioural or psychological approaches and psychosocial rehabilitation, possibly with the addition of pharmacological treatments, are indicated. Psychosocial rehabilitation includes engaging the young adult in meaningful and appropriate education or employment. This may need to commence slowly with minimal contact hours, building up over time.

Middle Adult Males and AOD Use

Middle adulthood – as its name suggests – spans the period between young adulthood and older adulthood.

From a bio-psycho-social perspective, middle adults generally tend to be established in employment, relationships, and families and in preferred social activities. Psychosocial stressors in this age group differ from those in other stages of life, hence also the patterns of substance use and their trajectories in this period.

Prevalence of Substance Use in Males in Middle Adulthood

General population surveys globally show that the prevalence of alcohol and other drugs in middle adulthood can vary substantially between countries. For example, in Australia, almost half of the middle adult age group reports consuming alcohol weekly, whereas rates of tobacco smoking are much less at around 20% (AIHW). Cannabis use is reported by less than 15% of middle adults in Australia, whereas in European countries such as Germany a much higher prevalence is reported with 42% of 25–29-year-olds and 26% of 40–59-year-olds using cannabis (Piontek, 2016). In general, for most countries, illicit drug use tends to decrease progressively with each decade of middle adulthood. It is important not to have in mind a stereotype of the substance misuser, because misuse of alcohol by the middle adult male may well be occurring concomitantly with a high-functioning career. Similarly, prescription medications – particularly opioids and benzodiazepines – may occur in this age group without being immediately obvious. It is therefore worthwhile screening middle adults for alcohol and drug use, both prescribed and illicit, whenever the opportunity arises.

Characteristics of Substance Use in Males in Middle Adulthood

By middle adulthood, men are at different points in the spectrum of substance use. Some men are abstinent or engage in minimal substance use (less than monthly). Others may be engaging in episodic use of substances, often to relieve stress or to celebrate an occasion. Still others may be suffering from a substance use disorder. A bio-psycho-social assessment of these men will often reflect the pattern of their substance use. At the less severe end of the spectrum, men are engaged in relationships, work, and other meaningful activities, and any alcohol or other drug use that is more than minimal interferes too much with these responsibilities. Those who engage in episodic heavy substance use may find that their relationships and work are impacted to a lesser or greater degree. Some men may not be cognizant of the impact their alcohol or drug use is having on their lives and those around them. The health professional therefore has an important role in making the connection between their substance use and absenteeism from work, or family disruption, or even perpetration of family violence (Choenni et al., 2017; see also Chapter 17).

Importantly, studies of the natural history of substance use disorders in males in middle adulthood show that the trajectory does not inevitably deteriorate; rather, a proportion improve over time (Tuithof, 2015). Those with severe substance use disorders, however, generally cannot maintain relationships or their work roles and their psychosocial stability progressively diminishes with a marital or relationship breakdown, deterioration of other meaningful relationships (e.g., with family, children, friends, colleagues), job losses, and other significant impacts.

Interventions for Males in Middle Adulthood with Substance Use Problems

Brief interventions can be effective for men at the less severe end of the spectrum of substance use. Discussion that reflects for the individual their pattern of use and associated complications and advice on reducing or ceasing drinking, smoking, or other substance use, together with exploration of potential strategies by which to do this, have been shown to be effective (Young et al., 2014).

Interventions for more severe substance use disorder, which typically has a relapsing–remitting– relapsing pattern, generally focus on prevention of relapse after a period of remission. To achieve remission, a period of substance withdrawal (colloquially referred to as 'detoxification') is often necessary. Depending on the severity of the dependence, this may occur in a non-residential or residential facility. Following this early phase, rehabilitation either in the form of counselling, day programme attendance, or – for the male with more severe dependence – residential rehabilitation is indicated.

Treatment for the complications of substance use disorder are also necessary at this point in life, such as treatment for hepatitis or liver cirrhosis, or other organ impairment secondary to heavy alcohol consumption or blood-borne virus infection from injecting drug use.

Mental health disorders are often an additional co-morbid condition and must be addressed as part of substance use treatment. In the first instance, a diagnosis must be made and a plan of management determined. In some men, the mental health disorder precedes the substance use disorder, while in other men it occurs as a consequence of the substance use disorder. It is difficult to gain improvements in mental health if heavy and persistent substance use continues. Therefore a focus on substance withdrawal and maintenance of abstinence is important to understanding the underlying mental health concerns.

Acquired brain injury may be a result of the direct toxic effect of alcohol, or secondary to hypoxic incidents (alcohol, opioids, other sedative drugs), and typically becomes evident in middle adulthood. Assessment of deficits and establishment of strategies to compensate for the cognitive deficiencies are required. For example, in more severe cases of poor working memory, reminder notes placed in key positions around the home might be considered. If attention is poor, then repeating tasks or instructions and writing them down may assist the individual to maintain focus.

Older Adult Males and AOD Use

Older adulthood, variably defined in the literature but here referring to those over 65 years old, is another phase in the lifespan with specific characteristics. Transition to retirement and loss of occupation can be a trigger for increased alcohol or other drug use, arising through social isolation or indeed the opposite, increased social contact with broadened social networks after retirement. Bereavement, physical health problems, social isolation, taking on the caregiving role of an unwell partner, and lack of religious affiliation can be drivers of substance use in older adults. Males might be differentially susceptible, expressly those from a generation in which they were the main 'breadwinners' (see Box 18.3).

Substance use and associated problems are often not detected in the older adult, as there is generally a tendency for substance use to be considered as being limited to younger people. Problems can arise as a result of the physiological changes that take place in older age that reduce tolerance to alcohol or other drugs and therefore present in masked ways, such as repeated falls, incontinence, dizzy spells, change in appetite or in behaviour, social withdrawal, mood

---

Box 18.3 Factors impacting substance use in older men

- Issues of transition to retirement
- Loss of 'breadwinner' role
- Loss of spouse
- Social isolation
- Socializing with others who use substances
- Physical health problems
- Sleep problems
- Depression and anxiety

---

swings, and suicidal ideation. Onset of mild cognitive decline may also be subtle and attributed to older age rather than to alcohol or other drug use. This can include memory difficulties, greater anxiety than is usual for the individual, difficulty making decisions, and loss of interest in usual activities. Substance use can also complicate prior brain injury, presenting as dementia secondary to alcohol or other drug use.

Prevalence of Substance Use in Males in Older Adulthood

Screening for alcohol and drug use in older adults tends not to be pursued as routinely as it is in the younger population, and as a result, prevalence estimates are likely to under-report alcohol and other drug use in this sub-population. The ageing population (65+ years) is estimated to double between 2001 and 2020 (Gossop and Moos, 2008). Alcohol and drug use in this age group increasingly require attention, because their prevalence is increasing. In part, this has arisen as a result of the increased life expectancy of baby boomers who started alcohol and other drug use in their teenage and early adult years. Combined with other health problems of ageing, however, the impacts of substance use in this age group can be significant.

Harmful alcohol consumption and tobacco smoking are estimated to be as high as 25% and 10%, respectively, in persons aged 65 years and over. Prescription medication use, especially opioids, benzodiazepines, antidepressants, and antipsychotics, also often occurs in this age group. Alcohol, tobacco, and other drug use in older people can lead to increased risk of stroke, high blood pressure, liver disease, and dementia. Falls and injuries occur in 30–60% of older adults each year, 10–20% resulting in injury, hospitalization, and/or death with

psychoactive and other drugs noted to be a significant contributing factor (NSW Ministry of Health, 2015; Rubenstein, 2006)

Characteristics of Substance Use in Males in Older Adulthood

In comparison to other age groups, relatively little is known about the patterns of use of substances among older men, especially poly-substance use. For some, heavy use of alcohol, tobacco, or other drugs has been occurring most of their lives and complications present in this stage of the lifespan. For others, there is new onset of heavy or problematic alcohol or other drug use in older age attributable to the transition to older adulthood and change of lifestyle and changing relationships. For example, sleep disturbance and sleep disorders are common in older men, and this can drive some forms of substance use such as alcohol, prescription medications, and cannabis.

Interventions for Males in Older Adulthood with Substance Use Problems

The approach to substance use problems in older adulthood is similar to those in middle adulthood but must take into account the context of the older male. There is still considerable stigma associated with substance use, particularly when it is problematic, and this influences the way health professionals engage the older male. In addition, there are many similarities between the effects of substance use and conditions of older age that occur for many men, such as increased fatigue, reducing physical stability with a propensity for falls, and difficulty sleeping as well as the general slowing of cognition, including memory (Dar, 2006) for which it takes time to discern the root cause. The approach therefore needs to be supportive, rather than confrontational, and is best positioned as part of an overall assessment of health and well-being rather than solely targeted at the substance use. For alcohol and tobacco in particular, the attitude that drinking and smoking are life's 'last little pleasures' is common and deeply entrenched in many older adult males, constituting a marker of reduced motivation to address drinking from a health-related perspective. In addition, a sense within the individual that they are approaching the end of life can impact motivation levels. Notwithstanding this, the frequency and quantity of drinking, cigarette smoking, and both prescribed and over-the-counter medications are usually best ascertained before asking about illicit substance use such as cannabis.

A screening tool validated across cultures that has been used in older adult population is the AUDIT (Lundin et al., 2015). The Michigan Alcohol Screening Test (MAST) is also sometimes used to screen for alcohol and there is a Geriatric Version for the older population. There are other screening tools, including the Alcohol, Smoking, and Substance Involvement Test (ASSIST) (Humeniuk et al., 2008), although this has not yet been validated in the older population. The screening tool for alcohol (Mayfield et al., 1974) has been adapted to include other drugs in addition to alcohol (CAGE-AID; Brown and Rounds, 1995).

Interventions follow the same continuum as described for the earlier life stages. It is important not to assume that there is nothing that can be done to change the patterns of alcohol or other drug use in the older adult male. Access to treatment services for the older person can pose problems as a result of difficulties with transport, stigma associated with having a substance use problem, or difficulty engaging with groups or services that cater more for the younger person. As a result, a published rigorous evidence base regarding the most effective approaches to this special population is relatively small.

Brief intervention has merit in its non-confrontational approach and its focus on reflecting on healthier lifestyle, although publications of trials in men older than 65 years are very few. Self-help groups such as Alcoholics Anonymous and Narcotics Anonymous as well as newer models such as SMART Recovery (Beck et al., 2017) can be helpful for older men, particularly if there are other similar aged men in the groups. No systematic studies have, however, explored the efficacy of these groups in older adults.

Pharmacotherapy for alcohol and drug use disorders similarly has not been extensively evaluated in men over 65, but they are likely at least as effective in the older male population as they are for younger individuals. Pharmacodynamic and pharmacokinetic considerations need to be taken into account given that muscle mass tends to decrease and body fat increases with age. Lipophilic drugs such as benzodiazepines or cannabinoids accumulate in the fat and their effects therefore endure longer. Hepatic metabolism and renal excretion also often decline in older age, and these can affect the rate of alcohol and drug metabolism.

Conclusions

Men differ from women in their patterns of alcohol and drug use. Across the lifespan, there are specific characteristics, hence the importance of stage-specific approaches to engaging the male in addressing their substance use, be it early or later in the substance-use spectrum. As a general rule, reduction in harmful drinking or drug use can be achieved, hence health professionals are encouraged to screen for substance use, and therein assist men to improve their health and well-being.

References

Adams, W. L. 1996. Alcohol use in retirement communities. *Journal of the American Geriatrics Society*, 44(9), 1082–5.

Adelman, W. P. 2004. Nicotine replacement therapy for teenagers: about time or a waste of time? *Archives of Pediatrics & Adolescent Medicine*, 158(3), 205–6.

Australian Institute of Health and Welfare [AIHW]. 2017. National Drug Strategy Household Survey 2016: detailed findings. Available from www.aihw.gov.au/reports/illicit-use-of-drugs/2016-ndshs-detailed/contents/table-of-contents.

Beck, A. K. et al. 2017. Systematic review of SMART Recovery: outcomes, process variables, and implications for research. *Psychol Addict Behav* 31(1), 1–20.

Brown, R. L. and Rounds, L. A. 1995. Conjoint screening questionnaires for alcohol and other drug abuse: criterion validity in a primary care practice. *Wis Med J*, 94(3), 135–40.

Choenni, V. et al. 2017. Association between substance use and the perpetration of family violence in industrialized countries: a systematic review. *Trauma Violence Abuse* 18(1), 37–50.

Dar, K. 2006. Alcohol use disorders in elderly people: fact or fiction? *Advances in Psychiatric Treatment*, 12(3), 173–81.

Degenhardt, L. et al. 2013. Global burden of disease attributable to illicit drug use and dependence: findings from the Global Burden of Disease Study 2010. *The Lancet*, 382(9904), 1564–74.

Diggs, O. N. et al. 2017. The association of harsh parenting, parent–child communication, and parental alcohol use with male alcohol use into emerging adulthood. *J Adolesc Health*, 61(6), 736–42.

Duff, G. and Munro, G. 2007. Preventing alcohol-related problems in community sports clubs: the good sports program. *Subst Use Misuse*, 42(12–13), 1991–2001.

Fergusson, D. M., McLeod, G. F., and Horwood, L. J. 2013. Childhood sexual abuse and adult developmental outcomes: findings from a 30-year longitudinal study in New Zealand. *Child Abuse & Neglect*, 37(9), 664–74.

Giedd, J. N. et al. 1999. Brain development during childhood and adolescence: a longitudinal MRI study. *Nature Neuroscience*, 2(10), 861.

Gogtay, N. et al. 2004. Dynamic mapping of human cortical development during childhood through early adulthood. *Proc Natl Acad Sci U S A*, 101(21), 8174–9.

Gossop, M. and Moos, R. 2008. Substance misuse among older adults: a neglected but treatable problem. *Addiction*, 103(3), 347–8.

Hawkins, J. D., Catalano, R. F., and Miller, J. Y. 1992. Risk and protective factors for alcohol and other drug problems in adolescence and early adulthood: implications for substance abuse prevention. *Psychological Bulletin*, 112(1), 64.

Hingson, R. et al. 2016. Alcohol-induced blackouts as predictors of other drinking related harms among emerging young adults. *Alcoholism: Clinical and Experimental Research*, 40(4), 776–84.

Humeniuk, R. et al. 2008. Validation of the alcohol, smoking and substance involvement screening test (ASSIST). *Addiction*, 103(6), 1039–47.

Ilomäki, J. et al. 2014. Alcohol consumption and tobacco smoking among community-dwelling older Australian men: the Concord Health and Ageing in Men Project. *Australasian Journal on Ageing*, 33 (3), 185–92.

Karpinski, J. P., Timpe, E. M., and Lubsch, L. 2010. Smoking cessation treatment for adolescents. *The Journal of Pediatric Pharmacology and Therapeutics*, 15(4), 249–63.

Kaynak, Ö. et al. 2014. Providing alcohol for underage youth: what

messages should we be sending parents? *J Stud Alcohol Drugs*, 75(4), 590–605.

Liang, W. and Chikritzhs, T. J. I. J. o. D. P. 2015. Age at first use of alcohol predicts the risk of heavy alcohol use in early adulthood: a longitudinal study in the United States. *Int J Drug Policy*, 26(2), 131–4.

Lundin, A., Hallgren, M., Balliu, N. and Forsell, Y. 2015. The use of alcohol use disorders identification test (AUDIT) in detecting alcohol use disorder and risk drinking in the general population: validation of AUDIT using schedules for clinical assessment in neuropsychiatry. *Alcoholism: Clinical and Experimental Research*, 39(1), 158–65.

Marino, E. N. and Fromme, K. 2018. Alcohol-induced blackouts, subjective intoxication, and motivation to decrease drinking: prospective examination of the transition out of college. *Addictive Behaviors*, 80, 89–94.

Mattick, R. P. et al. 2017. Parental supply of alcohol and alcohol consumption in adolescence: prospective cohort study. *Psychol Med*, 47(2), 267–78.

Mayfield, D., McLeod, G., and Hall, P. 1974. The CAGE questionnaire: validation of a new alcoholism screening instrument. *American Journal of Psychiatry*, 131(10), 1121–3.

NSW Ministry of Health. 2015. Older people's drug and alcohol project. Available from www.health.nsw.gov .au/aod/professionals/Publications/ opdap-fullreport.pdf.

Office for Natinoal Statistics. 2018. Adult drinking habits in Great Britain: 2017. E John – Statistical Bulletin. Office for National Statistics (ONS), backup.ons.gov.uk.

Olsson, C. A. et al. 2016. Drinking patterns of adolescents who develop alcohol use disorders: results from the Victorian Adolescent Health Cohort Study. *BMJ Open*, 6 2), e010455.

Piontek, D., Gomes de Matos, E., Atzendorf, J. and Kraus, L. 2016. *Brief Report Epidemiological Survey 2015. Table: Alcohol Consumption, Episodic Drunkenness and Evidence of Clinically Relevant Alcohol Consumption by Gender and Age in 2015*. Munich: IFT Institute for Therapy Research.

Resnick, M. D. et al. 1997. Protecting adolescents from harm: findings from the National Longitudinal Study on Adolescent Health. *JAMA*, 278(10), 823–32.

Rubenstein, L. Z. 2006. Falls in older people: epidemiology, risk factors and strategies for prevention. *Age and Ageing*, 35(suppl. 2), ii37–ii41.

Substance Abuse and Mental Health Services Administration. 2016. 2015 National survey on Drug Use and Health. Available from www .samhsa.gov/data/sites/default/files/ NSDUH-DetTabs-2015/NSDUH-DetTabs-2015/NSDUH-DetTabs-2015.pdf.

Swaim, R. C. and Stanley, L. R. 2018. Substance use among American Indian youths on reservations compared with a national sample of US adolescents. *JAMA Network Open*, 1(1), e180382.

Tuithof, M. 2015. Drinking Distilled. Onset, course and treatment of alcohol use disorders in the general population. PhD thesis, University of Amsterdam.

United Nations Office of Drugs and Crime [UNODC]. 2015. World drug report. Available from www .unodc.org/wdr2015/.

Young, M. M. et al. 2014. Effectiveness of brief interventions as part of the Screening, Brief Intervention and Referral to Treatment (SBIRT) model for reducing the nonmedical use of psychoactive substances: a systematic review. *Syst Rev*, 3(1), 50.

Zhu, J. X. and Rieder, M. J. P. 2012. Interventions for inhalant abuse among First Nations youth. *Paediatr Child Health*, 17(7), 391–2.

HIV and Mental Health in Men

Taylan Yukselen, Harriet Quigley, Lucy Blake, and Ian Paul Everall

We are almost into the fifth decade of the acquired immunodeficiency syndrome (AIDS) pandemic, and in that time the illness has gone from being a highly unpredictable series of life-threatening illnesses that is consequent upon being immune compromised with a high mortality rate to being a highly treatable one-tablet-a-day infection. This represents an enormous revolution in medical treatment. AIDS was first recognized in 1981 after early cases of kaposi sarcoma and pneumocystis carinii were reported in the USA in young immunocompromised homosexual men (David et al., 2012; Rosca et al., 2012). However, the disease has been thought to have existed since the mid-1970s (Des Jarlais et al., 1989). There then followed the AIDS pandemic of the early 1980s when the spread of the virus grew exponentially throughout the world. Since then, several breakthroughs have taken place. In 1983, a retrovirus, now called human immunodeficiency virus (HIV), was identified as the causative agent (Sharp and Hahn, 2011). This led to the synthesis of antiviral medication aimed at inhibiting enzymes unique to the virus, such as reverse transcriptase inhibitors, protease inhibitors, and most recently, integrase inhibitors. In 1996 it was shown that taking a combination of these medications called combination antiretroviral therapy (cART) provided significantly effective treatment and basically stopped viral replication and the ensuing damage to the immune system (Ghosn et al., 2018). Since the introduction of cART and with further advances in research, HIV and AIDS have become a chronic illness. There has been a significant reduction in mortality and morbidity as a result of increased viral suppression that markedly halts the disease progression and reduces the rate of human transmission, resulting in people living longer and healthier lives (Ghosn et al., 2018; David et al., 2012).

Despite encouraging advances in HIV treatment, and a dramatic reduction in new infections in the past decade, the Joint United Nations Programme on HIV and AIDS (UNAIDS) estimates that there are approximately 40 million people affected by the illness, with 1.8 million new infections in 2017 (UNAIDS, 1998). With increased life expectancy following the introduction of cART, people living with HIV now present with a new constellation of co-morbidities. These include those caused by traditional risk factors, such as smoking, alcohol consumption, and illicit drug use, in addition to those from chronic as well as HIV-specific risk factors such as toxic effects of long-term antiretroviral use, persistent immune activation, and inflammatory response (Ghosn et al., 2018).

HIV infection and associated immune deficiency are linked to a number of associated diseases, including opportunistic infections, different types of cancers, and illnesses related to chronic inflammation (Brew and Garber, 2018). Among all co-morbidities, as the virus targets the nervous system at an early stage, central nervous system (CNS) complications represent a large proportion of symptomatic infection, with reports suggesting up to 20% (Davis et al., 1992; Levy and Bredesen, 1988; Resnick et al., 1988). Therefore, HIV illness is particularly pertinent to both neurology and psychiatry; not only because of its economic and social burden but also its association with a variety of neuropsychiatric disorders. This chapter addresses HIV and its co-morbidities, with particular reference to men. First, we review the biology of HIV.

HIV Biology

HIV belongs to the human retrovirus family, and lentivirus subfamily. Unlike other members of retroviridae (e.g., HTLV-I and HTLV-II), it is a non-transforming cytopathic virus (Hauser, 2013; Robins and Kumar, 2010). There are two genetically different but related HIV forms: HIV-1 and HIV2, the former being the most common cause of HIV illness throughout the world (Hauser, 2013). HIV transmission occurs when there is an exchange of blood or bodily fluids that contain virus or virus-infected cells. The most common route of infection is sexual transmission, followed by parenteral inoculation (e.g., blood transfusion, intravenous drug use), then vertical transmission from mothers to their newborns (Robins and Kumar, 2010).

HIV Systemic Infection

HIV infects cells that have CD4 surface receptors (e.g., T lymphocytes, macrophages, monocytes, dendritic cells, and bone marrow-derived microglia, which are resident in the brain; Hauser, 2013; David et al., 2012) using its viral glycoproteins, such as external gp120 and transmembrane gp41. Once gp120 binds the CD4 it also binds co-receptors CCR5 (mostly on macrophages) or CXCR4 (mostly

on T cells) (Gendelman et al., 2012; Robins and Kumar, 2010) to activate gp41, which is responsible for the fusion to the host cell (Figure 19.1). Following the fusion, the virus' core enters the cytoplasm of the cell where its viral RNA is converted, by the viral enzyme reverse transcriptase, into a double-stranded DNA, which is then integrated into the host DNA by the viral enzyme integrase to form a provirus (David et al., 2012; Gendelman et al., 2012; Robins and Kumar, 2010). The provirus can stay dormant for years, causing a latent infection without any pathological effects. The viral cycle is completed when an infected immune cell is activated from either direct antigenic stimulation by either HIV or another infection, or cytokines that are released from other immune cells (Robins and Kumar, 2010). Cell activation upregulates transcription factors leading to viral replication and production of HIV proteins, which are toxic and lead to cell death. Untreated HIV

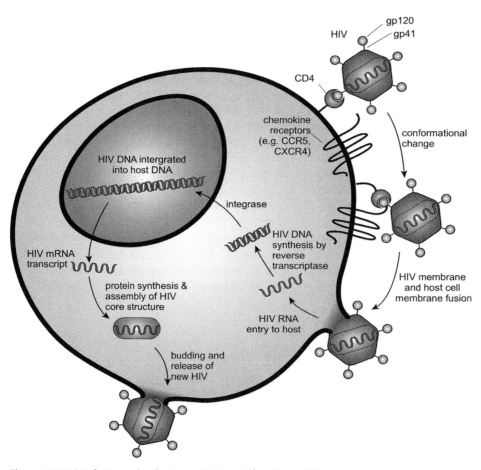

Figure 19.1 HIV infection and replication cycle (adapted from Fauci, 1996)

infection is characterized by profound immunodeficiency of CD4 expressing T cells. Abnormalities in other T cell, macrophage, and B cell functions also contribute to compromised immune function (Gendelman et al., 2012; Robins and Kumar, 2010). Moreover, due to low-level persistent T cell activation for prolonged periods, chronic inflammation also plays an important role in HIV pathogenesis and associated mortality and morbidity (Deeks et al., 2013).

Neuropathogenesis

HIV is neuro-invasive (Manji and Miller, 2004). It typically enters the CNS within two weeks after systemic infection (Gendelman et al., 2012) and crosses the blood–brain barrier (BBB), either whilst inside infected peripheral blood monocytes or by directly infecting astrocyte processes that are part of the BBB (Abutaleb et al., 2018; Hult et al., 2008; Meltzer et al., 1990). In the CNS, HIV-infected macrophages and/or monocytes secrete pro-inflammatory chemokines and cytokines (e.g., tumour necrosis factor alpha (TNF-α), interleukin 1β (IL-1β), interleukin 6 (IL-6), monocyte chemoattractant protein-1 (MCP-1), interferon γ (INF γ), and nitric oxide (NO)), leading to activation of the inflammation cascade. This then promotes increased permeability of the BBB and further migration of infected immune cells into the CNS (Gonzalez-Scarano and Martin-Garcia, 2005). Upon entering the brain parenchyma, although it does not directly infect neurons, HIV infect immune cells including perivascular macrophages and microglia (Abutaleb et al., 2018; Cosenza et al., 2002). CNS HIV triggers immune activation and further monocyte and/or macrophage infiltration, which in turn triggers viral replication and growth (Cohen et al., 2017; Gras and Kaul, 2010; Kaul and Lipton, 2006), resulting in synaptic and dendritic damage and neuronal loss. The extent of neuropathological changes does not always correlate with the severity of neuropsychiatric symptoms (Robins and Kumar, 2010). Although not entirely clear, two major mechanisms have been proposed to explain neuronal damage and loss, and white matter lesions. Direct neurotoxicity and neuronal apoptosis are caused by viral products (Brenneman et al., 1988; Hult et al., 2008; New et al., 1997; Price et al., 2006), while indirect neuronal loss is a result of chronic neuroinflammation and increased pro-inflammatory cytokines (Abutaleb et al., 2018).

HIV and Mental Health

Psychiatric aspects of HIV have become increasingly relevant in recent years. Mental health problems can occur as a result of the psychological reactions to and psychiatric manifestations of HIV infection (Cohen et al., 2017). Individuals with HIV continue to face substantial stigma, discrimination, and criminalization worldwide despite recent medical advances, increased awareness, and shifting social attitudes (Cohen et al., 2017; David et al., 2012). Resultant psychosocial consequences of infection can lead to severe emotional disturbance along the entire continuum of illness, from the time of diagnosis to the end of life (David et al., 2012). Moreover, clinical manifestations of HIV neuropathology may precipitate different psychiatric conditions and syndromes. Psychiatric problems, including substance misuse, are associated with an increased risk of HIV infection, and conversely some mental disorders occur as a direct result of HIV infection (WHO, 2008). The prevalence of psychiatric disorders among individuals who live with HIV is significantly higher than the general population (WHO, 2008; Lyketsos et al., 1996). Furthermore, the rate of specific psychiatric disorders is even higher in the most vulnerable and marginalized groups who are at increased risk of HIV: sex workers, men who have sex with men, drug users, and prisoners (Cohen et al., 2017; WHO, 2008). The most common psychiatric disorders in people with HIV are mood disorders (especially depression), anxiety and neurocognitive disorders, alcohol and substance misuse (especially injecting drugs and abuse of stimulants) (Cohen et al., 2017; WHO, 2008; Gendelman et al., 2012). Psychotic disorders and personality disorders are also relatively common. In addition, the risk of attempted or completed suicide is especially higher in HIV population (Alfonso and Cohen, 1997; WHO, 2008).

Before analysing each individual disorder, it is important to mention that psychiatric conditions play a very important role in both exposure to and transmission of HIV infection (Blank et al., 2002). They are highly relevant to risky behaviour (e.g., risky sexual acts, sharing needles), barriers to prevention of transmission (e.g., unprotected sex), adherence to treatment, and access to ongoing medical care. Therefore, understanding HIV and its mental health implications is as valuable as providing well-coordinated psychiatric care to those affected by it (Cohen et al., 2017).

HIV, Cognition, and Ageing

Since the introduction of combined antiretroviral therapy (cART), the life expectancy of people living with HIV has increased significantly. In 2013, infected individuals aged over 55 accounted for 26% of the 1.2 million people living with HIV (Zahr, 2018). This number has almost tripled since 2000 and is expected to increase to an estimated 7.5 million by 2020 (Autenrieth et al., 2018), reflecting a change in the perception of HIV from a terminal to a chronic illness.

The ageing brain infected with HIV is vulnerable to endogenous and exogenous insults that can result in accelerated brain ageing. These include cART toxicity, age-related cardiovascular and metabolic changes, coinfections (e.g., hepatitis C), higher rates of smoking, alcohol, and drug use, and chronic inflammation despite adequate virus-supressing treatment (Althoff et al., 2015; Kooij et al., 2016).

Telomeres are repetitive DNA sequences that are associated with maintaining the function of genome stability (Turner, Vasu, et al., 2019). Telomere length shortens with each cell division, and this shortening is related to ageing and age-related disease (Turner et al., 2019). Significant telomere shortening occurs during each HIV seroconversion (Gonzalez-Serna, Ajaykumar, et al., 2017). This may translate into accelerated cellular ageing, correlating with high viral load and the duration of HIV infection (Zanet, Thorne, et al., 2014).

HIV-Associated Neurocognitive Disorder (HAND)

HIV-associated neurocognitive disorder (HAND) was first recognized in the early 1980s following the first AIDS epidemic. Prior to development of antiretrovirals, severe cognitive impairment and rapidly progressing dementia accompanied by pathological brain changes, including cortical volume loss, encephalopathy, and leukoencephalopathy, were common and affected up to 60% of patients with HIV infection (Clifford and Ances, 2013; David et al., 2012; Nightingale et al., 2014). Despite improved life expectancy there has been a significant decrease in the incidence of severe neurocognitive impairment in people with HIV. Milder forms of neurocognitive impairment remain common; approximately 50–60% of infected individuals who have access to cARTs develop a degree of cognitive impairment over their illness course (Heaton et al., 2010; Nightingale et al., 2014; Saylor et al., 2016).

In the pre-HAART era, a number of risk factors were found to be associated with the development and progression of HIV-related neurocognitive disorder. These included decreased haemoglobin and body mass index, IV drug use, cocaine use, increased plasma viral load, and decreased CD4 count (Clifford et al., 2013; David et al., 2012; Gendelman et al., 2012). Extrapyramidal signs, premorbid abnormal scores on measures of psychomotor and executive functioning, and a history of depression were other proposed risk factors (De Ronchi et al., 2002; Stern et al., 2001). In the era of HAART/cART, serum viral load and CD4 count are less valid markers; cerebrospinal fluid (CSF) viral load and CSF chemokine concentration have been established as better predictors of cognitive impairment (David et al., 2012).

HAND refers to a spectrum of neurocognitive impairment of varying degrees, including asymptomatic neurocognitive impairment (ANI), mild neurocognitive disorder (MND), and HIV-associated dementia (HAD), and is diagnosed using neuropsychometric testing and functional status assessments (Clifford et al., 2013; Saylor et al., 2016). The diagnosis is made according to 'Frascati criteria', which was proposed in 2007 in the post-cART era, and categorizes the presentation of neurocognitive impairment. The Frascati criteria emphasize that the essential feature of HAND is neurocognitive disturbance (Gandhi et al., 2010). Table 19.1 details the revised criteria.

ANI and MND

ANI is defined by impairment of at least two cognitive domains without considerable interference in day-to-day functioning, whilst MND presents with a similar cognitive profile to ANI plus mild functional impairment. In clinical practice, assessment of functional ability is often challenging to assess objectively and measures imprecise (e.g., due to use self-report measures, educational and cultural biases); therefore distinction between ANI and MND is not always unequivocal (Clifford et al., 2013). Current evidence

Table 19.1 Frascati criteria for HIV-associated cognitive impairment (Antinori et al., 2007; Clifford et al., 2013)

HIV-associated asymptomatic neurocognitive impairment (ANI)

1. Acquired impairment in cognitive functioning,[*] involving at least two ability domains, documented by performance of at least 1.0 standard deviation (SD) below the mean for age-education-appropriate norms on standardized neuropsychological tests. The neuropsychological assessment must survey at least the following abilities: verbal/language; attention/working memory; abstraction/executive; memory (learning; recall); speed of information processing; sensory-perceptual, motor skills.
2. The cognitive impairment does not interfere with everyday functioning.
3. The cognitive impairment does not meet criteria for delirium or dementia.
4. There is no evidence of another pre-existing cause for the ANI.

HIV-1-associated mild neurocognitive disorder (MND)

1. Acquired impairment in cognitive functioning, [a] involving at least two ability domains, documented by performance of at least 1.0 SD below the mean for age-education-appropriate norms on standardized neuropsychological tests. The neuropsychological assessment must survey at least the following abilities: verbal/language; attention/working memory; abstraction/executive; memory (learning; recall); speed of information processing; sensory-perceptual, motor skills.
   Typically, this would correspond to an MSK (Memorial Sloan Kettering) scale stage of 0.5 to 1.0.
2. The cognitive impairment produces at least mild interference in daily functioning (at least one of the following):

   a. Self-report of reduced mental acuity, inefficiency in work, homemaking, or social functioning.
   b. Observation by knowledgeable others that the individual has undergone at least mild decline in mental acuity with resultant inefficiency in work, homemaking, or social functioning.

3. The cognitive impairment does not meet criteria for delirium or dementia.
4. There is no evidence of another pre-existing cause for the MND.

HIV-1-associated dementia (HAD)

1. Marked acquired impairment in cognitive functioning,[a] involving at least two ability domains; typically, the impairment is in multiple domains, especially in learning of new information, slowed information processing, and defective attention/concentration. The cognitive impairment must be ascertained by neuropsychological testing with at least two domains 2 SD or greater than demographically corrected means.
   Typically, this would correspond to an MSK scale stage of 2.0 or greater.
2. The cognitive impairment produces marked interference with day-to-day functioning (work, home life, social activities).
3. The pattern of cognitive impairment does not meet criteria for delirium (e.g., clouding of consciousness is not a prominent feature); or, if delirium is present, criteria for dementia need to have been met on a prior examination when delirium was not present.
4. There is no evidence of another, pre-existing cause for the dementia (e.g., other CNS infection, CNS neoplasm, cerebrovascular disease, pre-existing neurologic disease, or severe substance abuse compatible with CNS disorder).

[a] Neurocognitive testing should include evaluating at least five domains including attention-information processing, language, abstraction – executive, complex perceptual motor skills, memory (including learning and recall), simple motor skills or sensory perceptual skills (Clifford et al., 2013). Cognitive abilities such as basic visuo-perception, receptive language, and constructional praxis are relatively spared in people with HIV (Tierney et al., 2018).

suggests that ANI accounts for 70% of all forms of HAND (Heaton et al., 2010).

Detection of ANI is considered clinically relevant as individuals with ANI can transition to more severe forms of HAND (Saylor et al., 2016). Although it is difficult to predict, the first signs of progression generally include slowed mental processing and executive deficits followed by decline in episodic and semantic memory (David et al., 2012; Tierney et al., 2018). Progression is accelerated by underlying neurological conditions, early brain involvement after HIV infection, head injury, cerebral infections such as hepatitis C, and substance use (Chana et al., 2006; Durvasula et al., 2006; Justice et al., 2004; Letendre et al., 2006; Parsons et al., 2006). There are no clear prognostic or diagnostic indicators to determine the rate of progression (Sanmarti et al., 2014). In the pre-cART era, a low CD4 cell count, high plasma viral load, and CSF RNA levels were thought to be associated with developing HAD (David et al., 2012). These indicators have not been consistently associated with progression of neurocognitive impairment in cART-treated patients (Childs et al., 1999; Heaton et al., 2011; McArthur et al., 1997; Saylor et al., 2016).

HAD

HAD is the most severe form of HAND. Diagnosis requires impairment in two or more cognitive domains and significant functional decline (Antinori et al., 2007) (Table 19.2). The incidence of HAD fell from 7% in early 1990s (McArthur et al., 1993) to less than 1% in recent years (Heaton et al., 2010). The current prevalence remains stable, if not slightly higher due to increased longevity of patients with HIV who are treated with cART (Heaton et al., 2010). In the current cART era, HAD accounts for less than 5% of all HAND cases (Heaton et al., 2010).

The primary clinical presentation of HAD is progressive disabling cognitive impairment accompanied by behavioural changes (David et al., 2012). Motor deficits including bradykinesia and gait imbalance often follow (David et al., 2012; Saylor et al., 2016; Snider et al., 1983). Common features include impaired memory, poor concentration and attention, mental slowing, and confusion (Clifford et al., 2013). Behavioural changes include social withdrawal, apathy, lethargy, and psychomotor retardation (David et al., 2012). Initial clinical features are similar to depression and it is important to differentiate and exclude this diagnosis. For a more general discussion about depression in men, see Chapter 12. The course of HAD is steadily progressive (David et al., 2012). The pattern of cognitive dysfunction in the cART era is more cortical than subcortical, similar to other common neurodegenerative dementias such as Alzheimer's (compared historically to a predominantly subcortical AIDS-dementia complex; Clifford et al., 2013).

It is often difficult to correlate the neuropathological findings in HAD with the severity of cognitive symptoms (David et al., 2012). Changes are usually subtle and not specific to HIV infection. Historically, encephalitis and direct neuronal loss were thought to have a major role in HAD pathology, but with widespread use of cART, these are no longer sufficient to explain the neurological impairment (Saylor et al., 2016). Indeed, HIV-associated primary brain pathology has been reported in only 10% of HAD cases (Khanlou et al., 2009). Cortical neuronal loss does not appear to have any clinical pathological correlation, nor are there localized areas of pathology that can account for the cognitive deficits seen (Bell, 1998; Everall et al., 1995; Giometto et al., 1997; Petito et al., 2001). There are a variety of pathological changes that may contribute to HAD cognitive symptoms. These include synaptic and dendritic damage, reduced cortical synaptic density, extracellular beta-amyloid deposition (there are no neuritic plaques or tangles, as found in Alzheimer's disease), increased alpha-synuclein in substantia nigra, microgliosis, and astrocytosis (Achim et al., 2009; Everall et al., 1999; Khanlou et al., 2009; Scott et al., 2011). Lack of overt neuropathological findings specific to HIV infection suggest that HAND pathogenesis is driven by chronic inflammation in the CNS; systemic immune activation and activated monocytes are postulated to contribute to neuronal damage (Gannon et al., 2011; Saylor et al., 2016).

Diagnosis

Neuropsychological testing and functional assessments are necessary to diagnose and classify HIV-associated cognitive impairment. There is no specific biomarker, laboratory-based test, or diagnostic technology available to diagnose HAND (Antinori et al., 2007); laboratory investigations and imaging techniques have a role in excluding other causes of neurocognitive dysfunction, such as primary and

Table 19.2 Summary of Frascati Criteria (adapted from Clifford et al., 2013)

	Neurocognitive status	Functional status	Delirium/ other dementia
ANI	1 SD below mean, 2 cognitive domains	No impairment	No
MND	1 SD below mean, 2 cognitive domains	Minimal impairment	No
HAD	2 SD below mean, 2 cognitive domains	Marked impairment	No

degenerative dementias (Eggers et al., 2017). EEG might show diffuse slowing in advanced dementia. Brain MRI has limited diagnostic value unless there is cortical atrophy (Levy et al., 1986).

Treatment

Multiple mechanisms contribute to HAND pathology, requiring a multifaceted approach to management (Saylor et al., 2016). The mainstay of treatment is viral suppression, as HIV is the causative neuropathological factor. Early initiation of cART and adequate viral suppression within the CNS are correlated with better cognitive performance, slower illness progression, and partial reversal of neuronal injury (Gannon et al., 2011; Winston et al., 2010). cARTs that have better CNS penetration have theoretically better chance to reduce CNS viral load. Some non-retroviral drugs, including memantine, selegiline, rivastigmine, nimodipine, and psychostimulants, have been trialled, but have not proven beneficial (Eggers et al., 2017; Simioni et al., 2013). Adjunctive interventions complement the mainstay of treatment, for example preventing and treating co-infections such as HCV, addressing cardiac and metabolic risk factors, and adequate treatment of co-morbid psychiatric illness such as depression. In the future, treatments that supress systemic immune activation and associated inflammation could prove effective in reducing neuronal damage and cognitive decline.

Conclusions

CNS involvement of HIV remains an important problem and causes varying degrees of neurocognitive impairment. It has a considerable socioeconomic impact as well as increased mortality and morbidity. Widespread use of cART has reduced the incidence of the most severe forms. However, mild forms remain prevalent. The diagnosis is made on clinical grounds rather than definitive laboratory tests or neuroimaging. Early initiation of and effective treatment with cART slow down illness progression and improve cognitive functioning.

HIV and Substance Misuse

Intravenous drug use is recognized as one of the most significant risk factors for HIV infection (Centers for Disease Control and Prevention, 2000) and is more common in men than women (see Chapter 18).

Transmission of HIV by contaminated needles is a major route of infection in this population, and strategies targeting needle sharing and encouraging disinfection if sharing occurs have been shown to reduce the risk of viral transmission (McCoy et al., 1998). Alcohol consumption, smoking, inhaling, and ingesting drugs also increases the risk of contracting HIV. Drug misuse is also associated with high-risk sexual behaviour, which confers greater risk of exposure to the virus (Chesney et al., 1998). Moreover, adherence to antiretroviral therapy is affected by drug misuse (Bing et al., 1999), which contributes to disease progression and infectivity. HIV seropositive drug users have greater age-matched morbidity and mortality when compared to non-drug-using HIV seropositive individuals (Altice et al., 2010). Evidence suggests that drugs of abuse may increase HIV replication directly, as well as induce significant immunosuppression, raising the possibility that drugs themselves may increase sensitivity to infection, or hasten the progression of disease. Indeed, drug abuse is one of the risk factors for severe neurocognitive dysfunctions in HIV-positive individuals. Such effects may be drug-specific.

Cocaine

Cocaine mediates its effects on several pathways in cells infected with HIV-1, and many of these effects promote infectivity of disease and disease progression. Indeed, epidemiological studies of drug abusers with AIDS link use of cocaine in particular to increased incidence of HIV seroprevalence and progression to AIDS (Fiala et al., 1998). Cocaine promotes HIV-1 replication in peripheral blood mononuclear cells (PBMCs), macrophages, microglia, and astrocytes (Peterson et al., 1992; Reynolds et al., 2006). Cocaine, via IL-10 modulation, can also tilt the balance of cytokines towards the Th2 response, which is pro-inflammatory (Gardner et al., 2004). Cocaine upregulates the CCR5, HIV co-receptor, and reciprocally inhibits its ligands, thereby increasing virus infectivity. Cocaine also exacerbates neurotoxicity by interacting with viral protein products Tat and gp120, increasing neuronal apoptosis and augmenting the toxic responses that characterize HIV-associated neurocognitive disorders (HAND) (Gurwell et al., 2001). In addition, cocaine increases microvascular permeability, which leads to a HIV neuroinvasion through its direct effects on brain microvascular endothelial cells, as well as its paracrine effects on the BBB via release of pro-inflammatory cytokines (Buch et al., 2011).

Methamphetamine (Meth)

Studies have demonstrated an association between meth use and HIV risk behaviours and links between meth use and HIV incidence (Hurt et al., 2010; Plankey et al., 2007). Moreover, HIV and meth appear to have combined adverse effects on frontal and striatal neuronal and glial markers (Chang et al., 2005); and rates of neurocognitive impairment are increased in HIV seropositive individuals who abuse meth versus those who are non-users (Rippeth et al., 2004). Neuroimaging studies have shown than individuals with HIV have decreased cortical and subcortical brain area volumes, but increased cortical volumes are seen in meth users, with overlapping effects found in those infected with HIV and who use meth (Jernigan et al., 2005). Neurocognitive impairment correlates with decreased regional brain volumes in HIV and increasing meth use. Loss of interneurons (including parvalbumin interneurons) is also associated with cognitive deficits (primarily memory) in HIV seropositive meth users (Chana et al., 2006). Levels of plasma virus are higher in HIV-infected meth users than non-meth users (Ellis et al., 2003; Marcondes et al., 2010); further studies have revealed a negative association between HAART adherence and meth use (Reback et al., 2003). It is possible that the host inflammatory response to HIV infection of the brain might be increased by meth use, as suggested by a gene-expression profiling study of brains from individuals with HIV infection (Masliah et al., 2004); upregulation of interferon inducible genes may in part explain the higher neurodegenerative and neurocognitive burden seen in this population (Everall et al., 2005).

Opioids

Opioid drugs of abuse have diverse immunomodulatory effects on almost all aspects of the immune system, including suppression of natural killer cells (Yeager et al., 1995), inhibition of antibody responses (Eisenstein et al., 2006) and phagocytic cell function and mobilization (Roy et al., 1991; Szabo et al., 1993). In vitro, opioids have been shown to affect rates of HIV replication when added to human lymphoid, monocytic, or microglial cultures (Peterson et al., 1994). Moreover, opioids effect chemokine receptor

expression and chemokine levels, with potential to alter HIV infectivity directly at the level of co-receptor expression or competition for the co-receptor (Steele et al., 2003), or by influencing cell trafficking to sites of infection. Modulation of cytokine levels by opioids, or indeed opioids directly operating as cytokines, may affect activations states of lymphocytes and macrophages, which can influence HIV replication. Opioids can also induce lymphocyte apoptosis (Reddy et al., 2012), which can lead to the release of HIV from infected cells, as well as reduce the accessibility of lymphocytes targeted by HIV.

Alcohol

Alcohol use has a strong, established association with HIV incidence, as well as with high-risk sexual behaviours that potentiate the transmission of sexually transmitted infections (STIs) (Scott-Sheldon et al., 2016). Alcohol use has been shown to influence HIV care and outcomes at every stage of the illness trajectory; it is associated with lower receipt of HIV testing, greater delay in engaging with medical care after testing positive, worse rates of retention in treatment, and non-adherence to treatment (Vagenas et al., 2015). Alcohol use has also been associated with a hastened rate of disease progression, as measured in patients by increased viral load and reduced CD4+ cell counts (Wu et al., 2011). Identified associations may be mediated by behavioural factors, or they may be direct, resulting from biological mechanisms such as the immunological effects of alcohol (Hahn and Samet, 2010), translocation of bacteria and bacterial products from the gut to cause HIV immune activation (Balagopal et al., 2008), interactions and competition with other drugs, and nutritional intake and metabolic deficiencies (Watzl and Watson, 1992).

Cannabinoids

Cannabinoids have been shown to modulate both the function and secretion of a number of cells in the immune system, as well as influence the balance between neuroinflammation and neurodegeneration. Exogenous cannabinoids act directly on such cells by activating endogenous cannabinoid receptors, of which there are two types, cannabinoid receptor 1 (CB1) and cannabinoid receptor 2 (CB2), the latter being mainly expressed in immune tissues. Endogenous cannabinoids (endocannabinoids) can also modulate immune function through cannabinoid receptors, and exogenous cannabinoids may alter this homeostatic balance (Cabral and Staab, 2005). No studies to our knowledge have shown an association between cannabis use in humans and increased susceptibility to HIV infection, greater vulnerability to opportunistic infections, or accelerated disease progression in HIV seropositive individuals. That said, an association between cannabinoid-induced immune dysregulation, greater susceptibility to infection, decreased host resistance, and alteration of illness course in response to a variety of other infectious agents has been demonstrated both in vitro and in vivo (Cabral et al., 2005). Cannabinoids that bind the CB2 receptor selectively could prove useful therapeutic agents for ablating neuroinflammatory processes, including HIV-associated neuropathology. There is preliminary evidence to suggest that cannabis use may accelerate neurocognitive impairment among HIV seropositive individuals (Cristiani et al., 2004). This may have particular relevance given reforms to the legal status of medical and recreational cannabis.

Treatment

Individuals who are HIV seropositive underuse substance use treatment, and factors associated with this include lower socioeconomic status, lower educational levels, and psychiatric co-morbidity (Durvasula and Miller, 2014). There is a scarcity of literature specifically focusing on substance misuse treatments in HIV seropositive individuals and almost none specific to men. Available models of psychotherapy and substance misuse treatment, including cognitive behavioural therapy (CBT) and motivational interviewing, have proven to be useful for improving adherence to HAART, as well as promoting harm reduction and reducing rates of misuse (Parsons et al., 2005). Directly observed treatment models, including opioid replacement therapy, have also proven to be effective in providing medical management and psychiatric intervention, as well as reducing high-risk behaviours (Ferrando and Batki, 2000).

Conclusions

Individuals who misuse substances often self-administer combinations of drugs that commonly include cocaine, marijuana, opioids, alcohol, and cigarette smoke, in varying doses, ratios, frequencies, and durations. This challenges epidemiological and biological approaches to determining the effects of specific drugs of misuse on HIV infection and progression, particularly as these drugs can have opposite effects on the immune system. It is difficult to examine HIV infectivity in vivo directly, due to a lack of small animal models. Nevertheless, there is convincing evidence to implicate dugs of misuse in increasing susceptibility to HIV infection, and hastening progression of disease, via both behavioural and biological mechanisms. The differences in the prevalence of HIV amongst individuals of different ethnicity, gender, sexual orientation, and socioeconomic and immigrant status emphasize that treatment interventions must be culturally responsive and appropriately contextualized.

Anxiety and Depression

The recognition of psychiatric disorders – in particular depression and anxiety – in HIV, is important. They arise more frequently than in the general population, although they often go undetected and consequentially untreated (Choi et al., 2016). Men in particular are less likely to seek help for mental health problems (Oliver et al., 2005). This is further compounded by the effect of the stigma and marginalization associated with living with HIV (Mental Health Foundation, 2016).

Not only do untreated depression and anxiety have a direct impact on individual quality of life (Schroecksnadel et al., 2008) but they can also have direct consequences on the progression of the HIV disease itself (Taylor et al., 2018). In turn it appears that suboptimally treated or managed HIV can also contribute to the increased incidence of anxiety and depression seen in the disorder (Jacobs et al., 2017). Furthermore, HIV is disproportionately high in the male population meaning (UNAIDS, 1998) that overall men are at a particularly high risk of developing a high disease burden when considering both their mental and physical health in this context.

Prevalence of Anxiety and Depression in Men with HIV

Depression is the second most common psychiatric disorder in people living with HIV (PLWH) after substance misuse, with an overall estimated prevalence of 20% in men who live with HIV (Hays et al., 2000). However, the prevalence rates amongst studies vary from 7.2% to 71.9%. These differences have been attributed to the use of different depression rating scales, questionnaires, and methodologies (Chaudhury et al., 2016).

The prevalence of anxiety symptoms in PLWH is considered to be higher than the general population (Kessler et al., 1994), but similarly to the literature on depression there is a high variance in the recorded prevalence among studies. Rates vary from 4.5% to 82.3%, with the differences likely accounted for by the different tools used to qualify the presence of anxiety and the different stages of illness captured (Blalock, 2005; Dew et al., 1997). However, when considering specific anxiety syndromes, one US study identified the prevalence rates in men to be similar to those in the general population (4% had social phobia, 3% had specific phobias, 2% had obsessive-compulsive disorder, 2% generalized anxiety disorder) with the prevalence of any anxiety disorder in men being 12% (Chaudhury et al., 2016; Morrison et al., 2002). PLWH can also suffer with high levels of anxiety symptoms in the context of a stress response immediately after diagnosis or following treatment failure. These symptoms can resolve with time and with the establishment of effective ART treatment (Alonzo and Reynolds, 1995; Chaudhury et al., 2016; European AIDS Clinical Society, 2017; Sewell et al., 2000).

Aetiology of Depression and Anxiety in HIV

As with all psychiatric disorders that manifest in PLWH, the aetiology of anxiety and depression is multifactorial in nature and it can be helpful to employ the 'biopsychosocial' model.

Biological Factors

a. Immunological Changes

Several neurobiological changes caused by HIV in the central nervous system have been found to relate to the development of depression- and anxiety-related symptomatology. Depression, anxiety, and stress have been linked to immune dysregulation in the body. Impaired cellular immunity (lower natural killer cell count and function and higher cytotoxic $CD8^+$ T-lymphocyte counts) have been found in PLWH with symptoms of depression and stress (McGuire et al., 2015).

Chronic elevation of cytokines (through activation of microglia and astrocytes; decreasing monoaminergic function; inducing neurotoxicity, especially in dopaminergic neurons; and reducing brain-derived neurotrophic factor) have also been found, compatible with 'cytokine induced sickness' (Chaudhury et al., 2016). Symptoms include general malaise and fatigue, sleep changes, loss of interest in usual activities, reduced oral intake and weight loss; synonymous to a number of those seen in depressive illness (Kelley et al., 2003).

Interleukin 1 has also been identified to play a key role in activating immune response, which in turn appears to affect the physiological and behavioural sequelae associated with 'sickness behaviour' (Kelley et al., 2003).

Other markers of immune activation such as elevated neopterin levels have been shown to predict depressive symptoms in HIV patients (Gostner et al., 2015), with higher neopterin CSF concentrations being found in HIV-infected patients with neuropsychiatric symptoms in comparison to those without. Moreover, depressed PLWH have shown elevated levels of tryptophan degradation (Gostner et al., 2015). Given that tryptophan is a precursor to serotonin, a key neurotransmitter implicated in the development of depression, the depletion of tryptophan by an activated immune system alters the synthesis of serotonin (Simoni et al., 2011). Overall these immunological changes alter the biochemical input to the hypothalamic–pituitary axis and glucocorticoid system, both of which have been implicated in the development of stress response-related mood disorders (McGuire et al., 2015; Spencer et al., 2015).

b. Side Effects of Antiretroviral Therapy (ART)

Several studies have focussed on the impact of different ART agents on the development of depression and anxiety, but a causal relationship remains uncertain. Efavirenz has been most commonly implicated with associated symptoms, including a reduction in sleep quality, depression, dizziness, and anxiety, but overall these were found to be mild in nature with discontinuation of therapy not being warranted (Gaida et al., 2016; Huang et al., 2018).

Frequent switching of ART regimens has been associated with higher levels of depression (Etherton et al., 2015; Sin and DiMatteo, 2014) and anxiety, which is likely driven by the anticipated downward trajectory associated with the difficulty in maintaining viral suppression. However, no consistent

Table 19.3 Psychiatric side effects of antiretroviral medications (adapted from Taylor et al., 2018; Turjanski, 2005)

Medication	Psychiatric side effects
Protease inhibitors	
• Amprenavir	• Mood changes
• Atazanavir	• Depression, insomnia
• Fosamprenavir	• None reported
• Indinavir	• Mood changes
• Lopinavir	• Mood changes, agitation, anxiety
• Nelfinavir	• None reported
• Ritonavir	• Anxiety
• Saquinavir	• Depression, anxiety, sleep disturbance
Nucleoside reverse transcriptase inhibitors	
• Abacavir	• Depression, anxiety, nightmares
• Didanosine	• Lethargy, anxiety, confusion, sleep disturbance, mood disorders, psychosis
• Emtricitabine	• Confusion, irritability, insomnia
• Lamivudine	• Insomnia, mood disorders
• Stavudine	• Mood disorders, sleep disturbance, delirium
• Zalcitabine	• Somnolence, impaired concentration, mood disorders
• Zidovudine	• Sleep disturbance, vivid dreams, agitation, mania, depression, delirium
Non-nucleoside reverse transcriptase inhibitors	
• Delavirdine	• None reported
• Efavirenz	• Agitation, hallucinations, depersonalization, nightmares, depression, suicidality, insomnia
• Etravirine	• Sleep disturbance
• Nevirapine	• Visual hallucinations, paranoia, nightmares and vivid dreams, depression
• Rilpivirine	• Depression, suicidality, sleep disturbance
Nucleotide reverse transcriptase inhibitors (NtRTI)	
• Tenofovir	• None reported
Integrase inhibitors	
• Dolutegravir, Elvitegravir, Raltegravir	• Depression, suicidality
Fusion or entry inhibitors	
• Enfuvirtide	• Anxiety and depression

associations have been found between depression or anxiety and HIV-specific clinical factors such as CD4 + T cell count and current viral load (Huang et al., 2018).

Psychological and Social Factors

High levels of pre- and post-diagnosis of trauma, adversity, and stigma are seen in PLWH. One US study identified that PLWH come from disproportionately marginalized groups, including the economically disadvantaged, ethnic and sexual minorities, and those with a history of substance use, sex work, and trauma (Simoni et al., 2011). Levels of historical physical and sexual abuse in both HIV+ men and women have been found to be between 30–50% (Gendelman et al., 2012). Therefore, individuals in these at-risk groups are often subject to discrimination and stressors associated with poor mental health outcomes, even before acquiring the compounding factor of HIV (Simoni et al., 2011).

Due to the association of HIV with these marginalized groups, the disease itself has become stigmatized. PLWH are often very aware of the perceived stigma of the disease, which in turn causes them to restrict their social activities and collude with the negative stereotypes associated with the condition, a notion termed as 'internalized stigma' (Strodl et al., 2015). This can further increase the risk of psychological distress, depression, and anxiety (Chaudhury et al., 2016).

Along with the high levels of historical trauma associated with the diagnosis of HIV, many common life events associated with living with the condition, such as bereavement and job loss, can also result in major depressive episodes (Gendelman et al., 2012).

Diagnosing Anxiety and Depression in HIV

Given the frequency with which depression and anxiety present in PLWH, along with the significant disability and associated poor treatment outcomes, regular screening for these disorders should become a routine part of clinical management. Table 19.4 outlines the guidance on how the screening process for depression should be undertaken (European AIDS Clinical Society, 2017).

The specific diagnostic criteria for both anxiety and depression are covered in Chapters 9 and 12 of this book and remain pertinent in the context of comorbid HIV. However, alongside the diagnostic criteria, it is also important to consider whether the disorder may be primary or secondary in its origin. This may be determined by considering past psychiatric history, onset of symptoms, and symptom profile.

A primary mental disorder is indicated when the onset of the disorder predates the HIV infection and does not appear to be physiologically related to the HIV or any associated illnesses or their treatment regimes. In addition, any substance misuse or substance withdrawal states should also be excluded.

A secondary mental disorder in this instance refers to a mental disorder that has resulted directly from the neurobiological changes associated with HIV or HIV-related treatment. It can also refer to the associated mental disturbance secondary to substance misuse disorders, which usually remit after around one month's sobriety, or even as quickly as a week in the case of cocaine or methamphetamine abuse.

Most studies suggest that in about 50% of cases of first-episode major depression seen in PLWH precede the date of seroconversion (Gendelman et al., 2012).

Treatment of Depression and Anxiety in HIV

To manage depression and/or anxiety in PLWH effectively, adequate treatment and support for both the mental and physical disorder need to be established. When considering treatment for the psychological disorder it can be helpful to use a biopsychosocial model.

Biological Treatments for Depression and Anxiety in HIV

a. Antidepressant Therapy

Depression: Antidepressants are recommended for the treatment of moderate or severe depression (alongside a combination of antidepressant medication and a high-intensity psychological intervention; e.g., CBT or interpersonal therapy (NICE, 2018)). However, they should also be considered in people with a past history of moderate or severe depression,

Table 19.4 Screening guidance for depression in PWLH (adapted from European AIDS Clinical Society, 2017)

Who to screen?	How to screen?	How to diagnose?
Due to high prevalence of depression, screening of all HIV-positive people is recommended. Screening should be considered for high-risk population, such as: • Past history of depression • Family history of depression • Old age • Adolescence • History of substance use • History of neurological disorder • History of other psychiatric problems • Use of Efavirenz • Suspicion of neurocognitive impairment	• Frequency every 1–2 years • Organic cause should be ruled out (e.g., hypothyroidism, Addison's, hypercortisolemia, vitamin deficiencies, etc.) • Standardized rating scales could be used (e.g., clinician rated Hamilton depression rating scale (HDRS) or patient-rated Beck depression inventory)	• Depression criteria according to ICD 10 • Symptoms should be evaluated regularly

Table 19.5 Drug–drug interactions between antidepressants and antiretroviral medications (adapted from University of Liverpool, 2019)

	Antidepressants	ATV/c	ATV/r	DRV/c	DRV/r	LPV/r	EFV	ETV	NVP	RPV	MVC	DTG	EVG/c	RAL
SSRI	Citalopram	↑[a]	↑[a]	↑	↑	↑[a]	↓	→	→	↓[b]	↕	↕	↑	↕
	Escitalopram	↑[a]	↑[a]	↑	↑	↑[a]	→	→	→	↑[b]	↕	↕	↑	↕
	Fluvoxamine	↑	↑	↑	↑	↑	E	↕	E	↕	↕	↕	↑	↕
	Fluoxetine	↑	↑	↑	↑	↑	↑	↕	↕	↕	↕	↕	↓	↕
	Paroxetine	↑↓?	↑↓?	↑↓?	↓39%	↑↓?	↓	↕	↑	↕	↕	↕	↑↓?	↕
	Sertraline	↑	↑↓	↑	↓49%	↑	↓39%	↓	↓	↓	↕	↕	↓7%	↕
SNRI	Duloxetine	↑	↑↓	↑↕	↑↓	↑↓	↕	↑	↑	↕	↕	↕	↑	↕
	Venlafaxine	↑	↑	↑	↑	↑	↕	↕	↕	↕	↕	↕	↑	↕
TCA	Amitriptyline	↑[a]	↑[a]	↑[a]	↑[a]	↑[a]	↓	↕	↑	↑[b]	↕	↕	↑[a]	↕
	Clomipramine	↑[a]	↑[a]	↑[a]	↑[a]	↑[a]	↓	↕	↑	↕[b]	↕	↕	↕	↕
	Desipramine	↑[a]	↑[a]	↑[a]	↑[a]	↓5%[a]	↑	↕	↑	↕[b]	↕	↕	↕	↕
	Doxepin	↑	↑	↑	↑	↑	↑	↑	↑	↕	↕	↕	↕	↕
	Imipramine	↑[a]	↑[a]	↑[a]	↑[a]	↑[a]	↑	↕	↑	↕[b]	↕	↕	↕[a]	↕
	Nortriptyline	↑[a]	↑[a]	↑[a]	↑[a]	↑[a]	↑	↑	↑	↕	↕	↕	↕[a]	↕
	Trimipramine	↑	↑	↑	↑	↑	↑	↕	↓	↕	↕	↕	↕	↕
		↑	↑	↑	↑	↑	→	→	↑	↕	↕	↕	↓	↕
TeCA	Maprotiline	↑	↑	↓	↕	↑	↓	↕	↓	↕	↕	↕	↕	↕
	Mianserine													↕
	Mirtazapine	↓32%	↓32%	↕	↕	↓57%	↓5%	↑	↑	↕	↕	↑	↑?	↕
Others	Bupropion	↕	↕	↕	↕	↓57%	↓5%	↑	↑	↕	E	↕	↕	↕
	Lamotrigine	↕	↓32%	↕	↕	↓50%	E↑	E↑	E↑	E	E		↕	↕
	Nefazodone	↑	↑	↑	↑	↑	→	→	↑	↕	E	↕	↑	↕

Table 19.5 (cont.)

Antidepressants	ATV/c	ATV/r	DRV/c	DRV/r	LPV/r	EFV	ETV	NVP	RPV	MVC	DTG	EVG/c	RAL
St John's wort	D	D	D	D	D	D	D	D	D	D	D	D	D?
Trazodone	↑[a]	↑[a]	↑	↑	↑[a]	↑	↑	↓	↔[b]	↑	↑	↑	↑

Notes:

↑, Potential elevated exposure of the antidepressant; ↓, Potential decreased exposure of the antidepressant; ↔, No significant effect; D, potential decreased exposure of ARV drug; E, potential elevated exposure of ARV drug; ATV/c, ATV co-formulated with COBI (300/150 mg qd); DRV/c, DRV co-formulated with COBI (800/150 mg qd).

SSRI, selective serotonin reuptake inhibitors; **SNRI**, serotonin and norepinephrine reuptake inhibitors; **TCA**, tricyclic antidepressants; **TeCA**, tetracyclic antidepressants.

Numbers refer to decreased AUC of the antidepressant as observed in drug–drug interactions studies.

[a] ECG monitoring is recommended.
[b] Caution as both drugs can induce QT interval prolongation.
[c] The US Prescribing Information recommends that co-administration should be avoided as there are insufficient data to make dosing recommendations.

Colour legend
No clinically significant interaction expected.
These drugs should not be co-administered.
Potential clinically significant interaction that is likely to require additional monitoring, alteration of drug dosage, or timing of administration.
Potential interaction likely to be of weak intensity. Additional action/monitoring or dosage adjustment is unlikely to be required.

Comment:
For additional drug–drug interactions and for more detailed pharmacokinetic interaction data and dosage adjustments, please refer to www.hiv-druginteractions.org (University of Liverpool).

Table 19.6 Depression and anxiety in HIV

(1) Depression is the second most common psychiatric disorder in PLWH after substance misuse, with an overall estimated prevalence of 20 to 40%.

(2) The aetiology of depression and anxiety in PLWH has been shown to be multifactorial and includes:

- the immunological changes associated with HIV infection
- the increased levels of stigma, trauma, and adversity seen in this cohort when compared to the general population
- The impact of different ART agents on the development of depression and anxiety but a causal relationship remains uncertain

(3) Screening of depression and anxiety disorders is recommended for all PLWH every 1–2 years.

(4) Untreated depression and anxiety are associated with increased morbidity and mortality in PLWH.

(5) To successfully manage depression and/or anxiety in PLWH, adequate treatment and support for both the mental and physical disorder need to be established and should include:

- Biological interventions:

  Antidepressant therapy – in particular citalopram/escitalopram.

  Mirtazapine is recommended in HIV-wasting and co-morbid depression

  Benzodiazepines can play a role in the short-term management (i.e., up to one month) of acute life stress

- Psychosocial interventions: CBT, counselling, HIV support groups

with a presentation of subthreshold depressive symptoms that have been present for a long period (typically at least two years) or in subthreshold depressive symptoms or mild depression that persists after other interventions (NICE, 2018).

Anxiety: Antidepressants are recommended in the treatment of anxiety disorders such as generalized anxiety disorder (GAD) when there is marked functional impairment that has not improved following a course of either individual guided self-help or a psychoeducational group (NICE, 2011).

First-line antidepressant agents in PLWH include selective serotonin reuptake inhibitors (SSRIs), in particular escitalopram and citalopram (due to the lack of interaction with CYP2D6 or CYP3A4) (Gendelman et al., 2012; Taylor et al., 2018). For details of potential interactions, see Table 19.7. Further treatments should follow standard protocols. However, since adverse effects are the leading cause of poor/non-adherence, it may be helpful to choose an agent with a side-effect profile that could be advantageous (e.g., using mirtazapine in the treatment of co-morbid HIV wasting and depression due to its effects on appetite; Gendelman et al., 2012; Taylor et al., 2018).

It is also recommended to start treatment at the lowest starting dose and titrate slowly upwards. An adequate medication trial is considered to be a six-week duration. For further details see Chapters 9 and 12.

b. Benzodiazepine Treatment

Benzodiazepines can play a role in the short-term management (i.e., up to one month) of acute life stress including high levels of anxiety associated with the progression to AIDS, or sudden failure of ART (Hinkin et al., 2001).

Lorazepam, oxazepam, and temazepam are the preferred agents in PLWH because they are metabolized by non-CYP450 pathways (Taylor et al., 2018).

c. ART Treatment

Effective ART has the potential to reduce illness related anxiety (European AIDS Clinical Society, 2017) as well the production of inflammatory cytokines (Jacobs et al., 2017), which in turn can help modulate the depressive like symptoms associated with 'Cytokine induced sickness' (Chaudhury et al., 2016).

Antidepressants and ART have the potential to interact via metabolic pathways, e.g., cytochrome

Table 19.7 Drug–drug interactions between antidepressants and antiretroviral medications

	Protease Inhibitors					Non-nucleoside analogues				Entry and integrase inhibitors				Nucleoside analogues			
	ATV/c	ATV/r	DRV/c	DRV/r	LPV/r	DOR	EFV	NVP	RPV	MVC	DTG	EVG/c/TAF	RAL	FTC	3TC	TAF	ZDV
Serotonin reuptake inhibitors																	
Citalopram	↑	↑	↑	↑	↑	↕	→	→	↕	↕	↕	↑	↕	↕	↕	↕	↕
Excitalopram	↑	↑	↑	↑	↑	↕	→	→	↕	↕	↕	↑	↕	↕	↕	↕	↕
Fluoxetine	↑	↑	↑	↑	↑	↕	↕	↕	↕	↕	↕	↑	↕	↕	↕	↕	↕
Fluvoxamine	↑	↑	↑	↑	↑	↕	↕	⇐	↕	↕	↕	↑	↕	↕	↕	↕	↕
Paroxetine	↑↓?	↑↓?	↑↓?	↑↓	↑↓?	↕	↕	↕	↕	↕	↕	↑↓?	↕	↕	↕	↕	↕
Sertraline	↑↓?	→	↑	↓49%	→	↕	↓39%	→	↕	↕	↕	↓7%	↕	↕	↕	↕	↕
Serotonin and noradrenaline reuptake inhibitors																	
Duloxetine	↑	↑↓	↑	↑↓	↑↓	↕	↕	↕	↕	↕	↕	↑	↕	↕	↕	↕	↕
Venlafaxine	↑	↑	↑	↑	↑	↕	→	→	↕	⇒	↕	↑	↕	↕	↕	↕	↕
Tricyclic antidepressants																	
Amitriptyline	↑	↑	↑	↑	↑	↕	↕	↕	↕	↕	↕	↑	↕	↕	↕	↕	↕
Clomipramine	↑	↑	↑	↑	↑	↕	→	→	↕	↕	↕	↑	↕	↕	↕	↕	↕
Desipramine	↑	↑	↑	↑	↑5%	↕	→	↕	↕	↕	↕	↑	↕	↕	↕	↕	↕
Imipramine	↑	↑	↑	↑	↑	↕	→	→	↕	↕	↕	↑	↕	↕	↕	↕	↕
Nortriptyline	↑	↑	↑	↑	↑	↕	↕	↕	↕	↕	↕	↑	↕	↕	↕	↕	↕

Tetracyclic antidepressants

Antidepressant													
Mianserin	↔	↔	←	←	←	←	→	→	↔	↔	↔	↔	↔
Mirtazapine	↔	↔	←	←	←	←	→	→	↔	↔	↔	↔	↔

Other antidepressants

Antidepressant													
Agomelatine	↔	↓	↓	↓	↔	↓	↔	↔	↓	↔	↔	↔	↔
Buproprion	↔	↓	↓	↓	↓	↓57%	↓	↓	↓	↓	↓55%	↑?	↓
Lamotrigine	↔	↓32%	↓	↓50%	↓	↓	→	→	↓	↓	↔	←	↓
Reboxetine	←	←	←	←	←	←	→	→	↓	↔	↔	←	↔
Trazodone	←	←	←	←	←	←	→	→	↓	↔	↔	←	↔
Vortioxetine	←	←	←	←	←	↓	↓	↓	↓	↔	↔	↔	↔
St John's Wort	⇓	⇓	⇓	⇓	⇓	⇓	⇓	⇓	⇓	⇓	⇓	⇒	⇓

*Abbreviations
ATV Atazanavir
DRV Darunavir
LPV Lopinavir
/c cobistat
/r ritonavir

EFV Efavirenz
DOR Doravirine
ETV Etravirine
NVP Nevirapine
RPV Ripivirine

MVC Maraviroc
DTG Dolutegravir
EVG Elvitegravir
RAL Raltegravir
FTC Emtricitabine

TAF Tenofovir
3TC Lamivudine
ZDV Zidovudine

↔ No significant effect, ↑ increased antidepressant levels, ↓ decreased antidepressant levels, ⇑ increased HIV drug level, ⇓ decreased HIV drug level

P450. Table 19.5 outlines the potential interactions that may occur between different agents. Efavirenz has been most commonly implicated in adverse psychiatric effects associated with ART. At present HIV guidelines suggest avoiding its use with patients with psychiatric illness (Taylor et al., 2018).

Psychosocial Treatments for Depression and Anxiety in HIV

Psychological therapy, in particular self-guided or group CBT, is recommended as the first-line treatment for mild–moderate depression and anxiety (NICE, 2018, 2011). Individual psychological therapy is recommended in combination with antidepressant therapy.

PLWH can suffer high levels of stigmatization and social isolation, which are associated with higher levels of depression and anxiety. Various psychological interventions (e.g., counselling, CBT, self-help, or support groups) can play a role in tackling the self-stigma among PLWH as well as reducing social isolation (Li et al., 2017).

Conclusions

This chapter synthesizes a number of complex issues that affect men living with HIV. These include the biology of the virus and its effects on the brain both immunologically and neuropathologically that may contribute to mental health problems, the complicating effects of ageing and substance use, and the significant overrepresentation in this population of depression, anxiety, and cognitive impairment. The outlook for the population living with HIV in this fourth decade of the epidemic is far brighter with effective and fairly simple antiretroviral treatment regimens, but mental health problems may well persist due to the factors highlighted in this chapter and for ongoing effects of stigma.

References

Abutaleb, A., Kattakuzhy, S., Kottilil, S., O'Connor, E., and Wilson, E. 2018. Mechanisms of neuropathogenesis in HIV and HCV: similarities, differences, and unknowns. *J Neurovirol, 24*(6), 670–8.

Achim, C. L., Adame, A., Dumaop, W., Everall, I. P., Masliah, E., and Neurobehavioral Research, C. 2009. Increased accumulation of intraneuronal amyloid beta in HIV-infected patients. *J Neuroimmune Pharmacol, 4*(2), 190–9.

Alfonso, C. A. and Cohen, M. A. 1997. The role of group therapy in the care of persons with AIDS. *J Am Acad Psychoanal, 25*(4), 623–38.

Alonzo, A. A. and Reynolds, N. R. 1995. Stigma, HIV and AIDS: an exploration and elaboration of a stigma trajectory. *Soc Sci Med, 41*(3), 303–15.

Althoff, K. N., McGinnis, K. A., Wyatt, C. M., et al. 2015. Comparison of risk and age at diagnosis of myocardial infarction, end-stage renal disease, and non-AIDS-defining cancer in HIV-infected versus uninfected adults. *Clin Infect Dis, 60*(4), 627–38.

Altice, F. L., Kamarulzaman, A., Soriano, V. V., Schechter, M., and Friedland, G. H. 2010. Treatment of medical, psychiatric, and substance-use comorbidities in people infected with HIV who use drugs. *Lancet, 376*(9738), 367–87.

Antinori, A., Arendt, G., Becker, J. T., et al. 2007. Updated research nosology for HIV-associated neurocognitive disorders. *Neurology, 69*(18), 1789–99.

Autenrieth, C. S., Beck, E. J., Stelzle, D., Mallouris, C., Mahy, M., and Ghys, P. 2018. Global and regional trends of people living with HIV aged 50 and over: estimates and projections for 2000–2020. *PLoS One, 13*(11), e0207005.

Balagopal, A., Philp, F. H., Astemborski, J., et al. 2008. Human immunodeficiency virus-related microbial translocation and progression of hepatitis C. *Gastroenterology, 135*(1), 226–33.

Bell, J. E. 1998. The neuropathology of adult HIV infection. *Rev Neurol (Paris), 154*(12), 816–29.

Bing, E. G., Kilbourne, A. M., Brooks, R. A., Lazarus, E. F., and Senak, M. 1999. Protease inhibitor use among a community sample of people with HIV disease. *J Acquir Immune Defic Syndr Hum Retrovirol, 20*(5), 474–80.

Blalock, A. C., S. S., McDaniel, J. S. 2005. *Anxiety Disorders and HIV Disease.* Cambridge: Cambridge University Press.

Blank, M. B., Mandell, D. S., Aiken, L., and Hadley, T. R. 2002. Co-occurrence of HIV and serious mental illness among Medicaid recipients. *Psychiatr Serv, 53*(7), 868–73.

Brenneman, D. E., Westbrook, G. L., Fitzgerald, S. P., Ennist, D. L., Elkins, K. L., Ruff, M. R., and Pert, C. B. 1988. Neuronal cell killing by the envelope protein of HIV and its prevention by vasoactive intestinal peptide. *Nature, 335*(6191), 639–42.

Brew, B. J. and Garber, J. Y. 2018. Neurologic sequelae of primary HIV infection. In: Brew, B. J. (ed.), *Handbook of Clinical Neurology,* vol. 152. Cambridge, MA: Elsevier, pp. 65–74.

Buch, S., Yao, H., Guo, M., Mori, T., Su, T. P., and Wang, J. 2011. Cocaine and HIV-1 interplay: molecular mechanisms of action and addiction. *J Neuroimmune Pharmacol*, 6(4), 503–15.

Cabral, G. A. and Staab, A. 2005. Effects on the immune system. *Handb Exp Pharmacol*, 168, 385–423.

Centers for Disease Control and Prevention. 2000. HIV/AIDS Surveillance Report: US HIV and AIDS cases reported through December 1999. Centers for Disease Control and Prevention. https://ci.nii.ac.jp/naid/10010139231/

Chana, G., Everall, I. P., Crews, L., et al. 2006. Cognitive deficits and degeneration of interneurons in HIV+ methamphetamine users. *Neurology*, 67(8), 1486–9.

Chang, L., Ernst, T., Speck, O., and Grob, C. S. 2005. Additive effects of HIV and chronic methamphetamine use on brain metabolite abnormalities. *Am J Psychiatry*, 162(2), 361–9.

Chaudhury, S., Bakhla, A., and Saini, R. 2016. Prevalence, impact, and management of depression and anxiety in patients with HIV: a review. *Neurobehavioral HIV Medicine*, 7, 15–30.

Chesney, M. A., Barrett, D. C., and Stall, R. 1998. Histories of substance use and risk behavior: precursors to HIV seroconversion in homosexual men. *Am J Public Health*, 88(1), 113–16.

Childs, E. A., Lyles, R. H., Selnes, O. A., et al. 1999. Plasma viral load and CD4 lymphocytes predict HIV-associated dementia and sensory neuropathy. *Neurology*, 52(3), 607–13.

Choi, S. K., Boyle, E., Cairney, J., Collins, E. J., Gardner, S., Bacon, J., and Rourke, S. B. 2016. Prevalence, recurrence, and incidence of current depressive symptoms among people living with HIV in Ontario, Canada: results from the Ontario HIV Treatment Network Cohort Study. *PLoS One*, 11(11), e0165816.

Clifford, D. B. and Ances, B. M. 2013. HIV-associated neurocognitive disorder. *Lancet Infect Dis*, 13(11), 976–86.

Cohen, M. A. et al. (eds.). 2017. *Comprehensive Textbook of AIDS Psychiatry: A Paradigm for Integrated Care, 2nd Edition*. Oxford: Oxford University Press.

Cosenza, M. A., Zhao, M. L., Si, Q., and Lee, S. C. 2002. Human brain parenchymal microglia express CD14 and CD45 and are productively infected by HIV-1 in HIV-1 encephalitis. *Brain Pathol*, 12(4), 442–55.

Cristiani, S. A., Pukay-Martin, N. D., and Bornstein, R. A. 2004. Marijuana use and cognitive function in HIV-infected people. *J Neuropsychiatry Clin Neurosci*, 16(3), 330–5.

David, A. S. et al. 2012. *Lishman's Organic Psychiatry: A Textbook of Neuropsychiatry, Fourth Edition*. Oxford: Wiley-Blackwell.

Davis, L. E., Hjelle, B. L., Miller, V. E., et al. 1992. Early viral brain invasion in iatrogenic human immunodeficiency virus infection. *Neurology*, 42(9), 1736–9.

De Ronchi, D., Faranca, I., Berardi, D., Scudellari, P., Borderi, M., Manfredi, R., and Fratiglioni, L. 2002. Risk factors for cognitive impairment in HIV-1-infected persons with different risk behaviors. *Arch Neurol*, 59(5), 812–18.

Deeks, S. G., Tracy, R., and Douek, D. C. 2013. Systemic effects of inflammation on health during chronic HIV infection. *Immunity*, 39(4), 633–45.

Des Jarlais, D. C., Friedman, S. R., Novick, D. M., et al. 1989. HIV-1 infection among intravenous drug users in Manhattan, New York City, from 1977 through 1987. *JAMA*, 261(7), 1008–12.

Dew, M. A., Becker, J. T., Sanchez, J., et al. 1997. Prevalence and predictors of depressive, anxiety and substance use disorders in HIV-infected and uninfected men: a longitudinal evaluation. *Psychol Med*, 27(2), 395–409.

Durvasula, R. and Miller, T. R. 2014. Substance abuse treatment in persons with HIV/AIDS: challenges in managing triple diagnosis. *Behav Med*, 40(2), 43–52.

Durvasula, R. S., Myers, H. F., Mason, K., and Hinkin, C. 2006. Relationship between alcohol use/abuse, HIV infection and neuropsychological performance in African American men. *J Clin Exp Neuropsychol*, 28(3), 383–404.

Eggers, C., Arendt, G., Hahn, K., et al. 2017. HIV-1-associated neurocognitive disorder: epidemiology, pathogenesis, diagnosis, and treatment. *J Neurol*, 264(8), 1715–27.

Eisenstein, T. K., Rahim, R. T., Feng, P., Thingalaya, N. K., and Meissler, J. J. 2006. Effects of opioid tolerance and withdrawal on the immune system. *J Neuroimmune Pharmacol*, 1(3), 237–49.

Ellis, R. J., Childers, M. E., Cherner, M., Lazzaretto, D., Letendre, S., Grant, I., and Group, H. I. V. N. R. C. 2003. Increased human immunodeficiency virus loads in active methamphetamine users are explained by reduced effectiveness of antiretroviral therapy. *J Infect Dis*, 188(12), 1820–6.

Etherton, M. R., Lyons, J. L., and Ard, K. L. 2015. HIV-associated neurocognitive disorders and antiretroviral therapy: current concepts and controversies. *Curr Infect Dis Rep*, 17(6), 485.

European AIDS Clinical Society. 2017. European AIDS Clinical Society guidelines, v9.0. https://doi.org/10.1111/hiv.12878

Everall, I., Barnes, H., Spargo, E., and Lantos, P. 1995. Assessment of neuronal density in the putamen in human immunodeficiency virus (HIV) infection. Application of stereology and spatial analysis of quadrats. *J Neurovirol*, 1(1), 126–9.

Everall, I., Salaria, S., Roberts, E., et al. 2005. Methamphetamine stimulates interferon inducible genes in HIV infected brain. *J Neuroimmunol, 170* (1–2), 158–71.

Everall, I. P., Heaton, R. K., Marcotte, T. D., et al. 1999. Cortical synaptic density is reduced in mild to moderate human immunodeficiency virus neurocognitive disorder. HNRC Group. HIV Neurobehavioral Research Center. *Brain Pathol, 9*(2), 209–17.

Fauci, A. S. 1996. Host factors and the pathogenesis of HIV-induced disease. *Nature, 384*(6609), 529–34.

Ferrando, S. J., and Batki, S. L. 2000. Substance abuse and HIV infection. *New Dir Ment Health Serv, 87,* 57–67.

Fiala, M., Gan, X. H., Zhang, L., et al. 1998. Cocaine enhances monocyte migration across the blood–brain barrier. Cocaine's connection to AIDS dementia and vasculitis? *Adv Exp Med Biol, 437,* 199–205.

Gaida, R., Truter, I., Grobler, C., Kotze, T., and Godman, B. 2016. A review of trials investigating efavirenz-induced neuropsychiatric side effects and the implications. *Expert Rev Anti Infect Ther, 14*(4), 377–88.

Gandhi, N. S., Moxley, R. T., Creighton, J., et al. 2010. Comparison of scales to evaluate the progression of HIV-associated neurocognitive disorder. *HIV Ther, 4*(3), 371–9.

Gannon, P., Khan, M. Z., and Kolson, D. L. 2011. Current understanding of HIV-associated neurocognitive disorders pathogenesis. *Curr Opin Neurol, 24*(3), 275–83.

Gardner, B., Zhu, L. X., Roth, M. D., Tashkin, D. P., Dubinett, S. M., and Sharma, S. 2004. Cocaine modulates cytokine and enhances tumor growth through sigma receptors. *J Neuroimmunol, 147*(1–2), 95–8.

Gendelman, H. E. (eds.). 2012. *The Neurology of AIDS, 3rd Edition.* Oxford: Oxford University Press.

Ghosn, J., Taiwo, B., Seedat, S., Autran, B., and Katlama, C. 2018. *Hiv. Lancet, 392*(10148), 685–97.

Giometto, B., An, S. F., Groves, M., et al. 1997. Accumulation of beta-amyloid precursor protein in HIV encephalitis: relationship with neuropsychological abnormalities. *Ann Neurol, 42*(1), 34–40.

Gonzalez-Scarano, F. and Martin-Garcia, J. 2005. The neuropathogenesis of AIDS. *Nat Rev Immunol, 5*(1), 69–81.

Gonzalez-Serna, A., Ajaykumar, A., Gadawski, I., Munoz-Fernandez, M. A., Hayashi, K., Harrigan, P. R., and Cote, H. C. F. 2017. Rapid decrease in peripheral blood mononucleated cell telomere length after HIV seroconversion, but not HCV seroconversion. *J Acquir Immune Defic Syndr, 76*(1), e29–e32.

Gostner, J. M., Becker, K., Kurz, K., and Fuchs, D. 2015. Disturbed amino acid metabolism in HIV: association with neuropsychiatric symptoms. *Front Psychiatry, 6,* 97.

Gras, G. and Kaul, M. 2010. Molecular mechanisms of neuroinvasion by monocytes-macrophages in HIV-1 infection. *Retrovirology, 7,* 30.

Gurwell, J. A., Nath, A., Sun, Q., Zhang, J., Martin, K. M., Chen, Y., and Hauser, K. F. 2001. Synergistic neurotoxicity of opioids and human immunodeficiency virus-1 Tat protein in striatal neurons in vitro. *Neuroscience, 102*(3), 555–63.

Hahn, J. A., and Samet, J. H. 2010. Alcohol and HIV disease progression: weighing the evidence. *Curr HIV/AIDS Rep, 7*(4), 226–33.

Hauser, S. L. (ed.) 2013. *Harrison's Neurology in Clinical Practice, 3rd Edition.* Sydney: McGraw Hill Education.

Hays, R. D., Cunningham, W. E., Sherbourne, C. D., et al. 2000. Health-related quality of life in patients with human immunodeficiency virus infection in the United States: results from the HIV Cost and Services Utilization Study. *Am J Med, 108*(9), 714–22.

Heaton, R. K., Clifford, D. B., Franklin, D. R., Jr., et al. 2010. HIV-associated neurocognitive disorders persist in the era of potent antiretroviral therapy: CHARTER Study. *Neurology, 75*(23), 2087–96.

Heaton, R. K., Franklin, D. R., Ellis, R. J., et al. 2011. HIV-associated neurocognitive disorders before and during the era of combination antiretroviral therapy: differences in rates, nature, and predictors. *J Neurovirol, 17*(1), 3–16.

Hinkin, C. H., Castellon, S. A., Atkinson, J. H., and Goodkin, K. 2001. Neuropsychiatric aspects of HIV infection among older adults. *J Clin Epidemiol, 54 Suppl 1,* S44–52.

Huang, X., Meyers, K., Liu, X., et al. 2018. The double burdens of mental health among AIDS patients with fully successful immune restoration: a cross-sectional study of anxiety and depression in China. *Front Psychiatry, 9,* 384.

Hult, B., Chana, G., Masliah, E., and Everall, I. 2008. Neurobiology of HIV. *Int Rev Psychiatry, 20*(1), 3–13.

Hurt, C. B., Torrone, E., Green, K., Foust, E., Leone, P., and Hightow-Weidman, L. 2010. Methamphetamine use among newly diagnosed HIV-positive young men in North Carolina, United States, from 2000 to 2005. *PLoS One, 5*(6), e11314.

Jacobs, E. S., Keating, S. M., Abdel-Mohsen, M., et al. 2017. Cytokines elevated in HIV elite controllers reduce HIV replication in vitro and modulate HIV restriction factor expression. *J Virol, 91*(6).

Jernigan, T. L., Gamst, A. C., Archibald, S. L., et al. 2005. Effects of methamphetamine dependence and HIV infection on cerebral morphology. *Am J Psychiatry, 162*(8), 1461–72.

Justice, A. C., McGinnis, K. A., Atkinson, J. H., et al. 2004.

Psychiatric and neurocognitive disorders among HIV-positive and negative veterans in care: Veterans Aging Cohort Five-Site Study. *AIDS*, 18 Suppl 1, S49–59.

Kaul, M. and Lipton, S. A. 2006. Mechanisms of neuroimmunity and neurodegeneration associated with HIV-1 infection and AIDS. *J Neuroimmune Pharmacol*, 1(2), 138–51.

Kelley, K. W., Bluthe, R. M., Dantzer, R., Zhou, J. H., Shen, W. H., Johnson, R. W., and Broussard, S. R. 2003. Cytokine-induced sickness behavior. *Brain Behav Immun*, 17 Suppl 1, S112–18.

Kessler, R. C., McGonagle, K. A., Zhao, S., et al. 1994. Lifetime and 12-month prevalence of DSM-III-R psychiatric disorders in the United States. Results from the National Comorbidity Survey. *Arch Gen Psychiatry*, 51(1), 8 19.

Khanlou, N., Moore, D. J., Chana, G., et al. 2009. Increased frequency of alpha-synuclein in the substantia nigra in human immunodeficiency virus infection. *J Neurovirol*, 15(2), 131–8.

Kooij, K. W., Wit, F. W., Schouten, J., et al. 2016. HIV infection is independently associated with frailty in middle-aged HIV type 1-infected individuals compared with similar but uninfected controls. *AIDS*, 30(2), 241–50.

Letendre, S. L., Woods, S. P., Ellis, R. J., et al. 2006. Lithium improves HIV-associated neurocognitive impairment. *AIDS*, 20(14), 1885–8.

Levy, R. M. and Bredesen, D. E. 1988. Central nervous system dysfunction in acquired immunodeficiency syndrome. *J Acquir Immune Defic Syndr*, 1(1), 41–64.

Levy, R. M., Rosenbloom, S., and Perrett, L. V. 1986. Neuroradiologic findings in AIDS: a review of 200 cases. *AJR Am J Roentgenol*, 147(5), 977–83.

Li, J., Mo, P. K., Wu, A. M., and Lau, J. T. 2017. Roles of self-stigma, social

support, and positive and negative affects as determinants of depressive symptoms among HIV infected men who have sex with men in China. *AIDS Behav*, 21(1), 261–73.

Lyketsos, C. G., Hutton, H., Fishman, M., Schwartz, J., and Treisman, G. J. 1996. Psychiatric morbidity on entry to an HIV primary care clinic. *AIDS*, 10(9), 1033–9.

Manji, H. and Miller, R. 2004. The neurology of HIV infection. *J Neurol Neurosurg Psychiatry*, 75 (suppl. 1), i29–35.

Marcondes, M. C., Flynn, C., Watry, D. D., Zandonatti, M., and Fox, H. S. 2010. Methamphetamine increases brain viral load and activates natural killer cells in simian immunodeficiency virus-infected monkeys. *Am J Pathol*, 177(1), 355–61.

Masliah, E., Roberts, E. S., Langford, D., et al. 2004. Patterns of gene dysregulation in the frontal cortex of patients with HIV encephalitis. *J Neuroimmunol*, 157(1–2), 163–75.

McArthur, J. C., Hoover, D. R., Bacellar, H., et al. 1993. Dementia in AIDS patients: incidence and risk factors. Multicenter AIDS Cohort Study. *Neurology*, 43(11), 2245–52.

McArthur, J. C., McClernon, D. R., Cronin, M. F., Nance-Sproson, T. E., Saah, A. J., St Clair, M., and Lanier, E. R. 1997. Relationship between human immunodeficiency virus-associated dementia and viral load in cerebrospinal fluid and brain. *Ann Neurol*, 42(5), 689–98.

McCoy, C. B., Metsch, L. R., Chitwood, D. D., Shapshak, P., and Comerford, S. T. 1998. Parenteral transmission of HIV among injection drug users: assessing the frequency of multiperson use of needles, syringes, cookers, cotton, and water. *J Acquir Immune Defic Syndr Hum Retrovirol*, 18 (suppl. 1), S25–9.

McGuire, J. L., Kempen, J. H., Localio, R., Ellenberg, J. H., and Douglas, S. D. 2015. Immune markers predictive of neuropsychiatric symptoms in HIV-infected youth.

Clin Vaccine Immunol, 22(1), 27–36.

Meltzer, M. S., Skillman, D. R., Gomatos, P. J., Kalter, D. C., and Gendelman, H. E. 1990. Role of mononuclear phagocytes in the pathogenesis of human immunodeficiency virus infection. *Annu Rev Immunol*, 8, 169–94.

Mental Health Foundation. 2016. Survey of people with lived experience of mental health problems reveals men less likely to seek medical support. www .mentalhealth.org.uk/news/survey-people-lived-experience-mental-health-problems-reveals-men-less-likely-seek-medical.

Morrison, M. F., Petitto, J. M., Ten Have, T., et al. 2002. Depressive and anxiety disorders in women with HIV infection. *Am J Psychiatry*, 159 (5), 789–96.

New, D. R., Ma, M., Epstein, L. G., Nath, A., and Gelbard, H. A. 1997. Human immunodeficiency virus type 1 Tat protein induces death by apoptosis in primary human neuron cultures. *J Neurovirol*, 3(2), 168–73.

NICE. 2011. NICE Clinical Guidance (CG113) – Generalised anxiety disorder and panic disorder in adults: management. www.nice.org .uk/guidance/cg113

NICE. 2018. NICE Clinical Guidance (CG90) – Depression in adults: recognition and management. www .nice.org.uk/guidance/cg90

Nightingale, S., Winston, A., Letendre, S., Michael, B. D., McArthur, J. C., Khoo, S., and Solomon, T. 2014. Controversies in HIV-associated neurocognitive disorders. *Lancet Neurol*, 13(11), 1139–51.

Oliver, M. I., Pearson, N., Coe, N., and Gunnell, D. 2005. Help-seeking behaviour in men and women with common mental health problems: cross-sectional study. *Br J Psychiatry*, 186, 297–301.

Parsons, J. T., Rosof, E., Punzalan, J. C., and Di Maria, L. 2005. Integration of motivational interviewing and cognitive behavioral therapy to improve HIV medication adherence and reduce substance use among HIV-positive men and women: results of a pilot project. *AIDS Patient Care STDS*, 19(1), 31–9.

Parsons, T. D., Tucker, K. A., Hall, C. D., Robertson, W. T., Eron, J. J., Fried, M. W., and Robertson, K. R. 2006. Neurocognitive functioning and HAART in HIV and hepatitis C virus co-infection. *AIDS*, 20(12), 1591–5.

Peterson, P. K., Gekker, G., Chao, C. C., et al. 1992. Cocaine amplifies HIV-1 replication in cytomegalovirus-stimulated peripheral blood mononuclear cell cocultures. *J Immunol*, 149(2), 676–80.

Peterson, P. K., Gekker, G., Hu, S., et al. 1994. Morphine amplifies HIV-1 expression in chronically infected promonocytes cocultured with human brain cells. *J Neuroimmunol*, 50(2), 167–75.

Petito, C. K., Roberts, B., Cantando, J. D., Rabinstein, A., and Duncan, R. 2001. Hippocampal injury and alterations in neuronal chemokine co-receptor expression in patients with AIDS. *J Neuropathol Exp Neurol*, 60(4), 377–85.

Plankey, M. W., Ostrow, D. G., Stall, R., Cox, C., Li, X., Peck, J. A., and Jacobson, L. P. 2007. The relationship between methamphetamine and popper use and risk of HIV seroconversion in the multicenter AIDS cohort study. *J Acquir Immune Defic Syndr*, 45(1), 85–92.

Price, T. O., Uras, F., Banks, W. A., and Ercal, N. 2006. A novel antioxidant N-acetylcysteine amide prevents gp120- and Tat-induced oxidative stress in brain endothelial cells. *Exp Neurol*, 201(1), 193–202.

Reback, C. J., Larkins, S., and Shoptaw, S. 2003. Methamphetamine abuse as a barrier to HIV medication adherence among gay and bisexual men. *AIDS Care*, 15(6), 775–85.

Reddy, P. V., Pilakka-Kanthikeel, S., Saxena, S. K., Saiyed, Z., and Nair, M. P. 2012. Interactive effects of morphine on HIV infection: role in HIV-associated neurocognitive disorder. *AIDS Res Treat*, *2012*article ID: 953678, 10pp.

Resnick, L., Berger, J. R., Shapshak, P., and Tourtellotte, W. W. 1988. Early penetration of the blood–brain-barrier by HIV. *Neurology*, 38(1), 9–14.

Reynolds, J. L., Mahajan, S. D., Bindukumar, B., Sykes, D., Schwartz, S. A., and Nair, M. P. 2006. Proteomic analysis of the effects of cocaine on the enhancement of HIV-1 replication in normal human astrocytes (NHA). *Brain Res*, 1123(1), 226–36.

Rippeth, J. D., Heaton, R. K., Carey, C. L., et al. 2004. Methamphetamine dependence increases risk of neuropsychological impairment in HIV infected persons. *J Int Neuropsychol Soc*, 10(1), 1–14.

Robin, S. L. and Kumar, V. 2010. *Robbins and Cotran Pathological Basis of Disease, 8th Edition*. Philadelphia, PA: Saunders Elsevier.

Rosca, E. C., Rosca, O., Simu, M., and Chirileanu, R. D. 2012. HIV-associated neurocognitive disorders: a historical review. *Neurologist*, 18 (2), 64–7.

Roy, S., Ramakrishnan, S., Loh, H. H., and Lee, N. M. 1991. Chronic morphine treatment selectively suppresses macrophage colony formation in bone marrow. *Eur J Pharmacol*, 195(3), 359–63.

Sanmarti, M., Ibanez, L., Huertas, S., et al. 2014. HIV-associated neurocognitive disorders. *J Mol Psychiatry*, 2(1), 2.

Saylor, D., Dickens, A. M., Sacktor, N., et al. 2016. HIV-associated neurocognitive disorder – pathogenesis and prospects for treatment. *Nat Rev Neurol*, 12(5), 309.

Schroecksnadel, K., Sarcletti, M., Winkler, C., et al. 2008. Quality of life and immune activation in patients with HIV-infection. *Brain Behav Immun*, 22(6), 881–9.

Scott, J. C., Woods, S. P., Carey, C. L., Weber, E., Bondi, M. W., Grant, I., and Group, H. I. V. N. R. C. 2011. Neurocognitive consequences of HIV infection in older adults: an evaluation of the 'cortical' hypothesis. *AIDS Behav*, 15(6), 1187–96.

Scott-Sheldon, L. A., Carey, K. B., Cunningham, K., Johnson, B. T., Carey, M. P., and Team, M. R. 2016. Alcohol use predicts sexual decision-making: a systematic review and meta-analysis of the experimental literature. *AIDS Behav*, 20 (suppl. 1), S19–39.

Sewell, M. C., Goggin, K. J., Rabkin, J. G., Ferrando, S. J., McElhiney, M. C., and Evans, S. 2000. Anxiety syndromes and symptoms among men with AIDS: a longitudinal controlled study. *Psychosomatics*, 41 (4), 294–300.

Sharp, P. M. and Hahn, B. H. 2011. Origins of HIV and the AIDS pandemic. *Cold Spring Harb Perspect Med*, 1(1), a006841.

Simioni, S., Cavassini, M., Annoni, J. M., et al. 2013. Rivastigmine for HIV-associated neurocognitive disorders: a randomized crossover pilot study. *Neurology*, 80(6), 553–60.

Simoni, J. M., Safren, S. A., Manhart, L. E., et al. 2011. Challenges in addressing depression in HIV research. assessment, cultural context, and methods. *AIDS Behav*, 15(2), 376–88.

Sin, N. L. and DiMatteo, M. R. 2014. Depression treatment enhances adherence to antiretroviral therapy: a meta-analysis. *Ann Behav Med*, 47 (3), 259–69.

Snider, W. D., Simpson, D. M., Nielsen, S., Gold, J. W., Metroka, C. E., and Posner, J. B. 1983. Neurological complications of acquired immune deficiency syndrome: analysis of 50 patients. *Ann Neurol*, 14(4), 403–18.

Spencer, S. J., Emmerzaal, T. L., Kozicz, T., and Andrews, Z. B. 2015. Ghrelin's role in the hypothalamic–pituitary–adrenal axis stress response: implications for mood disorders. *Biol Psychiatry*, 78(1), 19–27.

Steele, A. D., Henderson, E. E., and Rogers, T. J. 2003. Mu-opioid modulation of HIV-1 coreceptor expression and HIV-1 replication. *Virology*, 309(1), 99–107.

Stern, Y., McDermott, M. P., Albert, S., et al. 2001. Factors associated with incident human immunodeficiency virus-dementia. *Arch Neurol*, 58(3), 473–9.

Strodl, E., Stewart, L., Mullens, A. B., and Deb, S. 2015. Metacognitions mediate HIV stigma and depression/anxiety in men who have sex with men living with HIV. *Health Psychol Open*, 2(1), 2055102915581562.

Szabo, I., Rojavin, M., Bussiere, J. L., Eisenstein, T. K., Adler, M. W., and Rogers, T. J. 1993. Suppression of peritoneal macrophage phagocytosis of Candida albicans by opioids. *J Pharmacol Exp Ther*, 267 (2), 703–6.

Taylor, D., Barnes, T., and Young, A. H. 2018. *The Maudsley Prescribing Guidelines in Psychiatry, 13th Edition*. New York: Wiley-Blackwell.

Tierney, S., Woods, S. P., Verduzco, M., Beltran, J., Massman, P. J., and Hasbun, R. 2018. Semantic memory in HIV-associated neurocognitive disorders: an evaluation of the 'cortical' versus 'subcortical' hypothesis. *Arch Clin Neuropsychol*, 33(4), 406–16.

Turjanski, N. L. G. G. 2005. Psychiatric side-effects of medications: recent developments. *Advances in Psychiatric Treatment*, 11, 58–70.

Turner, K. J., Vasu, V., and Griffin, D. K. 2019. Telomere biology and human phenotype. *Cells*, 8(1).

UNAIDS (The United Nations Joint Programme of HIV/AIDS). 2018. Report on the global HIV/AIDS epidemic, June 1998. Geneva: UNAIDS.

University of Liverpool. 2019. HIV drug interactions, antidepressants. www.hiv-druginteractions.org/prescribing-resources.

Vagenas, P., Azar, M. M., Copenhaver, M. M., Springer, S. A., Molina, P. E., and Altice, F. L. 2015. The impact of alcohol use and related disorders on the HIV continuum of care: a systematic review : alcohol and the HIV continuum of care. *Curr HIV/AIDS Rep*, 12(4), 421–36.

Watzl, B. and Watson, R. R. 1992. Role of alcohol abuse in nutritional immunosuppression. *J Nutr*, 122 (suppl. 3), 733–7.

WHO. 2008. HIV/AIDS and mental health. Geneva: World Health Organization.

Winston, A., Duncombe, C., Li, P. C., et al. 2010. Does choice of combination antiretroviral therapy (cART) alter changes in cerebral function testing after 48 weeks in treatment-naive, HIV-1-infected individuals commencing cART? A randomized, controlled study. *Clin Infect Dis*, 50(6), 920–9.

Wu, E. S., Metzger, D. S., Lynch, K. G., and Douglas, S. D. 2011. Association between alcohol use and HIV viral load. *J Acquir Immune Defic Syndr*, 56(5), e129–30.

Yeager, M. P., Colacchio, T. A., Yu, C. T., Hildebrandt, L., Howell, A. L., Weiss, J., and Guyre, P. M. 1995. Morphine inhibits spontaneous and cytokine-enhanced natural killer cell cytotoxicity in volunteers. *Anesthesiology*, 83(3), 500–8.

Zahr, N. M. 2018. The aging brain with HIV infection: effects of alcoholism or hepatitis C comorbidity. *Front Aging Neurosci*, 10, 56.

Zanet, D. L., Thorne, A., Singer, J., et al. 2014. Association between short leukocyte telomere length and HIV infection in a cohort study: no evidence of a relationship with antiretroviral therapy. *Clin Infect Dis*, 58(9), 1322–32.

Chapter

20

Cardiovascular Disease and Mental Health in Men

David R. Thompson and Chantal F. Ski

The concept of, and link between, the heart and mind has been postulated for centuries and there is now a growing recognition of the connection between mental and cardiovascular health: that cardiovascular disease (CVD) and mental health problems are not only common companions, but that each can lead to the other (Chaddha et al., 2016; Cohen et al., 2015). For example, depression and anxiety are common in people with CVD and are consistently associated with lower quality of life, poorer somatic symptoms, higher mortality, and higher healthcare costs, with between 1 in 2 (Westermair et al., 2018) to 1 in 3 (Norlund et al., 2018) people with CVD meeting the criteria for an anxiety and/or depressive disorder and 1 in 5 (Westermair et al., 2018) receiving mental health care.

CVD and Mental Health

The association between CVD and depression, and between both of these and mortality and morbidity, is well established, though the underlying mechanisms – biological and behavioural – are complex and multi-factorial (Dhar and Barton, 2016; Hare et al., 2014).

Both CVD and mental health disorders are prevalent, burdensome, and costly conditions. CVD is the leading cause of death worldwide, being responsible for 17.7 million deaths (a third of all global deaths) every year (World Health Organization, 2018a), with men having higher rates of both cardiovascular morbidity and mortality and a shorter life expectancy than women (Benjamin et al., 2018).

Mental health disorders are the leading causes of disability worldwide, with nearly 30% of people around the world experiencing a mood, anxiety, or substance-use disorder in their lifetime (Steel et al., 2014). Mortality is significantly higher among people with mental health disorders (particularly among those with psychoses, mood disorders, and anxiety), accounting for eight million deaths each year, and ten

years of potential life lost per person (Walker et al., 2015). Depression alone is the leading cause of ill health and disability worldwide, with more than 300 million people living with it (World Health Organization, 2018b) (see also Chapter 12).

Many people have CVD and depression, thus increasing their risk of death and morbidity and diminishing their quality of life (Cohen et al., 2015). Anxiety and its associated disorders are also common in people with CVD, being linked with the onset and progression of CVD and to adverse cardiovascular outcomes, including death (Celano et al., 2016; Tully et al. 2016). There is a bi-directional relationship between depression and anxiety and CVD: i.e., depression and anxiety can increase the risk of developing CVD and CVD can increase the risk of developing depression and anxiety (Chaddha et al., 2016).

To add to this disease burden are other common co-morbidities, especially diabetes. Worldwide, prevalence rates of diabetes, as well as CVD and mental health problems, are increasing rapidly, and many people with diabetes also have CVD and mental health problems, with at least 10% of people with diabetes having a major depressive disorder and 17% moderate-to-severe depressive symptomatology (Lloyd et al., 2018). As these diseases often occur

> **Box 20.1 The increasing burden of CVD and mental health**
>
> - CVD and mental health issues are prevalent, burdensome, and costly
> - CVD is the leading cause of death worldwide
> - Mental health disorders are the leading cause of disability worldwide
> - Mortality is significantly higher among people with mental health disorders
> - Many people have CVD and mental health disorders

together and can lead to a vicious circle, with each being a risk factor for the other, such co-morbidity adversely affects treatment adherence and ability to self-care, quality of life, health status, healthcare costs, and outcome.

CVD and Mental Health in Men

Despite the abundance of evidence of a clear relationship between CVD and mental health, many men with CVD are not assessed for mental health problems, even though depression and CVD affect millions of men – many experiencing both at the same time – with nearly 1 in 10 men feeling some depression or anxiety every day and 4 in 10 with daily feelings of anxiety or depression taking medications for these or talking to a mental health professional (Blumberg et al., 2015).

In men with a parental history of CVD, poor emotional control in adolescence is significantly predictive of long-term CVD risk even when adjusting for lifestyle-related factors (Potjik et al., 2015) Also, in men, depressed and exhausted mood is a strong predictor of all-cause and cardiovascular mortality risk (Ladwig et al., 2017) and depressive symptoms are associated with a higher resting heart rate and a lower heart rate variability (Jandackova et al., 2016). Men with a higher resting heart rate and higher blood pressure in late adolescence are more likely to have been diagnosed with obsessive-compulsive disorder, schizophrenia, or anxiety disorder later in life (Latvala et al., 2016).

People with severe mental illness such as schizophrenia, bipolar disorder, or other major depressive disorder have a 53% higher risk for having CVD, a 78% higher risk for developing CVD, and an 85% higher risk of death from CVD: the incidence of CVD increases with antipsychotic use, higher body mass index, and higher baseline prevalence of CVD (Correll et al., 2017). Importantly, it is estimated that life expectancy in people with severe mental illness is shorter by 10 to 17.5 years than among the general population, and CVD is a major contributor to early death (Correll et al., 2017).

In addition to depressive and anxiety disorders and severe mental illness, many – particularly older – people have other mental health issues such as dementia, with the incidence of vascular dementia being higher for men than for women in all age groups (Ruitenberg et al., 2001). Also, cognitive function is poor among frail and pre-frail men with CVD,

---

Box 20.2   CVD and mental health in men

- Men have higher rates of both cardiovascular morbidity and mortality and a shorter life expectancy than women
- Nearly 1 in 10 men feel some depression or anxiety every day
- 4 in 10 men with daily feelings of anxiety or depression are taking medications for these or talking to a mental health professional
- In men with a parental history of CVD, poor emotional control in adolescence is significantly predictive of long-term CVD risk
- In men, depressed and exhausted mood is a strong predictor of all-cause and cardiovascular mortality risk

---

particularly in non-memory domains (Weinstein et al., 2018). Sleep apnoea is particularly common in older men and is associated with cardiovascular, metabolic, respiratory, and psychiatric disorders, including depression, anxiety disorders, and schizophrenia (Senaratna et al., 2016). These are likely to be compounded by other health conditions such as diabetes, hearing loss, and osteoarthritis. Furthermore, as people age, they are more likely to experience several conditions at the same time.

Other issues for consideration are that homeless people with mental illness have highly elevated CVD risk, particularly among men and those diagnosed with substance dependence (Gozdik et al., 2015), and that depression is a risk factor for suicide, a leading cause of death in men (World Health Organization, 2014). Gay men are particularly vulnerable to depression and suicidality as well as to alcohol and drug overuse, relationship problems, discrimination, and alienation; these carry implications for healthcare providers who have to navigate particular barriers such as stigma and family relationships (Lee et al., 2017). Aboriginal men are a notable group who experience significant health inequalities, including in terms of CVD and mental health, and face particular issues in accessing appropriate care, including having available culturally specific tools to assess their psychosocial stress and depression, contributing to their under-diagnosis and under-treatment (Brown et al., 2016).

Risk Factors

In addition to US guidelines (Lichtman et al., 2014) recognizing depression as a risk factor for poor prognosis among people with CVD, European guidelines (Piepoli et al., 2016) recognize that low socio-economic status, lack of social support, stress at work and in family life, hostility, depression, anxiety, and other mental disorders contribute to the risk of developing CVD and carry a worse prognosis of CVD; the absence of these factors are associated with a lower risk of developing CVD and a better prognosis of CVD. These psychosocial risk factors are associated with unhealthy lifestyle behaviours that could increase CVD risk and patients should be screened for and counselled about risk factors such as smoking, poor diet, overweight or obesity, and a sedentary lifestyle.

Diabetes is a major risk factor for CVD, and in men with diabetes erectile dysfunction is not uncommon and adversely affects mental health, self-image, and sexual relationships. Erectile problems may be due to organic causes or a side effect of medication but also due to tiredness, anxiety, or drinking too much alcohol. It is important therefore that any indications of this are ascertained early on (which can be difficult because of a reluctance due to the man feeling embarrassed), as it can have profound psychological consequences.

Assessment

In order to help men at high risk due to their mental health risk profile it is important to identify them. Suitable measures include the Patient Health Questionnaire (PHQ) 2 and 9 for depressive symptoms as recommended by the American Heart Association (Lichtman et al., 2008); the Generalized Anxiety Disorder Scale (GAD-7) for anxiety symptoms; or the Hospital Anxiety and Depression Scale (HADS) for both depression and anxiety (Pedersen et al., 2017).

However, questions remain about whether to screen actively for depression in patients with CVD. Proponents of screening point to the high prevalence of these disorders in the CVD populations; profound impact on quality of life and prognosis; and the availability of brief screening instruments and effective treatments (Lichtman et al., 2008). Opponents point to risks, including potential for over-treatment, as well as the absence of proven treatments for patients who screen positive (Ziegelstein et al., 2009). Although general screening for depression, for example, is controversial, interventions offer potentially significant benefits.

In the case of men with severe mental illness, it seems sensible to screen regularly for CVD risk factors and to treat these risk factors, encourage healthy lifestyles, and ensure appropriate use of antipsychotics with a low risk of worsening cardiovascular risk factors such as obesity, diabetes, and hypercholesterolemia (Galletly et al., 2016; Correll et al., 2017).

Interventions

Men with CVD may or may not have mental health issues and this may be influenced not only by the severity of and limitations incurred by the CVD but also by socio-economic factors such as health literacy, the man's psychological make-up, and susceptibility to distress. Depression and other mental health disorders reduce adherence to treatment, serve as a barrier to behaviour change and the adoption of a healthy lifestyle, and increase the likelihood that the man will not access or complete cardiac rehabilitation or secondary prevention programmes, thereby diminishing the man's quality of life and increasing his risk of hospitalization and mortality.

Men are less likely than women to seek help for mental health problems and are more likely to use unhelpful coping strategies (Fogarty et al., 2015), likely due in part to the stigma imposed by dominant cultural masculine norms that discourage emotional expression and help-seeking as signs of weakness (Seidler et al., 2016). Such behaviours are likely to be amplified within male-dominated workplaces (Peters et al., 2018).

In order to be effective, interventions require a friendly and positive interaction to enhance a man's ability to cope and adhere to recommended lifestyle changes and treatments. Such empowerment means gauging the man's experiences, thoughts, attitudes, beliefs, worries, knowledge, and understanding and their motivation and commitment. This is likely to be enhanced by including the man's partner or family member who can reinforce information, correct misconceptions, dispel myths, and allay fears. Behavioural interventions such as motivational interviewing are designed to increase motivation and self-efficacy by helping set realistic, incremental goals in combination with self-monitoring of the chosen behaviour. The focus of such interventions should be on coping and empowerment strategies and include measurable and feasible goal setting and pacing.

Specialized psychological interventions have additional beneficial effects in terms of distress, depression, and anxiety (Richards et al., 2018). These interventions include individual or group counselling regarding psychosocial risk factors and coping with illness, stress management programmes, meditation, autogenic training, biofeedback, breathing, yoga, and/or muscular relaxation. Multimodal behavioural interventions, integrating health education, physical exercise, and psychological therapy, for psychosocial risk factors and coping with illness, are recommended in men with established CVD and mental health symptoms in order to improve their mental health. Whatever approach is taken, interventions should be designed to reach men and tailored to address contextual factors, health concerns, or health behaviours by gender, race, or ethnicity and to take account of considerations such as cultural sensitivity (Garbers et al., 2018). Also, low socio-economic status, low health literacy, and low awareness of health resources may result in impeded recognition of cardiac symptoms, fewer contacts with the healthcare system, and low adherence to recommended lifestyle and medication.

Consideration should be given to men's preferences, personal circumstances, and technical skills. Interventions should be evidence-based and needs-led. Tailoring and adapting the content and delivery of interventions to the capacity of the individual man has the potential to exert the most impact. For instance, text-based materials may be seen as too strenuous or time-consuming to read, and telephone calls may be offered as an alternative to written feedback.

In order to have a significant impact on men's health, innovative psychosocial and educational interventions are needed that address barriers to health promotion and preventative healthcare. Such interventions could take place in community-based settings and be delivered by male community healthcare workers who provide culturally appropriate health education and support. It is important that healthcare workers recognize issues such as financial worries, cultural, racial, ethnic, and linguistic backgrounds, rural and remote locations, family circumstances, social networks, and even sleep difficulties. Other considerations include involving actively the man's partner/spouse and addressing time and travel restrictions as barriers for working men.

Gender-sensitive interventions are needed for men, as notions of masculine social roles and sexual orientation can determine social norms and traditions to support men's self-care and self-management. For instance, it is important to recognize that a prevalent masculine culture of invulnerability, toughness, autonomy, and stoicism (Clarke and Bennett, 2013) implies that help-seeking is synonymous with weakness in men. Thus, negotiating gender norms to support men in distress is important but can be tricky (Keohane and Richardson, 2018), and it is important to facilitate support in ways that do not undermine a man's masculinity further and that he is enabled to retain a sense of normality, autonomy, and control. Healthcare providers need to be able to identify those men at risk, assess the level of risk, and manage the situation accordingly. A relationship of trust is central to asking for, offering, and accepting help.

Men, particularly those who are young, are heavy users of technology for connecting with friends and finding information and support. The challenge for online mental health services is to design interventions specifically suitable for men that are action-based and focus on shifting behaviour and stigma, rather than just increasing knowledge (Ellis et al., 2013). In considering the use of new technologies, the term 'mental health' is seen as highly stigmatized and disliked by men in the workplace, but tools that self-assess, track, and 'fix' mood are highly valued; app characteristics such as brevity of interactions, minimal onscreen text, and a solutions-oriented approach are deemed most suitable (Peters et al., 2018).

Whatever interventions are instituted, it is essential to ensure that systems are in place for referral where necessary, routine follow-up, monitoring, and evaluation.

Depression and Anxiety

Depression, anxiety, and other mental disorders may increase the risk of non-adherence to prescribed treatments and health-promoting practices and may contribute to the increased mortality and morbidity seen in people with CVD and co-morbid mental disorders (Mensah and Collins, 2015). However, there are many pharmacological and behavioural therapies available to treat depression and anxiety, though the evidence base varies (Hare et al., 2014). There is some evidence to support the effectiveness of selective serotonin reuptake inhibitors (SSRIs), though less than one-quarter of people with depressive symptoms are treated with anti-depressants (Nielsen et al., 2015).

Psychological interventions are likely to improve a person's function, quality of life, and general health (Richards et al., 2018), though it is recognized that psychological problems are under-reported and under-treated. People with anxiety disorders are less likely to receive any mental health care than people with depressive disorders (Westermair et al., 2018), which is surprising given that anxious patients with CVD consult their family doctor more often (Nielsen et al., 2015).

Patients who are screened at 'moderate to high' risk of depression have higher levels of depression and anxiety, and lower levels of well-being and social support at follow-up, than those at 'no to low' risk of depression. Importantly, screening and referral alone is insufficient to achieve optimal disease management: a collaborative care approach with integrated pathways to primary care is necessary (Ski et al., 2017). A promising approach is one that takes a patient-preference, stepped-care approach in which depressed patients participate in decision-making on whether to initiate medications and/or psychotherapy and receive frequent follow-up assessments with decisions as to whether to intensify, switch, or maintain therapies (Davidson et al., 2013; Huffman et al., 2014) .

Mental e-health services such as guided internet-based CBT (iCBT) may improve access to acceptable, effective, and cost-effective interventions to reduce symptoms of anxiety and depression (Arnberg et al., 2014). Given that anxiety disorders are common and impose a considerable burden on quality of life (Cohen et al., 2015), attention should be focused on alleviating these. Apart from pharmacotherapy, CBT is a front-line option, with novel approaches such as Panic Attack Treatment in Comorbid Heart Diseases (PATCHD) showing promise (Tully et al., 2016). Another promising and less intensive and costly approach, for depression at least, is the use of behavioural activation, a simpler psychological treatment than CBT (Richards et al., 2016).

Psychological interventions can improve psychological symptoms and reduce mortality in people with CVD but there remains considerable uncertainty regarding the magnitude of these effects and the specific techniques most likely to benefit people with different presentations of CVD (Richards et al., 2018).

> **Box 20.3** Interventions for men with CVD and mental health issues
>
> - Consider men's preferences, personal circumstances, and health literacy
> - Depression and other mental health disorders reduce adherence to treatment and serve as a barrier to behaviour change and the adoption of a healthy lifestyle
> - Interventions should be needs-led, menu-driven, and evidence-based
> - Many pharmacological and behavioural therapies are available
> - Use creative ways to reach out and engage with men

Diet and Weight

Poor diet is not uncommon in men with CVD and mental health issues. Certain groups of people, notably Hispanic, Black, and Aboriginal men, have higher rates of overweight and obesity and they may need prevention strategies that begin in adolescence and emerging adulthood in order to exert an impact on cumulative risk factors (Garbers et al., 2018).

People with depression are well known to have alterations in their dietary preferences and appetite, resulting in weight gain or weight loss. Although vegetarian diets have been associated with decreased risk of CVD death, caution is warranted as vegetarian men have more depressive symptoms (Hibbeln et al., 2018). There is growing evidence that diets that contain eicosapentaenoic acid (EPA)-predominant formulations (>50% EPA) are clinically beneficial for people with depression (Hallahan et al., 2016).

Common barriers to healthy eating include easy access to cheap unhealthy foods and not having the time and motivation to cook/prepare healthy foods. To help overcome this, men should be educated about the benefits of eating a healthy diet, including improvements in overall health, body image, and energy levels, and encouraged to choose healthy meal and snack options, including at least five portions of fresh fruit and vegetables each day, and to aim to maintain a healthy weight, stop smoking, and avoid excessive alcohol use. The major challenge is to help people change their diet and maintain that healthy diet and a healthy weight (Piepoli et al., 2016).

Smoking

Cessation of smoking and other substances is notoriously difficult, especially in men with CVD and mental health problems. This may also require extra attention as people with depressive and anxiety symptoms are more often current smokers compared to people without mental health problems (Nielsen et al., 2015). The best advice to offer men is not to smoke and if they do not smoke, not to start. They should be advised of the risks to their health and that quitting will lower their risk of CVD. They should be reminded that passive secondary smoking carries significant risk too. Brief interventions with advice to stop smoking and nicotine replacement therapy are effective and should be offered to men who do smoke (Piepoli et al., 2016).

Alcohol Use

Whilst many men drink alcohol in moderation, binge-drinking prevalence rates are highest in young adults and are associated with elevated blood pressure and other cardiovascular risk factors among young men (Piano et al., 2018). Thus, it is vital that an open and honest dialogue about alcohol consumption be initiated and maintained and that men make an informed decision about their level of alcohol intake and how this might influence their long- and short-term health. Men with mental health problems should be screened for alcohol habits, since risky drinking habits may affect the outcome of treatment (Strid et al., 2017).

Sedentary Lifestyle and Physical Inactivity

Physical activity among people with mental health disorders require particular attention, more contacts, and persistence, especially with regard to smoking cessation and regular physical activity. Physical activity can help maintain a healthy weight and lower cholesterol and blood pressure and men should be recommended to engage in moderate-intensity exercise for about 30 minutes per day.

People with severe mental illness spend on average eight hours per day being sedentary during waking hours, and are significantly more sedentary than healthy controls: their mean amount of moderate or vigorous physical activity is significantly lower than healthy controls (Vancampfort et al., 2017). Given the health benefits of physical activity and its low levels in people with severe mental illness, interventions targeting the prevention of physical inactivity and sedentary behaviour are warranted.

Despite evidence that physical activity and exercise are broadly as effective as drug interventions in preventing CVD and reducing mortality (Naci and Ioannidis, 2013), people with severe mental illness face a range of barriers to engaging in physical activity and exercise, including high levels of perceived stress, low mood, and a lack of self-confidence and of social support (Firth et al., 2016). Thus, creative strategies need to be adopted to overcome these barriers. These include education on the benefits of physical activity such as improvements in body image, fitness, and overall health, and group activities such as sports, yoga, dance, and Tai Chi. Community-based lifestyle interventions such as health counselling and exercise training appear to improve self-rated health and well-being and diminish depression in middle-aged men at increased risk of CVD (Engberg et al., 2017). Providing men with professional support to identify and achieve their exercise goals may enable them to overcome psychological barriers, and maintain motivation towards regular physical activity.

Physical exercise is an opportunity for men who have CVD and mental health problems. It can improve the person's body image, coping strategies with stress, quality of life, and independence in activities of daily living. The major challenge is for the therapist to be aware of characteristics of major depression, such as loss of interest, motivation, and energy, generalized fatigue, a low self-worth and self-confidence, and physical health problems that may interfere with participation in exercise. Thus, motivational strategies may need to be incorporated to enhance exercise and adherence (Knapen et al., 2015).

Box 20.4 Simple healthy tips for men with CVD and mental health issues

- Eat plenty of fruit and vegetables and maintain a healthy weight
- Do not smoke and limit alcohol consumption
- Take regular physical activity
- Avoid stressful situations
- Get support from a loved one

Work Stress

In men with cardiometabolic disease, job strain is a significant contributor to risk of death, independent of conventional risk factors and their treatment, and measured lifestyle factors (Kivimäki et al., 2018). In order to address this work stress in men, interventions such as consultation, rehabilitation, job redesign, and even retirement may need to be considered. For instance, work reorganizations aimed at improving autonomy and increasing control at work may result in improved social support and a reduction in physiological stress responses. Hence, a reduction of work stress in managers and supervisors may have beneficial health effects on the target individuals and may also improve perceived social support in their subordinates.

Partners

People living with a partner may have less distress than their single-living counterparts as the partner can share the emotional burden and provide social support. They can also bolster confidence, instil hope, and encourage the person to seek healthcare, attend cardiac rehabilitation and adhere to lifestyle and medications (Piepoli et al., 2016).

While family and friends are often the preferred source of support for many, there is a fear of placing undue worry on loved ones. The role of female partners/spouses in caring for men and serving as their primary source of support (Johnson et al., 2012) has the potential to place an undue burden on them. Hence they need support themselves.

Cardiac Rehabilitation

Encouraging men to attend a cardiac rehabilitation programme that integrates counselling for psychosocial risk factors and exercise is effective in reducing anxiety, distress, and stress, and may be home- or community-based (Hare et al., 2014, Pedersen et al., 2017). However, engaging men in health-promoting activities can be challenging, and novel approaches such as the HAT TRICK programme, a 12-week face-to-face, gender-sensitized intervention for overweight and inactive men focusing on physical activity, healthy eating, and social connectedness appears promising (Caperchione et al., 2017).

Conclusions

CVD and mental health are inextricably linked and impose a huge personal and economic burden on

Box 20.5 Key messages for men with CVD and mental health issues

- Treating depression and anxiety improves outcomes, including quality of life, adherence, and stress
- Physical activity increases fitness and improves cardiovascular and mental health
- Stopping smoking is the most effective way to prevent CVD
- Dietary habits influence the risk of CVD and other chronic diseases such as cancer
- Involving partners is likely to enhance health outcomes

men, their loved ones, and society as a whole. They are increasingly appearing against a background of economic recession, erosion, and disintegration of more disadvantaged and rural communities and disruption of family and community networks. Men with CVD and mental health issues are often marginalized, disadvantaged, under-diagnosed, and under-treated and face personal, health, social, sexual, and work issues, such as withdrawal from friends, sleep problems, and spiralling depression. It is important that they are offered access and take up appropriate services to help them cope and improve their quality of life. This often entails designing and providing more nuanced, sensitive, innovative, and flexible services that are tailored to their individual needs if men are to discuss their mental health with their healthcare provider. A host of support, intervention, and treatment services are available, including drug therapy and CBT, though mindfulness, meditation, yoga, transcendental meditation, slow breathing exercises, and exercise are also excellent options.

A major challenge for mental health services is to redesign systems that integrate mental disorders with other chronic diseases such as CVD and create parity between mental and physical health conditions, including treatment and prevention. This will necessitate a more creative approach to reach out and engage with men with CVD and mental health issues. Contemporary approaches that show promise include community-based or personally directed, interactive technology-based interventions that are solution-oriented and exclude direct engagement with a healthcare provider, such as push-out engagement (e.g., through email contacts, text messages, push notifications in apps) rather than the pull-in approach that requires men to seek out a website or app (Garbers et al., 2018).

References

Armstrong, N. M., Meoni, L. A., Carlson, M. C., et al. 2014. Cardiovascular risk factors and risk of incident depression throughout adulthood among men: the Johns Hopkins Precursors Study. *Journal of Affective Disorders*, 214, 60–6.

Arnberg, F. K., Linton, S. J., Hultcrantz, M., et al. 2014. Internet-delivered psychological treatments for mood and anxiety disorders: a systematic review of their efficacy, safety, and cost-effectiveness. *PLoS One*, 9(5), e98118

Benjamin, E. J., Virani, S. S., Callaway, C. W., et al. 2018. Heart disease and stroke statistics – 2018 update: a report from the American Heart Association. *Circulation*, 137, e67–e492.

Blumberg, S. J., Clarke, T. C., and Blackwell, D. L. 2015. *Racial and Ethnic Disparities in Men's Use of Mental Health Treatments. NCHS Data Brief, no 206.* Hyattsville, MD: National Center for Health Statistics.

Brown, A., Mentha, R., Howard, M., et al. 2016. Men, heart and minds: developing and piloting culturally specific psychometric tools assessing psychosocial stress and depression in central Australian Aboriginal men. *Social Psychiatry and Psychiatric Epidemiology*, 51, 211–23.

Caperchione, C. M., Bottorff, J. L., Oliffe, J. L., et al. 2017. The HAT TRICK programme for improving physical activity, healthy eating and connectedness among overweight, inactive men: study protocol of a pragmatic feasibility trial. *BMJ Open*, 7, e016940.

Celano, C.M., Daunis, D.J., Lokko, H.N., et al. 2016. Anxiety disorders and cardiovascular disease. *Current Psychiatry Reports*, 18(11), 101.

Chaddha, A., Robinson, E. A., Kline-Rogers, E., et al. 2016. Mental health and cardiovascular disease. *American Journal of Medicine*, 129, 1145–8.

Clarke, L. H. and Bennett, E. 2013. 'You learn to live with all the things that are wrong with you': gender and the experience of multiple chronic conditions in later life. *Ageing and Society*, 33, 342–60.

Cohen, B. E., Edmondon, D., and Kronish, I. M. 2015. State of the art review: depression, stress, anxiety, and cardiovascular disease. *American Journal of Hypertension*, 28, 1295–1302.

Correll, C. U., Solmi, M., Veronese, N., et al. 2017. Prevalence, incidence and mortality from cardiovascular disease in patients with pooled and specific severe mental illness: a large-scale meta-analysis of 3,211,768 patients and 1112,383,368 controls. *World Psychiatry*, 16, 163–80.

Davidson, K. W., Bigger, J. T., Burg, M. M., et al. 2013. Centralized, stepped, patient preference-based treatments for patients with post-acute coronary syndrome depression: CODIACS Vanguard randomized controlled trial. *JAMA Internal Medicine*, 173, 997–1004.

Dhar, A. K. and Barton, D. A. 2016. Depression and the link with cardiovascular disease. *Frontiers in Psychiatry*, 7, 33.

Ellis, L. A., Collin, P., Hurley, P. J., et al. 2013. Young men's attitudes and behaviour in relation to mental health and technology: implications for the development of online mental health services. *BMC Psychiatry*, 13, 119.

Engberg, E., Liira, H., Kukkonen-Harjula, K., et al. 2017. The effects of health counselling and exercise training on self-rated health and well-being in middle-aged men: a randomized trial. *Journal of Sports Medicine and Physical Fitness*, 57, 916–22.

Firth, J., Rosenbaum, S., Stubbs, B., et al. 2016. Motivating factors and barriers towards exercise in severe mental illness: a systematic review and meta-analysis. *Psychological Medicine*, 46, 2869–81.

Fogarty, A. S., Proudfoot, J., Whittle, E. L., et al. 2015. Men's use of positive strategies for presenting and managing depression: a qualitative investigation. *Journal of Affective Disorders*, 188, 179–87.

Galletly, C., Castle, D., Dark, F., et al. 2016. Royal Australian and New Zealand College of Psychiatrists clinical practice guidelines for the management of schizophrenia and related disorders. *Australian and New Zealand Journal of Psychiatry*, 50, 410–72.

Garbers, S., Hunersen, K., Nechiltilo, M, et al. 2018. Healthy weight and cardiovascular health promotion interventions for adolescent and adult young males of color: a systematic review. *American Journal of Men's Health*, 12, 1328–51.

Gozdik, A., Salehi, R., O'Campo, P., et al. 2015. Cardiovascular risk factors and 30-year in homeless adults with mental illness. *BMC Public Health*, 15, 165.

Hallahan, B., Ryan, T., Hibbeln, J. R., et al. 2016. Efficacy of omega-3 highly unsaturated fatty acids in the treatment of depression. *British Journal of Psychiatry*, 209, 192–201.

Hare, D.L., Toukhasti, S.R., Johansson, P., et al. 2014. Depression and cardiovascular disease: a clinical review. *European Heart Journal*, 35, 1365–72.

Hibbeln, J. R., Northstone, K., Evans, J., et al. 2018. Vegetarian diets and depressive symptoms among men. *Journal of Affective Disorders*, 225, 13–17.

Huffman, J. C., Mastromauro, C. A., Beach, S. R., et al. 2014. Collaborative care for depression and anxiety disorders in patients with recent cardiac events: the Management of sadness and Anxiety in Cardiology (MOSAIC) randomized clinical trial. *JAMA Internal Medicine*, 174, 927–35.

Jandackova, V. K., Britton, A., Malik, M., et al. 2016. Heart rate variability and depressive symptoms: a cross-lagged analysis over a 10-year period in the Whitehall II study. *Psychological Medicine*, 46, 2121–31.

Johnson, J. L., Oliffe, J. L., Kelly, M. T., et al. 2012. Men's discourses of help-seeking in the context of depression. *Sociology, Health and Illness*, 34, 345–61.

Keohane, A. and Richardson, N. 2018. Negotiating gender norms to support men in psychological distress. *American Journal of Men's Health*, 12, 160–71.

Kivimäki, M., Pentti, J., Ferrie, J. E., et al. 2018. Work stress and risk of death in men and women with and without cardiometabolic disease: a multicohort study. *Lancet Diabetes Endocrinology*, 6(9), 705–13.

Knapen, J., Vancampfort, D., Moriën, Y., et al. 2015. Exercise therapy improves both mental and physical health in patients with major depression. *Disability and Rehabilitation*, 37, 1490–5.

Ladwig, K. H., Baumert, J., Marten-Mittag, B., et al. 2017. Room for depressed and exhausted mood as a risk predictor for all-cause and cardiovascular mortality beyond the contribution of the classical somatic risk factors in men. *Atherosclerosis*, 257, 224–31.

Latvala, A., Kuja-Halkola, R., Rück, C., et al. 2016. Association of resting heart rate and blood pressure in late adolescence with subsequent mental disorders: a longitudinal population study of more than 1 million men in Sweden. *JAMA Psychiatry*, 73, 1268–75.

Lee, C., Oliffe, J. L., Kelly, M. T., et al. 2017. Depression and suicidality in gay men: implications for health care providers. *American Journal of Men's Health*, 11, 910–19.

Lichtman, J. H., Froelicher, E. S., Blumenthal, J. A., et al. 2014. Depression as a risk factor for poor prognosis among patients with acute coronary syndrome: systematic review and recommendations: a scientific statement from the American Heart Association. *Circulation*, 129, 1350–69.

Lichtman, J. H., Bigger, J. T. Jr., Blumenthal, J. A., et al. 2008. Depression and coronary heart disease: recommendations for screening, referral, and treatment: a science advisory from the American Heart Association Prevention Committee of the Council on Cardiovascular Nursing, Council on Clinical Cardiology, Council on Epidemiology and Prevention, and Interdisciplinary Council on Quality of Care and Outcomes Research: rendorsed by the American Psychiatric Association. *Circulation*, 118, 1768–75.

Lloyd, C. E., Nouwen, A., Satorius, N., et al. 2018. Prevalence and correlates of depressive disorders in people with Type 2 diabetes: results from the International Prevalence and Treatment of Diabetes and Depression (INTERPRET-DD) study, a collaborative study carried out in 14 countries. *Diabetic Medicine*, 35, 760–9.

Martin, L. A., Neighbors, H. W., and Griffith, D. M. 2013. The experience of symptoms of depression in men vs women. Analysis of the National Comorbidity Survey Replication. *JAMA Psychiatry*, 70, 1100–6.

Mensah, G. A. and Collins, P. Y. 2015. Understanding mental health for the prevention and control of cardiovascular diseases. *Global Heart*, 10, 221–4.

Naci, H. and Ioannidis, J. P. 2013. Comparative effectiveness of exercised and drug interventions on mortality outcomes: metaepidemiological study. *BMJ*, 347, f5577.

Nielsen, T. J., Vestergaard, M., Fenger-Grøn, M., et al. 2015. Healthcare contacts after myocardial infarction according to mental health and socioeconomic position: a population-based cohort study. *PLoS One*, 10(7), e0134557.

Norlund, F., Lissåker, C., Wallert, J., et al. 2018. Factors associated with emotional distress in patients with myocardial infarction: results from the SWEDEHEART registry. *European Journal of Preventive Cardiology*, 25, 910–20.

Pedersen, S. S., von Känel, R., Tully, P. J., et al. 2017. Psychosocial perspectives in cardiovascular disease. *European Journal of Preventive Cardiology*, 24, 108–15.

Peters, D., Deady, M., Gloziet, N., et al. 2018. Worker preferences for a mental health app within male-dominated industries: participatory study. *JMIR Mental Health*, 5(2), e30.

Piano, M. R., Burke, L., Kang, M., et al. 2018. Effects of repeated binge drinking on blood pressure and other cardiovascular health metrics in young adults: National Health and Nutrition Examination Survey, 2011–2014. *Journal of the American Heart Association*, 7, e008733.

Piepoli, M. F., Hoes, A. W., Agewall, S., et al. 2016. 2016 European guidelines on cardiovascular disease prevention in clinical practice. The Sixth Joint task Force of the European Society of Cardiology and Other Societies on Cardiovascular Disease Prevention in Clinical Practice (constituted by representatives of 10 societies and by invited experts). Developed with the special contribution of the European Association for Cardiovascular Prevention and Rehabilitation (EAPCR). *European Heart Journal*, 37, 2315–81.

Potjik, M. R., Janszky, I., Reijneveld, S. A., et al. 2015. Risk of coronary heart disease in men with poor emotional control: a prospective study. *Psychosomatic Medicine*, 78, 60–7.

Richards, D. A., Ekers, D., McMillan, D., et al. 2016. Cost and outcome of behavioural activation versus cognitive behavioural therapy for depression (COBRA): a randomised, controlled, non-inferiority trial. *Lancet*, 388, 871–80.

Richards, S. H., Anderson, L., Jenkinson, C. E., et al. 2018. Psychological interventions for coronary heart disease: Cochrane systematic review and meta-analysis. *European Journal of Preventive Cardiology, 25*, 247–59.

Ruitenberg, A., Ott, A., van Swieten, J. C., et al. 2001. Incidence of dementia: does gender make a difference? *Neurobiology of Aging, 22*, 575–80.

Seidler, Z. E., Dawes. A. J., Rice, S. M., et al. 2016. The role of masculinity in men's help-seeking for depression: a systematic review. *Clinical Psychology Review, 49*, 106–18.

Senaratna, C. V., English, D. R., Currier, D., et al. 2016. Sleep apnoea in Australian men: disease burden, co-morbidities, and correlates from the Australian longitudinal study on male health. *BMC Public Health, 16* (suppl. 3), 1029.

Ski, C. F., Worrall-Carter, L., Cameron, J., et al. 2017. Depression screening and referral in cardiac wards: a 12-month patient trajectory. *European Journal of Cardiovascular Nursing, 16*, 157–66.

Steel, Z., Marnane, C., Iranpour, C., et al. 2014. The global prevalence of common mental disorders: a systematic review and meta-analysis

1980–2013. *International Journal of Epidemiology, 43*, 476–93.

Strid, C., Andersson, C., and Öjehagen, A. 2017. The influence of hazardous drinking on psychological functioning, stress and sleep during and after treatment in patients with mental health problems; a secondary analysis of a randomised controlled intervention study. *BMJ Open, 8*, e019128.

Tully, P. J., Harrison, N. J., Cheung, P., et al. 2016. Anxiety and cardiovascular disease risk: a review. *Current Cardiology Reports, 18*, 120.

Tully, P. J., Sardhina, A., and Nardi, A. E. 2016. A new CBT model of Panic Attack Treatment in Comorbid Heart Diseases (PATCHD): how to calm an anxious heart and mind. *Cognitive Behavioral Practice, 24*, 329–41.

Vancampfort, D., Firth, J., Schuch, F. B., et al. 2017. Sedentary behavior and physical activity levels in people with schizophrenia, bipolar disorder and major depressive disorder: a global systematic review and meta-analysis. *World Psychiatry, 16*, 308–15.

Walker, E. R., McGee, R. E., and Druss, B. G. 2015. Mortality in mental

disorders and global disease implications: a systematic review and meta-analysis. *JAMA Psychiatry, 72*, 334–41.

Weinstein, G., Lutski, M., Goldbourt, U., et al. 2018. Physical frailty and cognitive function among men with cardiovascular disease. *Archives of Gerontology and Geriatrics, 78*, 1–6.

Westermair, A. L., Schaich, A., Willenborg, B., et al. 2018. Utilization of mental health care, treatment patterns, and course of psychosocial functioning in Northern German coronary artery disease patients with depressive and/or anxiety disorders. *Frontiers in Psychiatry, 9*, 75.

World Health Organization. 2014. *Preventing Suicide: A Global Imperative*. Geneva: WHO.

World Health Organization. 2018a. *Fact Sheets: Cardiovascular Diseases*. Geneva: WHO.

World Health Organization. 2018b. *Fact Sheets: Depression*. Geneva: WHO.

Ziegelstein, R. C., Thombs, B. D., Coyne, J. C., et al. 2009. Routine screening for depression in patients with coronary heart disease: never mind. *Journal of the American College of Cardiology, 54*, 886–90.

Chapter 2

Cancer and Mental Health

David W. Kissane

Cancer is a disease of ageing, as more DNA mutation errors eventually escape repair mechanisms, and present clinically with a variety of tumours. As the overall cure rate reaches close to 70% and is much higher in a range of specific cancers, many patients end up surviving two or three malignancies. Despite this treatment success, cancer is still deeply feared and viewed by society as a death threat. In many countries, cancer competes with heart disease for status as the leading cause of death in the community.

The impact of gender on cancer incidence is delivered through hormonal effects on cell division in gonads, lifestyle, and occupational exposure to carcinogens, and the impacts of alcohol, tobacco, obesity, radiation, chronic inflammation, infection, sunlight, immunosuppression, and simply ageing. Sex organs are pertinent, wherein ovarian, uterine, and the vast majority of breast cancers occur in women, while prostate and testicular cancers are found in the male. This chapter addresses cancer particularly as it impacts males.

Cancer as a Death Threat

Like Damocles' sword, a cancer diagnosis causes many to feel vulnerable, as if life is hanging by a thread. The term 'existential' is used to describe those universal challenges that are faced by all people as they grapple with the essential givens of our humanity (Yalom, 1980). Chief among these existential concerns are (1) death anxiety and living with uncertainty, (2) freedom to make our autonomous choices, (3) meaning and the value of life, and (4) existential aloneness, resultant from our individuality. Table 21.1 provides an outline of how these existential challenges are responded to successfully or become maladaptive and generate clinical presentations.

Table 21.1 Existential challenges met by men with cancer (Kissane, 2012)

Challenge	Adaptive response	Maladaptive response
Living with uncertainty and death anxiety	Courage, determination, and mature acceptance	Fear of cancer recurrence, panic and anxiety disorders
Transitions, loss, and change	Mourning and realignment focused on the living	Complicated grief, chronic anger, and poor adjustment
Autonomous choice that comes from personal freedom	Taking responsibility for opportunities, common-sense decision-making, treatment adherence	Feeling a burden, indecisive, non-adherence to recommended treatments
Dignity and integrity of the self	Robust self-esteem and retention of respect despite infirmity/frailty	Embarrassed, ashamed, avoidant
Loneliness	Connected and secure	Insecure, isolated, or alienated
Quality of family relationships	Mutually supportive and well-functioning family network	Dysfunctional or conflicted family
Meaning of life	Fulfilled by accomplishments and sense of leaving a legacy	Demoralization or clinically depressed
Mystery and the unknowable	Spiritually contented and at peace	Doubt, spiritual anguish, guilt, or loss of faith

The existential lens is an essential frame of reference for any clinician working in the oncology or palliative care setting. Being able to offer comprehensible descriptive words to a patient who is struggling to make sense of his angst, surprised at his guttural sense of panic, or feeling that his life has become pointless and lost its direction is a vital clinical skill (Kissane, 2012). Fear of cancer and its treatment journey can be ameliorated by well-presented oncology treatment plans, yet the discussion of prognosis alarms many and can quickly reduce hope, lower morale, and leave the man feeling trapped in a predicament he can no longer control (Kissane, 2014).

A common and disabling problem in oncology practice is the misunderstanding of prognosis. This arises from an interplay between the communication style of the cancer physician; the health literacy of the patient; use of coping mechanisms that may foster or restrict openness of discussion; and the patient's integration of all information into a coherent overall picture. Underestimates of the available future are as common as overestimates, depending on these interacting factors. Pessimism, magnification, and catastrophization are common thinking distortions that can increase existential fear when the prognosis is misunderstood.

Mental Health Morbidity

A large German study of the prevalence of mental disorders in 4020 patients with cancer used a structured clinical interview (CIDI-Oncology) and employed a random sample that was stratified by the national incidence of cancer (Mehnert et al., 2014). Overall, 32% of patients were diagnosed with

---

Box 21.1 Existential and mental health challenges due to cancer

- Cancer is feared in most cultures as a death threat
- Naming and explaining existential angst can ameliorate suffering
- Prognosis is often misunderstood, meriting correction
- Restoring hope and meaning counters demoralization
- Screening for distress and mental health disorders is recommended to avoid these passing unrecognized and undertreated

---

at least one mental disorder, with the prevalence of anxiety disorders 11.5%, adjustment disorders 11%, mood disorders 6.5%, and somatoform disorders 5.3%. Some 6% had two or more disorders, while co-morbidity with alcohol or nicotine dependence was high. Men were equally represented with women, although some specific cancers carried greater morbidity, depending on treatment, tumour aggression, and other risk factors. Cancer teaches people to be very observant and at times hypervigilant of symptoms, contributing to an elevated prevalence of somatic symptom disorders among survivors of cancer. Rates of mental disorders for specific male cancers are shown in Table 21.2, and a tumour-specific approach to mental morbidity is therefore adopted later in this chapter.

One set of studies of these psychiatric disorders in oncology deals with demoralization as a variation of the common adjustment disorder, where morale is lowered and coping is reduced, with resultant hopelessness, pointlessness, and loss of the meaning and purpose of life (Kissane, 2014). Studies informing ICD-11 have been examining the place of adjustment disorder alongside depressive and anxiety disorders, instead of being hierarchically below the threshold for the latter disorders (Glaesmer et al., 2015; Bachem and Casey, 2017). Latent class analysis has shown the unique features of loss of hope, meaning, and role in life, alongside a sense of poor coping, feeling trapped, and unable to be helped, which represent the primary phenomena of adjustment disorder with features of demoralization (Kissane et al., 2017; Bobevski et al., 2018). Interventions that restore meaning, hope, and morale employ the techniques of existential psychotherapy to ameliorate demoralization and sustain optimal engagement with life (Kissane, 2014).

Impact of Anti-Cancer Treatments

In addition to the existential challenge that a diagnosis of cancer brings, much of the risk for mental health disorders arises from the consequences of treatments delivered in an effort to cure the cancer. In some instances, these treatments damage functionality of the body (e.g., render the body infertile), mar body image (e.g., facial scarring and disfigurement), reduce a sense of masculinity (e.g., loss of a testicle), bring shame and embarrassment (e.g., stoma on the abdominal wall, incontinence), or impair fitness and

Table 21.2 Prevalence rates of major psychiatric disorders in specific male cancers (Mehnert et al., 2014)

Cancer type	Anxiety disorders % [95% CIs]	Adjustment disorders % [95% CI]	Mood disorders % [95% CIs]
Bladder cancer	7.6 [3.4 to 16.2]	13.9 [3.9 to 23.9]	5.1 [0.1 to 10.0]
Colorectal cancer	12.1 [8.8 to 16.4]	10.1 [6.6 to 13.5]	5.6 [3.2 to 8.0]
Head and neck	10.7 [5.0 to 21.4]	16.5 [7.7 to 25.3]	5.8 [0.0 to 11.7]
Lung cancer	8.8 [5.4 to 13.8]	6.4 [3.2 to 9.6]	5.1 [2.2 to 7.9]
Prostate cancer	6.0 [3.9 to 9.1]	6.2 [3.6 to 8.8]	3.7 [1.8 to 5.7]

CI = confidence interval, which shows the precision of prevalence estimation, the more narrow the band, the greater the precision. These are based on four-week prevalences.

activity (e.g., anaemia, refractory to transfusions). Such impacts challenge coping and the ability to adapt with courage. The resultant mental health morbidity is fully comprehensible and induces a compassionate response in clinicians. Psychotherapeutic interventions can do much to enhance coping, foster acceptance, and motivate patients to fight determinedly to re-establish well-being. The physician is truly a healer in assuaging the suffering that can otherwise overwhelm the strongest of men.

Specific Cancers in Men

Because the treatment of any cancer brings its own range of morbidities, both short-term treatment side effects and late effects that may arise some years into survivorship, each type of cancer needs to be considered individually. These are presented alphabetically below.

Bladder Cancer

Older men who have smoked are at risk of bladder cancer, most of which are transitional cell carcinomas – recently called urothelial cancers as they arise from the innermost wall of the bladder. Nearly 3000 new cases occur each year in Australia (Australian Cancer Council, 2016). They present with blood in the urine, and cystoscopy can be used to treat superficial cancers, including instillation of BCG. When cancer invades the muscle layer of the wall of the bladder, robot-assisted radical cystectomy is adopted, with reconstruction creating a urinary reservoir constructed from a length of bowel. Reconstructive options including a continent cutaneous reservoir needing a catheter to empty, an ileal neobladder, or the more traditional ileal conduit with

> **Box 21.2 Key impacts of specific cancers in men**
> - With bladder cancer, reconstruction of a bladder reservoir (ileal conduit, ileal neobladder, continent cutaneous reservoir) impacts body image and sexual function
> - With bowel cancer, the need for a stoma is associated with embarrassment, shame, social withdrawal, poorer sexual function, and greater risk for depression
> - Among cancers that occur in men, head and neck cancer has the highest rates of depression and other psychiatric disorders.
> - The burden of prostate cancer lies in treatment effects, including erectile dysfunction, urinary incontinence, and rectal symptoms.
> - Sperm banking is important with testicular cancer, where fertility may be a risk
> - Cancers associated with human papilloma virus (head and neck, anal and penile) can bring shame and relationship issues

external bag. Recurrent urinary infection is a common consequence.

The psychological impact of such bladder surgery includes altered body image; embarrassment and shame from skin irritation, leakage or nocturnal incontinence; delirium from urinary infection; and reduced quality of life (Poch et al., 2013; Karl et al., 2014). Sexual dysfunction is easily comprehensible with such changes; the prostate is removed with the bladder and perineal nerve function is generally interfered with. Of the mental health disorders found in men with bladder cancer, adjustment disorders (13.9%) are most common, followed by anxiety (7.6%) and then mood (5.1%) disorders (Mehnert et al., 2014).

Colorectal Cancer

The risk of bowel cancer in men is 1 in 11, making it the second most common form of male cancer (Cancer Council of Australia, 2016). It arises from a polyp growing on the inside of the mucosa of the colon or rectum, or human papilloma virus when anal cancer occurs. Bowel cancer is screened for by the faecal occult blood test done every two years once age 50 is reached, or by colonoscopy where a familial history is positive. Risk factors include inflammatory bowel disease, obesity, red or processed meat consumption, high alcohol intake and smoking. Surgical resection of segments of the bowel is the main treatment, supplemented by adjuvant chemotherapy if lymph nodes are involved.

Surgery for colon cancer typically involves hemicolectomy, which can include a temporary stoma or, when rectal cancer is present, either a low anterior resection or an abdomino-perineal resection with permanent ostomy can be undertaken. Systematic reviews have challenged the assumption that patients who escape a stoma have better quality of life (Pachler et al., 2005; Cornish et al., 2007). Laparoscopic surgery brings reduced short-term morbidity, without sacrificing any control over the cancer (Vennix et al., 2014). No difference in global quality of life outcomes has emerged from these laparoscopic approaches.

Some 20% of stoma patients experience a serious level of psychiatric disorder as they adjust to life with an ostomy. Practical handling of the stoma, anxiety, depression, and social isolation are major problems, while its potential impact on sexual functioning is clear (Sun et al., 2013). Leakage complications can cause deep shame and impede rehabilitation to employment and sporting activities, while flatus and odour cause embarrassment even to the seasoned veteran (Horner et al., 2010). An ostomy brings lower rates of sexual function and higher erectile dysfunction for men (Krouse et al., 2009). Negative body image and risk of inducing disgust in a partner inhibits intimate relations. An ostomy creates twice the risk of suicide in the post-operative period (Krouse et al., 2007). Patient-to-patient support can be helpful and stomal therapy nurses play a key supportive role.

The German epidemiological study of the four-week prevalence of psychiatric disorder in patients with colorectal cancer reported rates of mood disorder at 5.6%, anxiety disorder at 12.1%, and adjustment disorder at 10.1% (Mehnert et al., 2014). Nearly 22% of these patients had co-morbid alcohol or nicotine dependence. The need for a combination of psychotropic and psychotherapeutic support is very clear.

Head and Neck Cancer

Cancer involving the lip or mouth, pharynx or larynx, skin, and other parts of the head and neck account for 5% of all cancers, are more common in men and result from smoking and human papilloma virus infections. Treatment programmes are often arduous. Resultant disfigurement from surgery, functional impairment, and intrusion upon lifestyle result in stigma, with pronounced social consequences. In the German prevalence study of psychiatric disorders in cancer patients, rates of mood disorder in head and neck cancer were 5.8%, anxiety 10.7%, and adjustment disorder 16.5% (Mehnert et al., 2014).

A coordinated multidisciplinary approach is needed to support the adaptation of patients with head and neck cancer, including nutrition, speech and occupational therapy, social work and physiotherapy, as well as psycho-oncology services (Semple et al., 2013). Stepped care approaches are pragmatic in graduating the psychosocial response (Krebber et al., 2012). Couple and family support are often needed. Measurement of the level of shame and stigma found among these patients allows it to be a more specific focus of therapy (Kissane et al., 2013).

Lung Cancer

Cigarette smoking causes 85–90% of lung cancer, which develops in proportion to age of initiation, number of cigarette packs smoked, and years of smoking. It is clearly more common in men, and affects 1 man in 13 up to the age of 85 years (Cancer Council Australia, 2016). The mortality of lung cancer is 25 times higher in smokers compared to lifetime never-smoked. In the German epidemiological study, four-week prevalence rates of mood disorder in lung cancer were 5.1%, anxiety disorder 8.8%, and adjustment disorder 6.4% (Mehnert et al., 2014).

Prevention and smoking cessation programmes are clearly vital. Treatment options had not been very effective in lung cancer, which therefore carried a poor prognosis, until the recent arrival of immune therapies such as Nivolumab. These new therapies appear to be changing survival rates. The stigma of having smoked can lead some men to a fatalistic attitude. Supportive services need to address shame as they engage men in ongoing meaningful lives. Therapies that cultivate relaxation or mindfulness techniques, alongside anti-anxiety approaches are important to help patients overcome the challenge of breathlessness, especially in a palliative care setting.

Penile Cancer

Penile cancers are more common in regions of Africa and South America, with risk factors including human papilloma virus, infections, AIDS, smoking, and ultraviolet light exposure (Skeppner et al., 2008). Squamous cell carcinoma predominates. The general prevalence rate is 1 in 100,000 men. Presentations include ulcers and fissures. Fear is associated with delayed presentation. The mainstay of treatment has been radical amputation, although recent glanuloplasty techniques show promise, and include the use of grafts from the rectus abdominal muscles and skin from the thigh. Issues of shame, impact on quality of life, and sexual functioning are the main challenges to adaptation.

Prostate Cancer

This is the most common male cancer, affecting 1 man in 6 by the age of 85 years, with higher rates among African American men, and 63% of cases occurring after the age of 65 years (Cancer Council Australia, 2016). Only 5–10% have a familial basis and large-scale population studies have failed to show any reduction in death from prostate cancer when screening is used to assess prostate specific antigen (PSA). Many unnecessary treatments with resultant morbidities have occurred with PSA screening.

Treatment options for prostate cancer include (1) 'active surveillance', where the cancer is low-grade and indolent in nature, or other significant co-morbidities exist and overall life expectancy is less than 10 years; (2) robotic-assisted or laparoscopic 'radical prostatectomy' with nerve-sparing procedures, if the disease is localized and aggressive on histology scores (Gleason $\geq$7); (3) conventional external beam 'IMRT' (intensity-modulated radiation therapy) or 'brachytherapy' (seed implants), often associated with androgen blockade to reduce field size; (4) newer therapies that include cryotherapy

and proton beam treatments; (5) 'androgen ablation' therapy, if the disease is metastatic to bone or lymphatic system and while sensitive to anti-androgen therapies; and (6) chemotherapy and radioisotope treatments to palliate androgen-resistant secondaries.

Treatment side effects cause the morbidity associated with prostate cancer, and include erectile dysfunction and impotence, incontinence of urine, tenesmus and rectal discharge, pelvic pain, depression, anxiety, fatigue, and a sense of emasculation. Rates of sexual dysfunction can be >80%, incontinence >50%, and delayed effects from radiotherapy can end up spoiling quality of life. The smell of leaking urine and need for diapers is humiliating. Couple and intimate relations are clearly affected.

In the German epidemiology study of psychiatric disorders in prostate cancer, four-week prevalence rates of mood disorder were 3.7%, anxiety 6.0%, and adjustment disorder 6.2% (Mehnert et al., 2014). Supportive therapy and couple counselling are used in conjunction with appropriate psychotropics. Care to avoid drug interactions is illustrated by selective serotonergic reuptake inhibitors that use the 2D6 metabolic pathway competing with abiraterone, which inhibits Cyp 17 enzymes expressed in testes, adrenals, and prostate tumours, decreasing circulating levels of testosterone, where abiraterone is also metabolized by 2D6 pathways.

Sexual rehabilitation is practised in conjunction with prostatectomy surgery, with regular use of phosphodiesterase-5 (PDE-5) inhibitors such as sildenafil, tadalafil, and vardenafil to preserve cavernosal functionality and sustain erectile function. Twice-weekly penile injections during sexual rehabilitation, or the later use of vacuum erection devices and penile prostheses are examples of sexual therapies. Intimacy-enhancing couple therapy has shown more benefit to the partner than the patient himself (Manne et al., 2011).

Testicular Cancer

Generally found in younger men (< 40 years), germ-cell tumours of the testes account for more than 90% of testicular tumours and are divided into seminomas and non-seminomas; lymphoma can also occur in the testicle. Australian men have a risk of testicular cancer of 1 in 187 (Cancer Council of Australia, 2016). These tumours generally present as a painless lump or enlarged testicle. Elevated markers include α-foetoprotein (AFP), β-human chorionic gonadotropin (β-HCG), and lactate dehydrogenase (LDH). Orchidectomy (with implant) and chemotherapy have been the mainstay of treatment, with retroperitoneal lymph-node dissection being sometimes needed and bringing risk of ejaculatory dysfunction. Chemotherapy and consolidative radiotherapy are used. A cure rate close to 100% is anticipated.

Psychosocial issues related to testicular cancer include sexuality, sense of masculinity, fertility, and intimacy (Skoogh et al., 2013). Sperm banking is offered routinely, but low sperm counts can predate the diagnosis of testicular cancer. More recognition of late effects resultant upon curative treatment include secondary cancers and the vascular effects of any radiation therapy. Generally most young men adapt well to the treatment of testicular cancer.

Treatment of Depression, Anxiety, and Adjustment Disorders in Men's Cancers

Depression

In examining the prevalence rates of mood disorders (see Table 21.2), some are surprised at the lower rates of morbidity seen in prostate cancer, but this reflects the older age and indolent presentation of many patients. Where prostate cancer occurs in younger men and is aggressive, then mood disorder is noteworthy. Broad risk factors for the development of depression include a past history of depression and other psychiatric disorders, younger age, higher symptom burden, advanced disease, and poor social support.

Depression is frequently under-recognized and undertreated in oncology practices because clinicians often normalize the distress they see and avoid probing more deeply (Kissane, 2014). A major screening programme of 21,000 participants across three Scottish Cancer Centres revealed that 72% of depressed patients went unrecognized (Sharpe et al., 2014). When these individuals were treated in the SMaRT oncology collaborative care trials, treatment failure in the usual care arms involved inadequate dose titration of antidepressant medication by their general practitioners, or failure to move to second line and adjuvant regimens in more treatment-resistant cases (Sharpe et al., 2014; Walker et al., 2014). Depression in cancer care is associated with poorer adherence to anti-cancer treatments, poorer self-care,

and shorter survival (Mausbach et al., 2015; Satin et al., 2009; Pinquart and Duberstein, 2010).

First-line medications used to treat depression in oncology include selective serotonergic reuptake inhibitors (e.g., citalopram, with low 2D6 cytochrome enzyme interactions) and mirtazapine (benefitting sleep and appetite), while duloxetine (helpful as a co-analgesic for chronic cancer pain) or desvenlafaxine are examples of second-line agents (Li et al., 2017). Adjuvant therapy can employ risperidone or quetiapine when needed.

Psychotherapies used in the treatment of depression are as important as psychotropic medication, with meta-analytic evidence demonstrating their effectiveness (Faller et al., 2013; Hart et al., 2012). Elements of cognitive-behavioural therapy (Moorey and Greer, 2012), interpersonal psychotherapy, acceptance and commitment, problem-solving and meaning-centred therapies are all useful in treating depression in the context of cancer (Fujisawa and Uchitomi, 2017).

Anxiety

While the most common diagnostic categories identified among men with cancer will be Generalized Anxiety Disorder (GAD) and Panic Disorder (PD), occasional patients will present with a needle phobia, or fear of the tunnel in MRI machines used for imaging. Quietly in the background of GAD or panic episodes will be death anxiety, but this will usually not be volunteered as a leading symptom. Even with the

---

Box 21.3 Medication and psychotherapeutic treatment in oncology

- Attention to drug interactions is important as anti-cancer treatments such as abiraterone for prostate cancer are metabolized by 2D6 cytochrome enzymes
- Key reasons for treatment resistance in depressive disorders include inadequate titration of dose or rotation to second line and use of adjuvant medications
- Combinations of supportive, cognitive-behavioural, emotion-focused, interpersonal, acceptance and commitment, existential and meaning-centred psychotherapy play a helpful role in ameliorating psychiatric disorders in the oncology setting

language of 'Fear of Recurrence' (FCR), symptomatology will often be framed around staging procedures, fear of what will be discovered, and fear of side effects of treatments, with the issue of human mortality kept in the background. Experienced psycho-oncologists have learnt that many patients welcome the opportunity to unpack what underlies their angst, and that naming death anxiety for what it is permits patients to begin to process it.

The existential model of 'living in the moment because one day we all die' can be developed with patients who carry a lot of fear. A meta-cognitive position can allow a person to observe the cost that FCR brings, to better appreciate the burden of anticipatory fear, and to see the futility of anticipatory grief. Cultivating an attitude that empowers 'living in the moment' risks intellectualization, and so much empathic acknowledgement and emotional support is needed in parallel. Supportive psychotherapy is thus an essential ingredient of all therapy in cancer care (Lederberg and Holland, 2011). Working with ambivalence, ambiguity, and denial is grist for the mill. Cognitive reframing of any evident-thinking distortions proves helpful, recognizing that the yardstick is not the 'rationality'

of a thought, but how realistic and how unhelpful it might be (Kissane et al., 1997).

Adjustment Disorder

This is a common diagnosis in patients with cancer, often with specifiers like 'anxious mood' or 'demoralization' (Kissane et al., 2017). Strong evidence exists for the benefit of psychotherapy in alleviating this distress (Faller et al., 2013). Family-centred models of care make a further contribution, especially towards the end-of-life (Kissane and Bloch, 2002; Schuler et al., 2012).

Conclusion

Cancer is part of the inescapable experience of life for one person in three and one family in two. Historically, ignorance and fear was dealt with through use of denial and non-mention of the word 'cancer'. Today, much progress has been achieved in guiding psychological adaption and helping people to face this illness with courage. There are many medications and healing counselling techniques that ameliorate suffering and help men to sustain their focus on living life out fully. The battle against cancer is, indeed, a worthy one.

References

Bachem, R. and Casey, P. 2017. Adjustment disorders: a diagnosis whose time has come. *Journal of Affective Disorders*, 227, 243–53.

Bobevski, I., Kissane, D. W., Vehling, S., et al. 2018. Latent class analysis differentiation of adjustment disorder and demoralization, more severe depressive-anxiety disorders, and somatic symptoms in a cohort of patients with cancer. *Psycho-Oncology*. 27(11), 2623–30. doi:10.1002/pon.4761

Cancer Council of Australia. 2016. Understanding Testicular Cancer. Accessed at www.cancer.org.au/about-cancer/types-of-cancer/testicular-cancer.html.

Cornish, J. A., Tilnet, H. S., Heriot, A. G., Lavery, I. C., Fazio, V. W., and Tekkis, P. P. 2007. A meta-analysis of quality of life for abdominoperitoneal excision of

rectum versus anterior resection for rectal cancer. *Annals of Surgical Oncology*, 14, 2056–68.

Faller, H., Schuler, M., Richard, M., Heckl, U., Weis, J., and Küffner, R. 2013. Effects of psycho-oncologic interventions on emotional distress and quality of life in adult patients with cancer: systematic review and meta-analysis. *Journal of Clinical Oncology*, 31, 782–93.

Fujisawa, D. and Uchitomi, Y. 2017. Depression in Cancer Care. In: M. Watson and D. W. Kissane (eds.) *Management of Clinical Anxiety and Depression*. 23–41. Oxford: Oxford University Press.

Glaesmer, H., Romppel, M., Brahler, E., Hinz, A., et al. 2015. Adjustment disorder as proposed for ICD-11: dimensionality and symptom differentiation. *Psychiatry Research*, 229, 940–8.

Hart, S. L., Hoyt, M. A., Diefenbach, M., et al. 2012. Meta-analysis of

efficacy of interventions for elevated depressive symptoms in adults diagnosed with cancer. *Journal of National Cancer Institute*, 104, 990–1004.

Horner, D. J., Wendel, C. S., Skeps, R., et al. 2010. Positive correlation of employment and psychological well-being for veterans with major abdominal surgery. *American Journal of Surgery*, 200, 585–90.

Karl, A., Buchner, A., Becker, A., et al. 2014. A new concept for early recovery after surgery for patients undergoing radical cystectomy for bladder cancer: results from a prospective randomized study. *Journal of Urology*, 191, 335–40.

Kissane, D. W., Miach, P., Bloch, S., Seddon, A., and Smith, G. C. 1997. Cognitive-existential group therapy for patients with primary breast cancer. *Psycho-Oncology*, 6, 25–33.

Kissane, D. W. and Bloch, S. 2002. *Family Focused Grief Therapy:*

A Model of Family-Centred Care during Palliative Care and Bereavement. Buckingham: Open University Press.

Kissane, D. W. 2012. The relief of existential suffering. *Archives of Internal Medicine*, 172(19), 1501–5.

Kissane, D. W. 2014. Unrecognised and untreated depression in cancer care. *The Lancet Psychiatry*, 1(5), 320–1.

Kissane, D. W. 2014. Demoralization – A life-preserving diagnosis to make in the severely medically ill. *Journal of Palliative Care*, 30, 255–8.

Kissane, D. W., Bobevski, I., Gaitanis, P., et al. 2017. Exploratory examination of the utility of demoralization as a specifier for adjustment disorder and major depression. *General Hospital Psychiatry*, 46, 20–4.

Kissane, D. W., Patel, S. G., Baser, R. E., et al. 2013. Preliminary evaluation of the reliability and validity of the shame and stigma scale in head and neck cancer. *Head and Neck*, 35, 172–83.

Krebber, A. M., Leemans, C. R., de Bree, R., et al. 2012. Stepped care targeting psychological distress in head and neck and lung cancer patients: a randomized clinical trial. *BMC Cancer*, 12, 1–8.

Krouse, R. S., Grant, M., Wendel, C. S., et al. 2007. A mixed-methods evaluation of health-related quality of life for male veterans with and without intestinal stomas. *Disease of Colon and Rectum*, 50, 2054–66.

Krouse, R. S., Grant, M., Rawl, S. M., et al. 2009. Coping and acceptance: the greatest challenge for veterans with intestinal stomas. *Journal of Psychosomatic Research*, 66, 227–33.

Lederberg, M. S., Holland, J. C. 2011. Supportive psychotherapy in cancer care: an essential ingredient of all therapy. In: M. Watson and D. W. Kissane (eds.) *Handbook of Psychotherapy in Cancer Care*. 3–14. Chichester: Wiley-Blackwell.

Li, M., Rosenblat, J., and Rodin, G. 2017. Psychopharmacologic management of anxiety and depression. In: M. Watson and D. W. Kissane (eds.) *Management of Clinical Anxiety and Depression*. 78–107. Oxford: Oxford University Press.

Manne, S. L., Kissane, D. W., Nelson, C. J., Mulhall, J. P., Winkel, G., and Zaider, T. 2011. Intimacy-enhancing psychological intervention for men diagnosed with prostate cancer and their partners: a pilot study. *Journal of Sexual Medicine* 8(4), 1197–1209.

Mausbach, B. T., Schwab, R. B., and Irwin, S. A. 2015. Depression as a predictor of treatment adherence to adjuvant endocrine therapy (AET) in women with breast cancer: a systematic review and meta-analysis. *Breast Cancer Research and Treatment*, 152, 239–46.

Mehnert, A., Brahler, E., Faller, H., et al. 2014. Four-week prevalence of mental disorders in patients with cancer across major tumor entities. *Journal of Clinical Oncology*, 32, 3540–6.

Moorey, S. and Greer, S. 2012. *Oxford Guide to CBT for People with Cancer*. Oxford: Oxford University Press.

Pachler, J. and Wille-Jorgensen, P. 2005. Quality of life after rectal resection for cancer, with or without permanent colostomy. *Cochrane Database Systematic Review*, CD004323.

Pinquart, M. and Duberstein, P. R. 2010. Depression and cancer mortality: a meta-analysis. *Psychological Medicine*, 40, 1797–1810.

Poch, M. A., Stegemann, A. P., and Rehman, S., et al. 2013. Short-term patient reported health-related quality of life (HRQL) outcomes after robot-assisted radical cystectomy. *British Journal of Urology International*, 113, 260–5.

Satin, J. R., Linden, W., and Phillips, M. J. 2009. Depression as a predictor of disease progression and mortality in cancer patients. *Cancer*, 115, 5349–61.

Schuler, T. A., Zaider, T. I., and Kissane, D. W. 2012. Family grief therapy: a vital model in oncology, palliative care and bereavement. *Family Matters*, 90, 77–86.

Semple, C., Parahoo, K., Norman, A., et al. 2013. Psychosocial interventions for patients with head and neck cancer. *Cochrane Database Systematic Review*, CD009441.

Sharpe, M., Walker, J., Hansen, C. H., et al. 2014. Integrated collaborative care for comorbid major depression in patients with cancer (SMaRT Oncology-2): a multicentre randomised controlled effectiveness trial. *Lancet*, 384, 1099–1108.

Skeppner, E., Windahl, T., Andersson, S. O., Fugl-Meyer, K. S. 2008. Treatment-seeking, aspects of sexual activity and life satisfaction in men with penile carcinoma. *European Urology*, 54, 631–9.

Skoogh, J., Steineck, G., Johansson, B., Wilderang, U., and Stierner, U. 2013. Psychological needs when diagnosed with testicular cancer: findings from a population-based study with long-term follow-up. *British Journal of Urology International*, 111, 1287–93.

Sun, V., Grant, M., McMullen, C. K., et al. 2013. Surviving colorectal cancer: long-term, persistent ostomy-specific concerns and adaptations. *Journal of Wound Ostomy*, 40, 61–72.

Vennix, S., Pelzers, L., Bouvy, N., et al. 2014. Keyhole laparoscopic or open surgery for rectal cancer. *Cochrane Database of Systematic Reviews*, CD005200.

Walker, J., Holm Hansen, C., Martin, P., et al. 2014. Integrated collaborative care for major depression comorbid with a poor prognosis cancer (SMaRT Oncology-3): a multicentre randomised controlled trial in patients with lung cancer. *Lancet Oncology*, http://dx.doi.org/10.1016/S1470-2045(14)70343-2.

Yalom, I. D. 1980. *Existential Psychotherapy*. New York: Basic Books.

Chapter

22

Dementia

Terence W. H. Chong and Nicola T. Lautenschlager

Dementia is an increasing challenge across the globe. The 2015 World Alzheimer Report by Alzheimer's Disease International describes the global impact of dementia, which is summarized below (Prince et al., 2015). The prevalence of dementia is increasing worldwide with 47 million people with dementia in 2015, estimated to rise to 131 million by 2050. Dementia is the leading contributor to disability and need for care in older people, with a population-attributable fraction of 25% for disability. In people aged over 60 years globally, dementia is the ninth leading cause of Disability Adjusted Life Years (DALYs) lost and the eighth leading case of Years Lived with Disability. The global cost of dementia in 2015 was estimated to be US$818 billion. The rate of population ageing is relatively greater in low- to middle-income countries and this is compounded by a relative lack of resources. As a result, low- to middle-income countries will be impacted more dramatically by dementia compared to high-income countries. A recent review and accompanying editorial has concluded with 'a call to action' for greater research attention to the impact of sex in Alzheimer's disease to help improve outcomes with an acknowledgment that insufficient attention has hitherto been paid to sex-specific issues in dementia more broadly (Mielke et al., 2018 and Nebel et al., 2018). This chapter provides an overview of dementia, with a focus on males.

Definition

The DSM-5 has relabelled dementia as 'major neurocognitive disorder' (APA, 2013), although our experience is that most patients, families, clinicians, and organizations continue to refer to the condition as 'dementia'. The DSM-5 diagnostic criteria are summarized in Box 22.1.

The ICD-10 defines dementia as

a syndrome due to disease of the brain, usually of a chronic or progressive nature, in which there is

---

Box 22.1 Summary of DSM-5 criteria for major neurocognitive disorder

A. Evidence of significant cognitive decline based on:

 1. Concern of the individual, knowledgeable informant, or clinician and
 2. A substantial impairment in cognitive performance

B. The cognitive deficits interfere with independence in everyday activities

C. The cognitive deficits do not exclusively occur in the context of delirium

D. The cognitive deficits are not better explained by another mental disorder

---

disturbance of multiple higher cortical functions, including memory, thinking, orientation, comprehension, calculation, learning capacity, language, and judgement. Consciousness is not clouded. The impairments of cognitive function are commonly accompanied, and occasionally preceded, by deterioration in emotional control, social behaviour, or motivation. (WHO, 2019)

The most common cause of dementia is Alzheimer's disease, followed by vascular dementia, although there is some geographical variation in the relative prevalence of these two conditions. Other causes of dementia include Dementia with Lewy Bodies, Fronto-temporal Dementia, and Alcohol-related Dementia.

Regional estimates of dementia prevalence in adults aged 60 years and over are reported to range from 4.6% in Central Europe to 8.7% in North Africa and the Middle East, while the prevalence in all other regions are found within the range of 5.6% to 7.6% (Prince et al., 2015). It is still unclear as to whether sex has an effect on an individual's risk of developing dementia; however, most studies have found a higher prevalence of dementia in women compared to men across the age spectrum (Rocca et al., 2014). One postulated reason for this difference is that women have a longer life expectancy than men (Rocca et al., 2014).

A recent review of fourteen studies looking at dementia prevalence trends and incidence reported stable or declining prevalence and incidence of dementia, and that no single factor could account for this change (Wu et al., 2017). The authors describe that factors such as education, vascular risk, body mass index, and smoking could explain some of the reduction, and this emphasizes the importance of future research to investigate possible factors that may be relevant to reducing the prevalence and incidence of dementia. In this review, sex differences were noted in three of these studies: the Cognitive Functioning and Ageing Study (CFAS) in the UK, the Framingham Study in the USA, and the Bordeaux Study in France (Wu et al., 2017).

The CFAS study recruited adults aged 65 years and above in 1989–94 (n=5156) and compared them to a cohort recruited in 2008–11 (n=5288) and found a 20% drop in incidence that was mainly attributed to a reduction in incidence for males across all age groups (Matthews et al., 2016). It was unclear what factors caused this sex difference.

The Framingham study determined the five-year incidence of dementia for 5205 adults aged 60 years and above across five epochs with the first epoch being late 1970s–early 1980s and the fifth epoch being late 2000s–early 2010s (Satizabal et al., 2016). An average 20% per decade decline in the incidence of dementia was found and it was postulated that education levels and vascular risk factors accounted for some of the reduction. The reduction in women occurred earlier and across all epochs, while the reduction in men only occurred in the last epoch, with no explanation for this sex difference being able to be identified (Satizabal et al., 2016 and Wu et al., 2017).

In the Bordeaux study, two different populations of adults aged 65 years and above were recruited in 1988–9 (n=1469) and 1999–2000 (n=2104) and were followed up for ten years (Grasset et al., 2016). A significant decrease in incidence was shown for women but not men with a Hazard Ratio of 0.64. The reasons for the sex difference were postulated as possible gender differences in improvement in levels of education and risk factors, as well as a greater reduction in disability (instrumental activities of daily living) amongst French women compared to men during the ten-year period (Grasset et al., 2016).

Risk Factors

Given that there are still no disease-modifying treatments available despite more than 200 drugs having entered at least Phase II trials between 1984 and 2014 (Schneider et al., 2014), there is increasing focus towards the possibility of dementia risk reduction (Chong et al., 2016). Approximately 40% of an individual's risk of dementia is potentially modifiable (Livingston et al., 2020). Globally, the most significant modifiable risk factors and their population attributable fraction (PAF) in order of magnitude are shown in Box 22.2 (Livingston et al., 2020).

In western nations (Australia, Europe, United Kingdom, and the United States), the most significant modifiable risk factors in order of magnitude are (Norton et al., 2014 and Ashby-Mitchell et al., 2017) physical inactivity, mid-life obesity, mid-life hypertension, low educational attainment, smoking, depression and diabetes mellitus. Modelling performed by Norton and colleagues (2014) predicted that relative reductions of 10% per decade in each of these seven modifiable risk factors would result in an 8.3% reduction in dementia prevalence worldwide by 2050.

There are some relevant sex differences in these risk factors. Male older adults are generally more physically active than female older adults, while overall, the majority of both sexes still do not meet the levels recommended by physical activity guidelines (Keadle et al., 2016 and Booth et al., 2000). The prevalence of overweight and obesity is higher in females than males (Ng et al., 2014). In contrast, male sex is associated with increased odds of being

---

Box 22.2 Population attributable fractions of modifiable risk factors for dementia

- Mid-life hearing loss, PAF = 8%
- Early life less education, PAF = 7%
- Later life smoking, PAF = 5%
- Later life depression, PAF = 4%
- Later life social Isolation, PAF = 4%
- Mid-life traumatic brain injury, PAF = 3%
- Later-life air pollution, PAF = 2%
- Mid-life hypertension, PAF = 2%
- Later-life physical inactivity, PAF = 2%
- Later-life diabetes, PAF = 1%
- Mid-life alcohol (>21 units/week), PAF = 1%
- Mid-life obesity (Body Mass Index ≥30), PAF = 1%

Note: Early life = < 45 years, Mid-life = 45–65 years of age and Later life = >65 years of age.

hypertensive (Theodore et al., 2015). Due to historical societal factors, lower educational attainment was more prevalent in females than males in the past, and this is relevant to the group of older adults currently at risk of developing dementia (Mielke et al., 2014). This educational difference is changing in many parts of the world, with a trend towards increasing educational attainment in females. This will potentially lead to a change in the risk-factor profile of older adults in the future. Smoking has historically been more prevalent in males than females, although this difference has narrowed over time and will also modify the future risk factor profile of older adults (Mielke et al., 2014). A consistent sex difference has been found in a systematic review and meta-analysis of global prevalence of common mental disorders, in that women had higher rates of mood disorders, including depression, compared to men (7.3% versus 4.0%; Steel et al., 2014). There is no evidence of any significant sex difference in the prevalence of diabetes mellitus (Guariguata et al., 2013).

A review by Nebel and colleagues (2018) also describes sex differences in other dementia risk factors, including sleep, marital status, and the ε4 allele of the APOE gene. Sleep apnoea is more prevalent in males and individuals with sleep apnoea perhaps contributing to cognitive impairment at an earlier age compared with those without. Men who have never married or are widowed are at greater risk of developing Alzheimer's disease than women with the same marital status. This difference may be related to women traditionally being responsible for their family's healthcare and single women being more likely to attend health professionals and be socially active. Finally, there is some evidence that females with the APOE ε4 allele are at increased risk of developing Alzheimer's disease or MCI than males, but the mechanism for this difference is not clear.

There is a an increasing consensus that personalized recommendations should be made for dementia risk reduction through

> increasing levels of education in young adulthood, increasing physical, cognitive and social activity throughout adulthood, reducing cardiovascular risk factors including diabetes in middle-age, through lifestyle and medication, treating depression, adopting a healthy diet and physical activity, avoiding pesticides and heavy air pollution and teaching avoidance of all potential dangers to brain health while enhancing potential protective factors. (Anstey et al., 2015, p. 194)

Throughout adulthood

Increase physical, cognitive and social activity
Treat depression
Follow healthy diet
Avoid pesticides and heavy air pollution

Young adulthood	**Middle age**
Increase levels of education	Decrease cardiovascular risk factors: diabetes, hypertension, stroke, obesity, smoking, hypercholesterolaemia

Figure 22.1 Suggested targets for personalized recommendations for dementia risk reduction. Reproduced with permission from *Medicine Today* (Curran et al., 2018)

This is shown diagrammatically in in Figure 22.1.

Given the breadth and scope of these risk factors, there are several levels at which intervention could occur. This could include a 'micro level', focusing on individuals and families within community and healthcare settings, all the way up to the 'macro level' of societal public policy and health initiatives.

Diagnosis and Assessment

Given the significant impact of dementia on an individual and their family, it is important that memory concerns are explored rather than being dismissed as an expected part of the process of ageing. This is especially important in men, as they are generally less likely to present to health professionals for help for cognitive or mental health concerns. Sometimes, they may be attending reluctantly at the request of a family member. This emphasizes the importance of assessing the concerns thoroughly in case there is not the opportunity for further appointments.

Early diagnosis provides benefits to individuals and their families, including early use of treatments that may slow cognitive decline and allow more time to plan for the future when considering the optimal living environment, organizing support services, addressing driving safety, organizing a will, power of attorney, and myriad other psychosocial issues.

Delays in presentation are a challenge to early and timely diagnosis of dementia. Studies have found average delays of between 8 and 52 months from first clinical signs of dementia to first medical consultation (Perry-Young et al., 2018). Our clinical experience is that men are often more reluctant to present with cognitive concerns than women, thus exacerbating this delay.

A recent systematic review and meta-ethnography described some key factors that delay seeking medical attention to assess signs of dementia, including (Perry-Young et al., 2018):

- Discounting the symptom as normal ageing, normal compared to others or compared to their usual self
- Deferring the review
- Misattributing the change to something else, for example, their medication affecting their cognition
- Interpersonal issues where the individual does not accept there is a problem while others do; and
- Cultural beliefs may affect interpretation of signs of dementia

The diagnosis of dementia remains a clinical diagnosis, informed by thorough history taking, cognitive assessment, physical examination, and investigations. The history is gathered from the patient and also from an informant, where possible. An informant history is particularly important given that some individuals are unaware of the presence or extent of their cognitive impairment and the impact on their functioning. An informant history must be gathered sensitively, especially as some families and cultures have quite well-defined gender roles that may be impacted by the older male in the family developing cognitive impairment. This will also have later consequences for the family if the older male has taken primary responsibility for tasks such as financial management and driving.

A comprehensive medical history, psychiatric history, and physical examination are pivotal to accurate diagnosis. Medical history and physical examination should focus on identifying causes of cognitive impairment, such as Parkinson's disease, vascular disease, or chronic liver disease from alcohol excess. Potentially reversible causes of cognitive impairment such as hypothyroidism and electrolyte disturbance should be excluded via history, examination, and investigation. A suggested list of investigations is included in Table 22.1 (adapted from Loi et al., 2017). The time course of cognitive changes is informative as a more rapid and fluctuating pattern may indicate delirium rather than dementia. The psychiatric history is important as some diagnoses may affect cognition, such as the concept of 'pseudodementia' where depression causes a syndrome of cognitive impairment that usually is reversible on recovery from depression. Current medications, including complementary or over-the-counter medications should also be enquired about as some may contribute to cognitive impairment, such as benzodiazepines and anticholinergic medications. Asking about family history provides some indication of genetic predisposition given that many causes of dementia can have some genetic contributions.

The pattern of the cognitive impairment is informative as it may facilitate the diagnostic process. Cognitive impairment may affect functions such as memory, attention, language, visuo-spatial, and executive function. Cognitive assessment occurs

Table 22.1 Suggested investigations in assessment of possible dementia

Test	Purpose/condition
Full blood count	Anaemia, infections
Electrolytes	Renal impairment, hyponatraemia
Liver function tests	Hepatitis, bile duct obstruction, alcohol
Thyroid function tests	Hypo- or hyperthyroidism
B12, folate, vitamin D	Deficiency
C-reactive protein (CRP) or Erythrocyte sedimentation rate (ESR)	Marker of infection, vasculitis, cancer, etc.
Urine	Infection
Magnetic Resonance Imaging (MRI) (or Computerized Tomography (CT) brain if MRI not available)	May help determine a cause for dementia or exclude pathology such as haemorrhage or tumour
Functional imaging such as Positron Emission Tomography (PET) or Single Photon Emission Computed Tomography (SPECT)	May help determine a cause for dementia but availability of scanners varies

Box 22.3 Important components of assessment of memory concerns

- Do not dismiss memory concerns as an expected part of the ageing process
- Take a thorough history from the individual and an informant
- Assess and investigate for other reversible causes of memory changes including delirium, other medical conditions, or other psychiatric conditions
- Use a recognized cognitive assessment tool to examine the pattern of cognitive changes
- Refer to a specialist service where available
- Consider gender in the process of assessment and how this may influence presentation, rapport, and subtype of dementia

throughout the interview with the individual and involves both observation and formal testing with assessment tools. It is important to perform cognitive testing sensitively as many individuals find this very confronting. Our clinical experience is that men from older generations may often feel insulted by the process of cognitive testing. This may damage already tenuous rapport with the individual, particularly if they are not aware of any problems and presented at the request of a family member. The main sex difference in healthy cognitive ageing that has been consistently shown is that women perform better in verbal memory function while men perform better in visuo-spatial function (Mielke et al., 2014).

Causes of Dementia

Alzheimer's disease is the most common cause of dementia and is typically characterized in the early stages by an insidious decline in the ability to lay down new memory. It progresses over time to cause more global impairment of cognition. Deposition of beta amyloid protein in plaques and tau protein in neurofibrillary tangles is hypothesized to lead to neuronal loss. The prevalence of Alzheimer's dementia is consistently found to be higher in women than men, while incidence studies are equivocal (Mielke et al., 2014).

Vascular dementia is the second most common cause of dementia and usually presents as a 'subcortical' picture characterized by general slowing of cognitive processes and a varied presentation that may include impairment across a range of cognitive

domains. Some studies have found that men are at greater risk of developing vascular dementia, but these findings are not consistent (Kalaria et al., 2008; Andersen et al., 1999).

Dementia with Lewy Bodies is the third most common cause of dementia and its core features include fluctuating cognition, visual hallucinations, Rapid Eye Movement (REM) sleep behaviour disorder, and Parkinsonism (McKeith et al., 2017). A recent review was unable to confirm previous findings that men are at greater risk of developing Dementia with Lewy Bodies and concluded that more research is needed (Jones and O'Brien, 2014).

Fronto-temporal dementia has a propensity to impact frontal and temporal lobe function leading to impairment in executive and language functions. This commonly presents as behavioural change and/or aphasia. Fronto-temporal dementia has an earlier age of onset compared to other dementias, typically commencing between the ages of 45 and 65 years, and there does not appear to be a sex difference in prevalence or incidence (Neary, Snowden, and Mann, 2005).

Alcohol-related dementia classically presents with an amnestic syndrome in the context of prolonged intake of excessive alcohol that persists despite abstinence. Alcohol-related dementia is more common in men than women (Ridley et al., 2013). There is some debate about how alcohol-related dementia differs from Wernicke–Korsakoff's Syndrome (Ridley et al., 2013).

Mild cognitive impairment (MCI) is described as an intermediate state that exists on the cognitive spectrum between healthy ageing and early dementia – a state characterized by mild objective cognitive impairment without significant impairment of function (Livingston et al., 2017). A proportion of individuals who have MCI will develop dementia, while others will revert to healthy cognition and others will have stable impairments. A review of epidemiological studies estimated the prevalence of MCI as around 10–20% of the population aged 65 years and above with some studies showing a higher prevalence in men, some showing a higher prevalence in women, and some showing no sex difference (Mielke et al., 2014). The same review described men having a higher incidence of non-amnestic MCI than women. This finding may be supportive of the higher prevalence and incidence of some of the non-Alzheimer's dementias in males, as non-amnestic MCI is thought to be prodromal for non-Alzheimer's dementias (Mielke et al., 2014).

Box 22.4 Subtypes of dementia as they affect men vs women

- Alzheimer's disease is the most common cause of dementia and is more prevalent in women than men
- It has been thought that Vascular dementia and Dementia with Lewy Bodies are more common in men than women; however, the findings have been inconsistent
- Alcohol-related dementia is more common in men than women
- There is no sex difference in the prevalence of Fronto-temporal dementia
- Findings on assessment, including the pattern of cognitive impairment, can help to determine the subtype of dementia

Table 22.2 Prevalence of NPI symptoms

NPI Symptom	Prevalence
Apathy	49%
Depression	42%
Aggression	40%
Anxiety	39%
Sleep disorder	39%
Irritability	36%
Appetite disorder	34%
Aberrant motor behaviour	32%
Delusion	31%
Disinhibition	17%
Hallucination	16%
Euphoria	7%

Some individuals will have a combination of different subtypes of dementia, for example, Alzheimer's dementia and Vascular dementia.

Behavioural and Psychological Symptoms of Dementia

Behavioural and Psychological Symptoms of Dementia (BPSD) are also referred to as neuropsychiatric symptoms of dementia and are highly prevalent. A recent systematic review and meta-analysis described the prevalence of these symptoms as reported in the Neuropsychiatric Inventory (NPI); these symptoms are summarized in Table 22.2 (Zhao et al., 2016).

BPSD has been shown to have a negative impact on outcomes such as institutionalization and quality of life in people with dementia as well as caregiver psychological outcomes such as carer burden and carer well-being (Fauth and Gibbons, 2014). The three NPI symptoms that caused the most distress to caregivers in a large caregiver survey were delusions, agitation/aggression, and irritability (Fauth and Gibbons, 2014).

Some sex differences in BPSD prevalence have been reported. A Swedish study of 3395 people with cognitive impairment in geriatric care settings found that men were more likely to have aggressive or regressive behaviours while women were more likely to have depressive symptoms (Lovheim et al., 2009). There was higher use of antipsychotics in men, higher use of antidepressants in women, and no sex difference in the use of anxiolytics, hypnotics, and sedatives

(Lovheim et al., 2009). Overall in the context of BPSD, men more often than women (Lovheim et al., 2009):

- hit other patients or staff
- made aggressive threats
- resisted being dressed or undressed
- were easily annoyed
- piled up or overturned chairs or other furniture
- stood at the outer door wanting to go out
- were unruly in bed
- were smeared with faeces
- urinated in the wrong place, such as in wastepaper baskets or on the floor; and
- were found lying in other patients' beds

These sex differences in BPSD confirm our clinical experience that men may have BPSD that is more challenging to their caregivers and their environment. It may also partly explain the relative greater use of antipsychotics as opposed to antidepressants in men with dementia.

Management

The management of dementia should involve a multidisciplinary team using a collaborative approach to work with the individual with dementia and their families and broader network as appropriate. Dementia may impact individuals through cognitive symptoms, neuropsychiatric symptoms, co-morbid physical health conditions, and impairment of function (Livingston et al., 2017). The interventions may be psychosocial and/or pharmacological and need to be tailored to the individual's needs. Like other aspects of the individual's context, gender is a factor that may influence how treatment is tailored to the individual.

Cognitive Symptoms

Over 200 medications have reached Phase II clinical trials over the three decades from 1984 to 2014 with only four medications currently available for treatment of dementia; none is disease modifying (Schneider et al., 2014). One of the hypotheses for this lack of success is that treating clinical dementia is targeting the condition too late. In the case of Alzheimer's disease, for example, amyloid pathology in the brain reaches a threshold around seventeen years before a clinical diagnosis can be made (Villemagne et al., 2014), and thus 'hippocampal damage is so profound by the time individuals present with AD dementia that attempting to slow their decline with an anti-amyloid agent may be analogous to starting statins in patients on a heart transplantation waiting list' (Chong et al., 2016). Another hypothesis is that Alzheimer's disease may be multifactorial and treatment needs to address amyloid, tau, inflammation, and other factors.

Currently, there are three cholinesterase inhibitors – donepezil, galantamine, and rivastigmine – which have evidence for the treatment of cognitive impairment in Alzheimer's dementia and Dementia with Lewy Bodies as well as hallucinations in the latter (Livingston et al., 2017). There is also an NMDA receptor antagonist, memantine, which has evidence for treatment of moderate-to-severe Alzheimer's dementia (Livingston et al., 2017). These medications provide modest benefit for cognition in some patients, putatively through enhancing cholinergic signalling and reducing glutamatergic neuro-excitation, respectively. There is ongoing research into potential new treatments.

There has been limited research into sex differences in the pharmacological treatment of dementia. A systematic review of randomized controlled trials of the cholinesterase inhibitors and memantine did not report any studies that considered the medications separately for men and women (Canevelli et al., 2017). Of the 48 trials identified, 2 studies examined the effect of sex on efficacy, showing no difference;

and no studies examined the effect of sex on safety and tolerability of these agents (Canevelli et al., 2017).

There is some evidence supporting the cognitive benefits in mild-to-moderate dementia with the use of group cognitive stimulation therapy and individual cognitive rehabilitation for specific functional goals, but individual cognitive stimulation has not been shown to be effective (Livingston et al., 2017). Again, exploration of sex-specific effects is lacking.

Behavioural and Psychological Symptoms of Dementia

Management of BPSD needs to be informed by thorough assessment of the BPSD, given that BPSD is a collection of quite different symptoms. The assessment process usually involves an attempt to 'understand the person and symptoms via a comprehensive assessment and analysis of the behaviour': including the Antecedents, Behaviour description and Consequences – the 'ABC model' (Laver et al., 2016). This can be aided by the use of tools such as behaviour charts. It is also important to consider the sex difference in the prevalence of different types of BPSD symptoms noted earlier.

First-line treatment of BPSD should be with psychosocial interventions that are tailored to the individual's preferences, needs, and presentation. The gender of the individual with dementia will also influence this. Pharmacological treatments for BPSD should be second line, and antipsychotic medication should only be used where there is significant distress and/or risk to the individual or others, and where a discussion with the individual and their family about the risks and benefits has occurred (Laver et al., 2016). This is due to the increased risk of cerebrovascular events and death that has been identified with antipsychotic medication use in people with dementia.

Caregivers

Caregivers often play an extremely important role in the lives of people with dementia. Their contribution can make a significant difference to the functioning of society as a whole, as the community would not have the resources needed to provide the care that is needed without family caregivers. There is consistent evidence that female carers experience worse outcomes compared with men, including higher levels of depression and caregiver burden (Pillemer et al.,

2018; Bedard et al., 2005). There is also evidence that a female caregiver providing support to a male person with dementia is associated with greater caregiver role burden than any other gender combination (Bedard et al., 2005). Care–recipient problem behaviours and dependence with instrumental activities of daily living are associated with increased caregiver role burden (Bedard et al., 2005). The former is particularly relevant to men who have dementia given the sex difference in BPSD, with men exhibiting more aggressive and regressive behaviours than women. Consequently, it is critical that the community and health and social support systems provide tailored support to caregivers.

The residential care setting is often a major adjustment for new residents as it represents a significant change from their home environment and removes much of their independence and flexibility in daily life routines and activities. The challenge of this adjustment is further compounded for new residents who have cognitive impairment as the change will cause more bewilderment with greater difficulties in learning and adapting to a new environment, people, and routines. Residential care settings have a higher proportion of female residents and this may have some implications for male residents. The design and tailoring of activities and the environment in general need to consider gender as one of the important attributes of residents.

The important and challenging role of carers should be recognized and supported.

Conclusions

Dementia is a global health challenge that results in significant morbidity and mortality as well as impact on carers, communities, service systems, and national resources. The causes of dementia and the

---

Box 22.5 Management of dementia

- Management should be multidisciplinary
- Management should be tailored to individual preferences and needs
- Sex and gender are factors that may impact on how management is tailored
- There are limited pharmacological interventions available for dementia
- Psychosocial interventions are first line for the management of BPSD

---

manifestations of dementia differ between individuals. This means that assessment and management of individuals with dementia need to be tailored to the person and their support network. Sex and gender are important factors that need to be considered when tailoring interventions. Male sex can influence the prevalence and incidence of dementia and its different subtypes as well as risk factors and risk-reduction strategies for dementia. Our clinical experience, supported by emerging evidence, suggests that men may present differently with dementia and approach to assessment may need to be adapted to these differences. Males with dementia tend to manifest more problematic BPSD than females and this may lead to greater carer burden, especially where the caregiver is female. The research on sex and gender differences in dementia is still limited and thus there is a need for future dementia research to focus on this area through sex- and gender-specific research, or at least through consideration of possible sex and gender effects when designing research studies. Consideration of sex and gender, amongst other factors, is an important component of providing person-centred care.

References

American Psychiatric Association. 2013. *Diagnostic and Statistical Manual of Mental Disorders*, 5th ed. Arlington, VA: American Psychiatric Publishing.

Andersen, K., Launer, L. J., Dewey M. E., et al. 1999. Gender differences in the incidence of AD and vascular dementia: The EURODEM Studies. *Neurology*, 53, 1992–7.

Anstey, K. J., Eramudugolla, R., Hosking, D. E., et al. 2015. Bridging the translation gap: from dementia risk assessment to advice on risk reduction. *Journal of Prevention of Alzheimers Disease*, 2, 189–98.

Ashby-Mitchell, K., Burns, R., Shaw, J., and Anstey, K. 2017. Proportion of dementia in Australia explained by common modifiable risk factors. *Alzheimer's Research and Therapy*, 9, 11.

Bedard, M., Kuzik, R., Chambers, L. et al. 2005. Understanding burden differences between men and women caregivers: the contribution of care–recipient problem behaviors. *International Psychogeriatrics*, 17, 99–118.

Booth, M. L., Owen, N., Bauman, A., Clavisi, O., and Leslie, E. 2000. Social-cognitive and perceived environment influences associated with physical activity in older

Australians. *Preventive Medicine*, 31, 15–22.

Canevelli, M., Quarata, F., Remiddi, F., et al. 2017. Sex and gender differences in the treatment of Alzheimer's disease: a systematic review of randomized controlled trials. *Pharmacological Research*, 115, 218–23.

Chong, T. W. H., Loi, S. M., Lautenschlager, N. T., and Ames, D. A. 2016. Therapeutic advances and risk factor management: our best chance to tackle dementia? *Medical Journal of Australia*, 204, 91–2.

Curran, E., Chong, T., and Lautenschlager, N. 2018. Dementia – how to reduce the risk and impact. *Medicine Today*, 19, 14–23.

Fauth, E. B. and Gibbons, A. 2014. Which behavioral and psychological symptoms of dementia are the most problematic? Variability by prevalence, intensity, distress ratings, and associations with caregiver depressive symptoms. *International Journal of Geriatric Psychiatry*, 29, 263–71.

Grasset, L., Brayne, C., Joly P., et al. 2016. Trends in dementia incidence: Evolution over a 10-year period in France. *Alzheimer's and Dementia*, 12, 272–80.

Guariguata, L., Whiting D. R., Hambleton, I., et al. 2013. Global estimates of diabetes prevalence for 2013 and projections for 2035. *Diabetes Research and Clinical Practice*, 103, 137–49.

Jones, S. A. V. and O'Brien, J. T. 2014. The prevalence and incidence of dementia with Lewy bodies: a systematic review of population and clinical studies. *Psychological Medicine*, 44, 673–83.

Kalaria, R. N., Maestre, G. E., Arizaga, R., et al. 2008. Alzheimer's disease and vascular dementia in developing countries: prevalence, management, and risk factors. *Lancet Neurology*, 7, 812–26.

Keadle, S. K., McKinnon, R., Graubard B. I., and Troiano, R. P. 2016.

Prevalence and trends in physical activity among older adults in the United States: a comparison across three national surveys. *Preventive Medicine*, 89, 37–43.

Laver, K., Cumming, R. G., Dyer, S. M., et al. 2016. Clinical practice guidelines for dementia in Australia. *Medical Journal of Australia*, 204, 191–3.

Livingston, G., Sommerlad, A., Orgeta, V., et al. 2017. Dementia prevention, intervention, and care. *Lancet*, 390, 2673–734.

Livingston, G., Huntley, J., Sommerlad, A., et al. 2020. Dementia prevention, intervention, and care: 2020 report of the Lancet Commission. *Lancet*, 396, 413–46.

Loi S., Chong, T., and Ames, D. 2017. Cognitive Screening for Dementia. In: S. Lautenbacher and S.J. Gibson (eds.) *Pain in Dementia*. Philadelphia: Wolters Kluwer Health.

Lovheim, H. Sandman, P., Karlsson, S., and Gustafson, Y. 2009. Sex difference in the prevalence of behavioral and psychological symptoms of dementia. *International Psychogeriatrics*, 21, 469–75.

Matthews, F. E., Arthur, A., Barnes, L. E., et al. 2016. A two-decade comparison of prevalence of dementia in individual aged 65 years and older from three geographical areas of England: results of the Cognitive Function and Ageing Study I and II. *Lancet*, 382, 1405–12.

McKeith, I. G., Boeve, B. F., and Dickson, D. W. 2017. Diagnosis and management of dementia with Lewy bodies. *Neurology*, 89, 88–100.

Mielke, M. M., Ferretti, M. T., Iulita, M. F., Hayden, K., and Khachaturian, A. S. 2018. Sex and gender in Alzheimer's disease – does it matter? *Alzheimer's and Dementia*, 14, 1101–3.

Mielke, M. M., Vemuri, P., and Rocca, W. A. 2014. Clinical epidemiology

of Alzheimer's disease: assessing sex and gender differences. *Clinical Epidemiology*, 6, 37–48.

Neary, D., Snowden, J., and Mann, D. 2005. Frontotemporal dementia. *Lancet Neurology*, 4, 771–80.

Nebel, R. A., Aggarwal, N. T., Barnes, L. L., et al. 2018. Understanding the impact of sex and gender in Alzheimer's disease: a call to action. *Alzheimer's and Dementia*, 14, 1171–83.

Ng, M., Fleming, T., Robinson, M., et al. 2014. Global, regional, and national prevalence of overweight and obesity in children and adults during 1980–2013: a systematic analysis for the Global Burden of Disease Study 2013. *Lancet*, 384, 766–81.

Norton, S., Matthews, F. E., Barnes, D. E., et al. 2014. Potential for primary prevention of Alzheimer's disease: an analysis of population-based data. *Lancet Neurology*, 13, 788–94.

Perry-Young, L., Owen, G., Kelly, S., and Owens, C. 2018. How people came to recognise a problem and seek medical help for a person showing early signs of dementia: a systematic review and meta-ethnography. *Dementia*, 17, 34–60.

Pillemer, S., Davis, J., and Tremont, G. 2018. Gender effects on components of burden and depression among dementia caregivers. *Aging and Mental Health*, 22(9), 1156–61.

Prince, M., Wimo, A., Guerchet, M., et al. 2015. World Alzheimer report 2015. The global impact of dementia: an analysis of incidence, prevalence, cost and trends. London: Alzheimer's Disease International. Available at www.alz .co.uk/research/ WorldAlzheimerReport2015.pdf (accessed September 2015).

Ridley, N. J., Draper, B., and Whithall, A. 2013. Alcohol-related dementia: an update of the evidence. *Alzheimer's Research and Therapy*, 5, 3.

Rocca, W. A., Mielke, M. M., Vemuri, P., and Miller, V. M. 2014. Sex and gender differences in the causes of dementia: a narrative review. *Maturitas*, 79, 196–201.

Satizabal, C. L., Beiser, A. S., Chouraki, V., et al. 2016. Incidence of dementia over three decades in the Framingham Heart Study. *New England Journal of Medicine*, 374, 523–32.

Schneider, L. S., Mangialasche, F., Andreasen, N., et al. 2014. Clinical trials and late-stage drug development for Alzheimer's disease: an appraisal from 1984 to 2014. *Journal of Internal Medicine*, 275, 251–83.

Steel, Z. Marnane, C., Iranpour, C., et al. 2014. The global prevalence of common mental disorders: a systematic review and meta-analysis 1980–2013. *International Journal of Epidemiology*, 43, 476–93.

Theodore, R. F., Broadbent, J., Nagin, D., et al. 2015. Childhood to early–midlife systolic blood pressure trajectories – Early life predictors, effect modifiers, and adult cardiovascular outcomes. *Hypertension*, 66, 1108–1115.

Villemagne, V. L., Burnham, S., Bourgeat, P., et al. 2014. Amyloid β deposition, neurodegeneration, and cognitive decline in sporadic Alzheimer's disease: a prospective cohort study. *Lancet Neurology*, 12, 357–67.

World Health Organization. 2019. *The ICD-10 Classification of Mental and Behavioural Disorders: Clinical Descriptions and Diagnostic Guidelines*. Geneva: World Health Organization. https://icd.who.int/browse10/2019/en#/F00-F09

Wu, Y., Beiser, A. S., Breteler, M. M. B., et al. 2017. The changing prevalence and incidence of dementia over time – current evidence. *Nature Reviews Neurology*, 13, 327–40.

Zhao, Q., Tan, L, Wang, H., et al. 2016. The prevalence of neuropsychiatric symptoms in Alzheimer's disease: a systematic review and meta-analysis. *Journal of Affective Disorders*, 190, 264–71.

Mental Health of Men in Later Life

Osvaldo P. Almeida

The world's population is ageing rapidly, with the proportion of people aged 60 years or over growing faster than any other age group. Estimates from the United Nations indicate that the number of people older than 60 years will rise from 962 million in 2017 to 2.1 billion in 2050 and 3.1 billion by 2100 (United Nations, 2017). The number of persons aged 80 years or above will triple by 2050 and will increase more than seven times by 2100 compared with 2017 (United Nations, 2015; 2017). Women continue to outnumber men in the older age groups, although the probability of survival to age 60 and 80 years is increasing more rapidly in men than women (United Nations, 2015). As a consequence, the life expectancy gap between men and women is expected to continue to narrow over the coming decades.

This increasing longevity is a welcome phenomenon, although its consequences require careful consideration. In Australia, 80% of all deaths occur among people aged 65 years or over (Australian Institute of Health and Welfare, 2017). Coronary heart disease, stroke, cancer, chronic respiratory diseases, and dementia are the leading causes of death among older men (Almeida et al., 2016b; Australian Institute of Health and Welfare, 2017), while cause-specific mortality varies around the globe according to socio-demographic index (GBD Causes of Death Collaborators, 2017). In fact, the risk of death seems to be modulated by several potentially modifiable factors in addition to socioeconomic status, such as smoking, alcohol intake, physical inactivity, obesity, diabetes, and hypertension, which suggests that further gains in longevity could be achieved by means of effective risk-reduction strategies (Stringhini et al., 2017). There is also substantial evidence that mental health disorders decrease the life expectancy of older men. For example, with alcohol use, affective and psychotic disorders more than doubled the mortality of participants aged 65–85 years in a large cohort study, and this increase in risk was largely

independent of age (Almeida et al., 2014). Existing data also suggest that mental health disorders are often associated with common chronic health conditions of older people, such as diabetes, cardiovascular diseases (e.g., ischaemic heart disease and stroke), and several neurodegenerative disorders like Parkinson's and Alzheimer's diseases (Almeida et al., 2012a; Almeida et al., 2016a; Almeida et al., 2016d; Chi et al., 2015; Hackett et al., 2014), and that these co-morbidities contribute to further undermine the quality of life and life expectancy of older people (Almeida et al., 2016b; 2017c; Almeida and Xiao, 2007; Ayerbe et al., 2013; Bosboom et al., 2013). As the Lancet Global Mental Health review has aptly summarized: there can be 'no health without mental health' (Prince et al., 2007).

Dementia, affective, and substance use disorders are the most prevalent mental health conditions of older men (Almeida et al., 2014). Chapter 22 of this book presents a detailed description of the causes and course of dementia in men, so this chapter will limit its focus to affective, anxiety, psychotic, and substance use disorders in later life.

Depression

Prevalence, Incidence, and Contributing Factors

Clinically significant symptoms of depression, as measured by a rating scale, affect about 8% of men and women aged 60 years or over living in the community, while the point prevalence of major depression in this group is close to 2% (Pirkis et al., 2009). The incidence rate of clinically significant depressive symptoms is 7 new cases per 100 person-years and, for major depression, 0.2 to 14 per 100 person-years (Buchtemann et al., 2012). In contrast, the estimated prevalence of major depression among older adults living in aged care facilities ranges from 14% to 42%

(Djernes, 2006). Sex does not seem to affect the prevalence or incidence of depression in later life.

The factors that contribute to the expression of depressive symptoms in old age are varied. The vascular hypothesis of depression proposed that changes in the course of a depressive disorder or the onset of symptoms in later life could be attributed to cardiovascular diseases or cardiovascular risk factors. The concept of 'vascular depression' gained popularity over the past two decades, but it is now seen as excessively narrow and limited (Almeida, 2008). In fact, the recurrence or emergence of depression in older age has been associated with numerous social, lifestyle, and clinical factors. Some of these factors may have occurred early in life (such as childhood physical or sexual abuse, limited education), while others may be more proximal (e.g., death of spouse, pain, loss of physical function). For example, exposure to physical abuse early in life may contribute to social isolation, misuse of substances, and a sedentary lifestyle. This, in turn, could render the person more vulnerable to certain health hazards (e.g., diabetes and hypertension), which may then lead to the development cardiovascular and cerebrovascular diseases, multiple morbidities, increasing frailty, and loss of function. These factors interact with each other and, independently or together, are believed to play a part in modulating the risk of depression in older age (Almeida, 2014; Figure 23.1). The development of effective preventive strategies relies on the validity of this model.

The risk factors for depression described above are relevant to all older adults, although prolonged widowhood seems to be a stronger predictor of depression in men than women (van Grootheest et al., 1999). Another risk factor that is particularly relevant to men is testosterone. Low concentration of testosterone in the serum has been associated with increased prevalence of depression in cross-sectional and longitudinal studies of older men (Almeida et al., 2008; Ford et al., 2016). A multicentre randomized controlled trial of testosterone replacement for men aged 65 years or older with hypogonadism (total testosterone < 9.5 nmol/L), but free of severe depressive symptoms (Patient Health Questionnaire, PHQ-9 < 20), showed that 1-year treatment with testosterone compared with placebo gel improved mood, albeit only modestly (Snyder et al., 2016). There is also preliminary evidence that testosterone treatment may improve the severity of depressive symptoms among non-elderly men with treatment-resistant depression (Pope et al., 2003); this seems to support the hypothesis that low total testosterone concentration contributes to cause depression and that testosterone replacement may have a role to play in alleviating symptoms. However, the quality of the data currently available remains suboptimal, and caution is required because of ongoing concerns about the potential adverse effects associated with testosterone treatment (Calof et al., 2005; Xu et al., 2013).

Clinical Presentation and Course of Symptoms

Depressive symptoms in older men may be the expression of a depressive disorder, dysthymia, an adjustment disorder, or bipolar disorder; or may result from a medical condition or use of a substance (see Chapters 12 and 14 for detailed descriptions of these syndromes). Consequently, and because of our reliance on the use of current diagnostic guidelines, the clinical presentation of people with depression seems to vary little with age. Nonetheless, somatic complaints and psychotic symptoms seem to be more frequent in late than early life (Hegeman et al., 2012). However, there is no compelling evidence that the clinical presentation of a depressive episode is influenced by sex. There is one exception to this generalization: self-harm behaviour is more violent and lethal among men than women (Bostwick et al., 2016) and, in later life, is consistently associated with the presence of clinically significant depressive symptoms (Lawrence et al., 2000; Snowdon et al., 2011).

Existing evidence suggests that the natural history of depression in later life is poor. Six-year data from the Longitudinal Ageing Study Amsterdam (LASA) showed that 32% of older adults with depression experienced persisting symptoms and 44% had

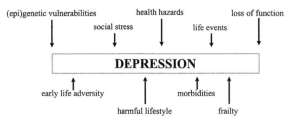

Figure 23.1 The figure depicts the multiplicity of risk factors that contribute, individually and together, to modulate the risk of depression. These risk factors are not necessarily independent from each other.

frequent recurrences. In 14% of participants the depression was short-lived (i.e., not present at subsequent annual assessments) and in 23% the symptoms remitted (Beekman et al., 2002). Two-year Australian data on 635 older men and women with clinically significant depressive symptoms showed that at least 25% of them remained depressed after two years – this proportion could be twice as high if the cases lost to follow-up had a poor outcome (Almeida et al., 2012b). These sobering findings should be balanced by two facts: (1) the chronicity of symptoms does not necessarily reflect treatment resistance – it may indicate suboptimal detection of cases and treatment (Mitchell et al., 2009); (2) depression in later life is very treatable (reviewed in greater detail below).

In older men, the presence of clinically significant symptoms of depression has been associated with a decline in measures of physical function and daily activities over the subsequent decade (Almeida et al., 2017b). Not surprisingly, frailty is more prevalent among older men with than without depression (Almeida et al., 2015), and this could explain why there is an 80% increase in the risk of death associated with major depression and minor depressive symptoms in later life (Cuijpers and Smit, 2002) – i.e., frailty may be the mediating factor linking depression to increased mortality in older men (Almeida et al., 2015).

There is also some concern that depression could increase the risk of cognitive decline and dementia in later life (Norton et al., 2014), although a recent longitudinal study found that when depression is associated with dementia, affective symptoms are more likely to represent a prodromal manifestation of dementia than a cause of it (i.e., only recent diagnosis of depression seems to be associated with increased risk of dementia; Almeida et al., 2017a).

Management

The optimal approach to the management of older people with a mental disorder should be guided by a detailed assessment of needs and, by necessity, involve professionals with complementary skills. In this context, targeting the treatment of symptoms in an older man with depression is but one aspect of management, which will often also involve education, management of co-morbidities, and interpersonal conflicts, development of risk-reduction programmes, assistance with socio-economic stressful factors, and

remediation of cognitive and functional deficits, among others. In this section, the focus of the discussion will be restricted to psychological and pharmacological treatments of depression, as well as electroconvulsive therapy (ECT).

Several psychotherapeutic approaches have been trialled for the treatment of mild-to-moderate symptoms of depression in later life: cognitive-behavioural therapy, non-directive supportive counselling, problem-solving, interpersonal therapy, psychodynamic treatment, and behavioural activation. A systematic review and meta-analysis of existing data indicated that structured interventions are slightly more efficacious than non-structured ones (e.g., supportive counselling), although their effect is modest (Cuijpers et al., 2008). A separate analysis of trials of behavioural activation showed that this approach may be particularly efficacious for the management of depression in older adults (Cuijpers et al., 2007) and may also help to reduce the proportion of people with subthreshold depression who develop clinically significant symptoms over time (Gilbody et al., 2017). There is no evidence that the outcomes of these interventions are affected by sex.

Data from randomized placebo-controlled trials of antidepressants in older age suggest that tricyclic (TCA) and selective serotonin inhibitors (SSRI) have similar efficacy, although adherence is lower among TCA users (Mottram et al., 2006). However, most of the trial data currently available have been derived from small studies of selective samples treated for 4 to 12 weeks, so that generalization of the findings remains uncertain (Tham et al., 2016). Dual action non-TCA antidepressants such as venlafaxine and duloxetine do not seem to offer additional benefits compared with other antidepressants. Preliminary evidence also suggests that adjunctive treatment with atypical antipsychotics (e.g., aripiprazole) may be particularly useful for people with psychotic depression, whilst certain B-vitamins and exercise may enhance treatment response to antidepressants. However, systematic data on this topic remain sparse.

ECT is an intervention commonly reserved to older people who fail to respond adequately to other treatment options (treatment-resistant) or who present with very severe depression (with or without psychotic symptoms or melancholia). A small number of trials has shown that ECT has excellent efficacy (about 80%) and, when administered appropriately, is safe and well-tolerated (Geduldig and Kellner, 2016). Its continuous use after remission of symptoms (maintenance ECT) may also contribute to decrease the risk of relapse of symptoms, although the quality of existing supportive data is suboptimal.

Finally, it seems opportune to consider the role of testosterone for the treatment of depressive symptoms in older men. Observational data suggest that older men with low serum concentration of testosterone have greater risk of experiencing depressive symptoms than other men (reviewed above), but data from randomized controlled trials remain scant. Pope and colleagues (2003) randomly assigned adult men with low testosterone who had remained depressed (major depressive episode) after four weeks of antidepressant treatment to either eight-week testosterone gel 1% (10 g/day; n=12) or placebo gel (n=10). Scores on the Hamilton Depression Rating Scale declined significantly more among men treated with testosterone than placebo, although one of the men treated with testosterone developed difficulties with micturition during the trial (Pope et al., 2003). It is unclear how many of the participants experienced remission of the depressive episode. Another small trial of hypogonadal adult men with subthreshold depressive symptoms (dysthymia or minor depression) found that those treated with testosterone gel showed greater decline in the severity of depressive symptoms after twelve weeks than their counterparts treated with placebo gel (Shores et al., 2009). However, the small differences between the groups disappeared after an additional open-label treatment period of twelve weeks. In summary, the role of testosterone for the treatment of older men with depression is yet to be determined. For a further discussion of these issues, the reader is referred to Chapter 12.

Box 23.1 Depression

- In later life depression is as common in men as in women: 8%
- Chronicity and recurrence of symptoms are common
- Depression decreases function and increases frailty and mortality
- Psychological and pharmacological interventions are efficacious and prevent relapse
- The role of testosterone in triggering and treating depressive symptoms remains unclear

---

Bipolar Disorder

The community prevalence of bipolar disorder (BD) among people aged 65 years or older is about 0.7%, with no obvious difference in frequency between men and women (Almeida et al., 2016b; Sajatovic et al., 2015). In aged care facilities, nearly 8% of residents have a recorded history of BD (Sheeran et al., 2012), and it is estimated that one in every four older adults in contact with mental health services may have BD (Sajatovic et al., 2004).

The clinical presentation and diagnosis of BD in later life is similar to that of their younger counterparts. By definition, it requires evidence of a current or past episode of hypomania (type II) or mania (type I) characterized by abnormally persistent elevated, expansive, or irritable mood, and increased goal-directed activity or energy (see detailed description in Chapter 14). Nonetheless, preliminary evidence suggests that as people with BD age, depressive episodes may become the predominant clinical manifestation of the disorder (Coryell et al., 2009). To date, no obvious clinical differences between older men and women with BD have been described.

Older men with BD have greater risk of developing dementia as they age, as well as greater risk of death (Almeida et al., 2016b). The increase in the risk of dementia is particularly pronounced among men with a recent (< 5 years) and long-standing (> 15 years) diagnosis of BD. In addition, a greater proportion of older men with BD onset before age 60 years have an established diagnosis of alcohol-use disorder – these men are also more likely to receive a new diagnosis of alcohol-use disorder during the following decade (Almeida et al., 2018c). There is also tentative evidence that older men with BD diagnosed for the first time before age 60 years are more likely to die a violent death (suicide or accident; Almeida et al., 2018b). Taken together, these findings suggest (but do not prove) that BD starting later in life has different clinical associations, and possibly course, compared with BD with onset in adult life.

The treatment of BD in older adults follows the same principles described for younger adults with BD, although the management of concurrent medical morbidities is a much more prominent concern in later than early life. Monotherapy with lithium, valproate, or an atypical antipsychotic are the preferred pharmacological options for the treatment of hypomanic or manic symptoms. Data from the GERI-BD trial showed that lithium and valproate lead to significant reductions in the severity of the symptoms of mania in later life (improvements were more pronounced with lithium than valproate), although side effects were a concern (Young et al., 2017). The treatment of depressive episodes in people with BD should include the use of lithium, lamotrigine, or quetiapine, or a combination of lithium or valproate with an SSRI, or olanzapine and a SSRI. Trial data for older adults with BD experiencing a depressive episode are all but nonexistent. Lastly, the recommended approach to the maintenance of BD in later life suggests the use of monotherapy with lithium (target concentration between 0.4 and 0.8 mmol/L), lamotrigine (not helpful for the prevention of manic episodes), valproate, olanzapine, quetiapine, risperidone, or aripiprazole (the last two for the prevention of manic episodes). ECT may be an effective alternative for treatment resistant cases of mania, depression, or mixed episodes (Perugi et al., 2017). At present, it is unclear whether testosterone plays a role in the expression of BD symptoms and their treatment in older men.

Anxiety Disorders

Anxiety disorders are much less frequent in older men than women, yet they affect nearly 8% of males aged 55 years or over in the USA (Reynolds et al., 2015). Specific phobias and post-traumatic stress disorder are the commonest diagnoses ascribed to older men (> 2%), although generalized anxiety disorder, social phobia, and panic disorder all have a one-year prevalence greater than 1% (Reynolds et al., 2015). It is unclear what the frequency of obsessive-compulsive symptoms in later life might be, but they are believed to be less frequent than other anxiety disorders.

Box 23.2 Bipolar disorder

- Bipolar disorder affects nearly 1% of older men
- Depressive episodes may become more frequent than manic episodes with increasing age
- Older men with bipolar disorder have greater risk of developing dementia
- The current management of affective episodes in later life follows the guidelines for adults
- The target serum concentration of lithium for maintenance in later life ranges from 0.4 to 0.8 mmol/L

In addition to sex, other factors thought to render older adults more vulnerable to experiencing symptoms of anxiety include childhood adversity (abuse, limited education), high neuroticism, multiple chronic diseases, functional decline in daily activities, social isolation, caring for a disabled person, fear of falling, and life events (Wolitzky-Taylor et al., 2010). Symptoms of anxiety may also be associated with other health disorders such as depression, dementia, or Parkinson's disease, psychotic disorders or the use of substances (e.g., SSRIs, dopamine agonists, decongestants, noradrenergic agonists, thyroid hormone, nicotine, alcohol, caffeine). Hence, the assessment of older men with symptoms of anxiety should include a detailed clinical history, physical and cognitive examination, and, if appropriate, laboratory investigations. Of note, it is currently unclear whether the serum concentration of testosterone has a direct, inverse, or no relationship with the expression of anxiety symptoms in older men (see also Chapters 9 and 10).

The general approach to the treatment of anxiety symptoms in later life should include a detailed diagnostic workup, management of contributing factors, education, and, if appropriate, specific psychological or pharmacological interventions. Structured psychological interventions, such as cognitive-behavioural therapy (CBT), seem capable of reducing the severity of anxiety symptoms in later life, although the number of studies available is small and their generalizability uncertain (Goncalves and Byrne, 2012). There is also evidence that eye-movement desensitization and reprocessing (EMDR) may be an inexpensive and efficacious form of treatment for post-traumatic stress disorder (Cusack et al., 2016), but supportive evidence for its use in later life is not available. A similar paucity of data occurs in relation to the pharmacological interventions for anxiety disorders in later life. Several agents have been trialled for the management of generalized anxiety disorder in older age: the largest study (n=273) showed that pregabalin is more efficacious than placebo, while pooled analyses indicate that duloxetine, venlafaxine, citalopram, escitalopram, and sertraline may also be helpful (Katzman et al., 2014). Obsessive-compulsive symptoms may be responsive to treatment with escitalopram, citalopram, or fluvoxamine (Katzman et al., 2014). However, more than half of older adults with an anxiety disorder will be using a benzodiazepine – these agents show some evidence of efficacy (Goncalves and Byrne, 2012), but their prolonged use may lead to the development of tolerance and abuse, and increased risk of falls, accidents, and cognitive impairment.

Psychotic Disorders

Delusions and hallucinations can arise in the context of multiple health conditions, such as delirium, psychosis induced by substances, or a medical illness, dementia, depressive or bipolar disorder, delusional or schizophreniform disorder or schizophrenia (see Chapter 5). In the case of delusional disorder and schizophrenia, psychotic symptoms express a primary psychopathological experience which, when arising later in life, affects predominantly women. Nonetheless, the schizophrenia-spectrum disorders (i.e., delusional disorder, schizophrenia, schizophreniform, and schizoaffective disorders) affect slightly over 1% of men aged 65 years or over living in the community (Almeida et al., 2014). Factors commonly associated with the onset of psychotic symptoms in later life include sensory impairment (particularly hearing loss), social isolation and cluster A personality traits (Almeida et al., 1995). The risk of dementia over twelve years for these individuals is three times greater than for the general population of older men (Almeida et al., 2018a).

The management of schizophrenia-spectrum disorders in later life is not as yet supported by compelling trial data, partly because recruiting into studies older people with limited insight into their psychotic experiences is challenging. Addressing possible contributing factors (such as hearing impairment) may be helpful (Almeida et al., 1993), while clinical experience suggests that treatment with atypical antipsychotics decreases the severity of symptoms (Scott et al., 2011). The results of a recently published randomized placebo-controlled trial showed that the severity of psychotic symptoms (onset $\geq$ 60 years) decreased with amisulpride treatment (100 mg daily; Howard et al., 2018). Treatment was well tolerated over a period of 36 weeks and nearly 25% of the randomized participants were male (Howard et al., 2018).

Substance-Use Disorders

Alcohol is the most frequently used substance in later life, and the prevalence of related disorders is particularly high among men (O'Connell et al., 2003). Four per cent of men aged 65 years or older living in the community have a recorded diagnosis of alcohol-use disorder (intoxication, harmful use or dependence; Almeida et al., 2018c), although suboptimal case-finding suggests that the true life-time prevalence may be higher. Moreover, the harmful use of alcohol may affect an even larger proportion of older men (about 16%), as current guidelines indicate that the regular weekly consumption of more than seven standard drinks is detrimental to health (Kucrbis et al., 2014). Alcohol consumption may also hinder the course and management of mental disorders (e.g., depressive or bipolar disorder) and facilitate the expression of self-harm behaviours (see below).

Approximately two in every three older men report having smoked tobacco regularly at some point during their lifetime, and 9% of them still smoke on a daily basis (Jamrozik et al., 2011). Smoking is associated with multiple health hazards and early death, with the risk increasing with the number of cigarettes smoked per day and with the number of years of smoking (Jamrozik et al., 2011). The prevalence of smoking is higher among older men with than without a mental health disorder, and this may contribute to complicate the clinical course of existing disorders and increase the risk of cognitive impairment, frailty, and mortality (Almeida et al., 2002; Jamrozik et al., 2011). Cessation of smoking, even late in life, is associated with health benefits, including improved mood and cognitive function (Almeida et al., 2011). The management of nicotine and alcohol use disorders in the elderly follows the same principles described for younger adults.

The misuse of prescribed and over-the-counter medications is an area of growing public health concern. Nearly half of community-dwelling men aged 70 years or over are using potentially inappropriate medicines and 35% are exposed to polypharmacy (five or more daily medications; Beer et al., 2011). Such misuse of medicines is associated with increased risk of health events (e.g., falls and cardiovascular events), hospital admission, and death (Beer et al., 2011). Opioid agents (often used to manage pain) and benzodiazepines are among the medications with a particularly high potential for misuse in later life (Kuerbis et al., 2014) – they should become consistent targets of risk-reduction interventions.

The use of illicit drugs (e.g., cannabis, cocaine, and heroin) seems much less frequent in late than early life, although recent trends suggest their use may be on the rise among the new generation of older adults (Taylor and Grossberg, 2012). Due to the lack of good-quality data, it is unclear how the recreational or potential medicinal use of these agents will affect the mental and physical health of older men, although existing evidence from studies with young adults suggests that physical and mental health complications should be expected (West et al., 2015).

Box 23.5 Substance Use

- The harmful and hazardous use of alcohol and smoking are common among older men
- Tentative evidence suggests that harm minimization and cessation strategies are associated with benefits in physical and mental health
- Polypharmacy and inappropriate, harmful, and hazardous use of prescription and over-the-counter medications in older age are an increasing public health problem
- Data on illicit substance use among older men remain scant

Suicide

Thoughts about death or dying are common in later life. In about 5% of older adults these thoughts take the form of intentional self-inflicted death (suicidal thoughts), which, when acted upon, become a suicide attempt or completed suicide (when death ensues; Almeida et al., 2012c). A large cross-sectional study of over 20,000 older men and women found that suicidal ideation was associated with male gender, higher education, smoking, poor social support, financial strain, no religious engagement, childhood abuse, poor perceived health, pain, history of past suicide attempt, or of suicide in the family, history of depression, and current symptoms of anxiety and depression (Almeida et al., 2012c). The risk factors associated with the highest population-attributable fraction of suicidal ideation were poor social support, past depression, pain and current depressive and/or anxiety symptoms, suggesting that the successful management of these factors could substantially decrease the number of older adults contemplating suicide. A clustered randomized controlled trial involving primary care providers showed that education and academic detailing targeting depressive symptoms decreases the prevalence of suicidal thoughts among older adults by about 20% over a period of two years (Almeida et al., 2012d), although it is unclear whether this would have had any impact on completed suicides.

The rate of suicide attempts is similar for men and women, although suicide completion is much higher among men (Lawrence et al., 2000). The reasons underlying this sex discrepancy are unclear, but may be partly mediated by the greater lethality of the suicide methods employed by men. The rates of suicide are particularly high among men aged 75 years or over and, according to psychological autopsy studies, are strongly associated with depressive symptoms in the days or weeks preceding death (Snowdon and Baume, 2002). A more recent investigation of older men using administrative health linkage data showed that, in addition to mental and substance use disorders, the presence of multiple medical co-morbidities is a very strong independent predictor of suicide among older men (Almeida et al., 2016c).

Behavioural and Psychological Symptoms Associated with Common Diseases of Older Men

Most chronic medical conditions are associated with increased prevalence of mental disorders. For example, depression and anxiety disorders are more prevalent in people with than without diabetes, chronic respiratory diseases, coronary heart disease, stroke, and Parkinson's and Alzheimer's diseases. These associations are not specific. For example, Parkinson's disease is associated with an increased prevalence and incidence of dementia and affective and psychotic disorders (Almeida et al., 2016a), which also occur more frequently among older adults who experience a stroke (Almeida and Xiao, 2007). What is clear, however, is that behavioural and psychological symptoms contribute to further undermine the quality of life and clinical outcomes of older adults with medical morbidities. Hence, the prevention and effective treatment of these symptoms are of critical importance.

Some psychological interventions have shown a small but significant beneficial effect in preventing depression among stroke patients (Hackett et al., 2008a), whereas the use of antidepressants (but not psychotherapy) reduces the severity and prevalence of clinically significant depressive symptoms (Hackett et al., 2008b). Unfortunately, however, there are limited data on how best to approach the prevention and treatment of older men with other concurrent medical morbidities. Available guidelines encourage the use of non-pharmacological strategies first (e.g., psychological interventions, physical activity, education) and warn about the paucity of data to guide the safe and effective use of pharmacological agents and other biological treatments.

Conclusions

As the world's population ages, the number of older men will continue to rise and, with them, the prevalence of health conditions that are common in later life. This demographic shift will place significant pressure on existing health services and public health expenditure. A particular challenge will be the development of strategies capable of decreasing the use of health services and increasing disability-free survival. Preventing and effectively managing mental health disorders will be a necessary key component of any such strategy.

References

Almeida, O. P. 2008. Vascular depression: myth or reality? *Int Psychogeriatr*, 20, 645–52.

Almeida, O. P. 2014. Prevention of depression in older age. *Maturitas*, 79, 136–41.

Almeida, O. P., Alfonso, H., Flicker, L., Hankey, G. J., and Norman, P. E. 2012a. Cardiovascular disease, depression and mortality: the Health In Men Study. *Am J Geriatr Psychiatry*, 20, 433–40.

Almeida, O. P. et al. 2012b. Anxiety, depression, and comorbid anxiety and depression: risk factors and outcome over two years. *Int Psychogeriatr*, 24, 1622–32.

Almeida, O. P. et al. 2012c. Factors associated with suicidal thoughts in a large community study of older adults. *Br J Psychiatry*, 201, 466–72.

Almeida, O. P., Ford, A. H., Hankey, G. J., Yeap, B. B., Golledge, J., and Flicker, L. 2018a. Risk of dementia associated with psychotic disorders in later life: the health in men study (HIMS). *Psychol Med*, 1–11.

Almeida, O. P., Forstl, H., Howard, R., and David, A. S. 1993. Unilateral auditory hallucinations. *Br J Psychiatry*, 162, 262–4.

Almeida, O. P. et al. 2011. 24-month effect of smoking cessation on cognitive function and brain structure in later life. *Neuroimage*, 55, 1480–9.

Almeida, O. P., Hankey, G. J., Yeap, B. B., Golledge, J., and Flicker, L. 2017a. Depression as a modifiable factor to decrease the risk of dementia. *Transl Psychiatry*, 7, e1117.

Almeida, O. P., Hankey, G. J., Yeap, B. B., Golledge, J., and Flicker, L. 2018b. Older men with bipolar disorder: clinical associations with early and late onset illness. *Int J Geriatr Psychiatry*, 33(12), 1613–19.

Almeida, O. P., Hankey, G. J., Yeap, B. B., Golledge, J., and Flicker, L. 2018c. Substance use among older adults with bipolar disorder varies according to age at first treatment contact. *J Affect Disord*, 239, 269–73.

Almeida, O. P., Hankey, G. J., Yeap, B. B., Golledge, J., Hill, K. D., and Flicker, L. 2017b. Depression among nonfrail old men is associated with reduced physical function and functional capacity after 9 years follow-up: the Health in Men Cohort Study. *J Am Med Dir Assoc*, 18, 65–9.

Almeida, O. P., Hankey, G. J., Yeap, B. B., Golledge, J., Norman, P. E., and Flicker, L. 2014. Mortality among people with severe mental disorders who reach old age: a longitudinal study of a community-representative sample of 37,892 men. *PLoS One*, 9, e111882.

Almeida, O. P., Hankey, G. J., Yeap, B. B., Golledge, J., Norman, P. E., and Flicker, L. 2015. Depression, frailty, and all-cause mortality: a cohort study of men older than 75 years. *J Am Med Dir Assoc*, 16, 296–300.

Almeida, O. P., Howard, R. J., Levy, R., and David, A. S. 1995. Psychotic states arising in late life (late paraphrenia). The role of risk factors. *Br J Psychiatry*, 166, 215–28.

Almeida, O. P., Hulse, G. K., Lawrence, D., and Flicker, L. 2002. Smoking as a risk factor for Alzheimer's disease: contrasting evidence from a systematic review of case-control and cohort studies. *Addiction*, 97, 15–28.

Almeida, O. P., McCaul, K., Hankey, G. J., Yeap, B. B., Golledge, J., and Flicker, L. 2016a. Affective disorders, psychosis and dementia in a community sample of older men with and without Parkinson's disease. *PLoS One*, 11, e0163781.

Almeida, O. P., McCaul, K., Hankey, G. J., Yeap, B. B., Golledge, J., and Flicker, L. 2016b. Risk of dementia and death in community-dwelling older men with bipolar disorder. *Br J Psychiatry*, 209, 121–6.

Almeida, O. P., McCaul, K., Hankey, G. J., Yeap, B. B., Golledge, J., and Flicker, L. 2016c. Suicide in older men: the Health in Men Cohort Study (HIMS). *Prev Med*, 93, 33–8.

Almeida, O. P., McCaul, K., Hankey, G. J., Yeap, B. B., Golledge, J., and Flicker, L. 2017c. Excessive alcohol consumption increases mortality in later life: a genetic analysis of the health in men cohort study. *Addict Biol*, 22, 570–578.

Almeida, O. P. et al. 2016d. Duration of diabetes and its association with depression in later life: The Health in Men Study (HIMS). *Maturitas*, 86, 3–9.

Almeida, O. P. et al. 2012d. A randomized trial to reduce the prevalence of depression and self-harm behavior in older primary care patients. *Ann Fam Med*, 10, 347–56.

Almeida, O. P., and Xiao, J. 2007. Mortality associated with incident mental health disorders after stroke. *Aust N Z J Psychiatry*, 41, 274–81.

Almeida, O. P., Yeap, B. B., Hankey, G. J., Jamrozik, K., and Flicker, L. 2008. Low free testosterone concentration as a potentially treatable cause of depressive symptoms in older men. *Arch Gen Psychiatry*, 65, 283–9.

Australian Institute of Health and Welfare. 2017. Older Australia at a glance. Canberra: Australian Institute of Health and Welfare and the Dept. of Health and Ageing. www.aihw.gov.au › older-people

Ayerbe, L., Ayis, S., Wolfe, C. D., and Rudd, A. G. 2013. Natural history, predictors and outcomes of depression after stroke: systematic review and meta-analysis. *Br J Psychiatry*, 202, 14–21.

Beekman, A. T., et al. 2002. The natural history of late-life depression: a 6-year prospective study in the community. *Arch Gen Psychiatry*, 59, 605–11.

Beer, C. et al. 2011. Quality use of medicines and health outcomes among a cohort of community dwelling older men: an observational study. *Br J Clin Pharmacol*, 71, 592–9.

Bosboom, P. R., Alfonso, H., and Almeida, O. P. 2013. Determining the predictors of change in quality of life self-ratings and carer-ratings for community-dwelling people with Alzheimer disease. *Alzheimer Dis Assoc Disord*, 27, 363–71.

Bostwick, J. M., Pabbati, C., Geske, J. R., and McKean, A. J. 2016. Suicide attempt as a risk factor for completed suicide: even more lethal

than we knew. *Am J Psychiatry*, 173, 1094–1100.

Buchtemann, D., Luppa, M., Bramesfeld, A., and Riedel-Heller, S. 2012. Incidence of late-life depression: a systematic review. *J Affect Disord*, 142, 172–9.

Calof, O. M. et al. 2005. Adverse events associated with testosterone replacement in middle-aged and older men: a meta-analysis of randomized, placebo-controlled trials. *J Gerontol A Biol Sci Med Sci*, 60, 1451–7.

Chi, S., Wang, C., Jiang, T., Zhu, X. C., Yu, J. T., and Tan, L. 2015. The prevalence of depression in Alzheimer's disease: a systematic review and meta-analysis. *Curr Alzheimer Res*, 12, 189–98.

Coryell, W., Fiedorowicz, J., Solomon, D., and Endicott, J. 2009. Age transitions in the course of bipolar 1 disorder. *Psychol Med*, 39, 1247–52.

Cuijpers, P., and Smit, F. 2002. Excess mortality in depression: a meta-analysis of community studies. *J Affect Disord*, 72, 227–36.

Cuijpers, P., van Straten, A.,, Andersson, G. and van Oppen, P. 2008. Psychotherapy for depression in adults: a meta-analysis of comparative outcome studies. *J Consult Clin Psychol*, 76, 909–22.

Cuijpers, P., van Straten, A., and Warmerdam, L. 2007. Behavioral activation treatments of depression: a meta-analysis. *Clin Psychol Rev*, 27, 318–26.

Cusack, K. et al. 2016. Psychological treatments for adults with posttraumatic stress disorder: a systematic review and meta-analysis. *Clin Psychol Rev*, 43, 128–41.

Djernes, J. K. 2006. Prevalence and predictors of depression in populations of elderly: a review. *Acta Psychiatr Scand*, 113, 372–87.

Ford, A. H. et al. 2016. Prospective longitudinal study of testosterone and incident depression in older men: The Health in Men Study. *Psychoneuroendocrinology, 64,* 57–65.

GBD Causes of Death Collaborators. 2017. Global, regional, and national age-sex specific mortality for 264 causes of death, 1980–2016: a systematic analysis for the Global Burden of Disease Study 2016. *Lancet, 390,* 1151–1210.

Geduldig, E. T., and Kellner, C. H. 2016. Electroconvulsive therapy in the elderly: new findings in geriatric depression. *Curr Psychiatry Rep, 18,* 40.

Gilbody, S. et al. 2017. Effect of collaborative care vs usual care on depressive symptoms in older adults with subthreshold depression: the CASPER Randomized Clinical Trial. *JAMA, 317,* 728–37.

Goncalves, D. C., and Byrne, G. J. 2012. Interventions for generalized anxiety disorder in older adults: systematic review and meta-analysis. *J Anxiety Disord, 26,* 1–11.

Hackett, M. L., Anderson, C. S., House, A., and Halteh, C. 2008a. Interventions for preventing depression after stroke. *Cochrane Database Syst Rev,* CD003689.

Hackett, M. L., Anderson, C. S., House, A., and Xia, J. 2008b. Interventions for treating depression after stroke. *Cochrane Database Syst Rev,* CD003437.

Hackett, M. L., Kohler, S., O'Brien, J. T., and Mead, G. E. 2014. Neuropsychiatric outcomes of stroke. *Lancet Neurol, 13,* 525–34.

Hegeman, J. M., Kok, R. M., van der Mast, R. C., and Giltay, E. J. 2012. Phenomenology of depression in older compared with younger adults: meta-analysis. *Br J Psychiatry, 200,* 275–81.

Howard, R. et al. 2018. Antipsychotic treatment of very late-onset schizophrenia-like psychosis (ATLAS): a randomised, controlled, double-blind trial. *Lancet Psychiatry, 5,* 553–63.

Jamrozik, K. et al. 2011. Women who smoke like men die like men who smoke: findings from two Australian cohort studies. *Tob Control, 20,* 258–65.

Katzman, M. A., et al. 2014. Canadian clinical practice guidelines for the management of anxiety, posttraumatic stress and obsessive-compulsive disorders. *BMC Psychiatry, 14* (suppl. 1), S1.

Kuerbis, A., Sacco, P., Blazer, D. G., and Moore, A. A. 2014. Substance abuse among older adults. *Clin Geriatr Med, 30,* 629–54.

Lawrence, D., Almeida, O. P., Hulse, G. K., Jablensky, A. V., and Holman, C. D. 2000. Suicide and attempted suicide among older adults in Western Australia. *Psychol Med, 30,* 813–21.

Mitchell, A. J., Vaze, A., and Rao, S. 2009. Clinical diagnosis of depression in primary care: a meta-analysis. *Lancet, 374,* 609–19.

Mottram, P., Wilson, K., and Strobl, J. 2006. Antidepressants for depressed elderly. *Cochrane Database Syst Rev,* CD003491.

Norton, S., Matthews, F. E., Barnes, D. E., Yaffe, K., and Brayne, C. 2014. Potential for primary prevention of Alzheimer's disease: an analysis of population-based data. *Lancet Neurol, 13,* 788–94.

O'Connell, H., Chin, A. V., Cunningham, C., and Lawlor, B. 2003. Alcohol use disorders in elderly people – redefining an age old problem in old age. *BMJ, 327,* 664–7.

Perugi, G., Medda, P., Toni, C., Mariani, M. G., Socci, C., and Mauri, M. 2017. The role of electroconvulsive therapy (ect) in bipolar disorder: effectiveness in 522 patients with bipolar depression, mixed-state, mania and catatonic features. *Curr Neuropharmacol, 15,* 359–71.

Pirkis, J. et al. 2009. The community prevalence of depression in older Australians. *J Affect Disord, 115,* 54–61.

Pope, H. G., Jr., Cohane, G. H., Kanayama, G., Siegel, A. J., and Hudson, J. I. 2003. Testosterone gel supplementation for men with refractory depression: a randomized, placebo-controlled trial. *Am J Psychiatry, 160,* 105–11.

Prince, M., et al. 2007. No health without mental health. *Lancet, 370,* 859–77.

Reynolds, K., Pietrzak, R. H., El-Gabalawy, R., Mackenzie, C. S., and Sareen, J. 2015. Prevalence of psychiatric disorders in U.S. older adults: findings from a nationally representative survey. *World Psychiatry, 14,* 74–81.

Sajatovic, M., Blow, F. C., Ignacio, R. V., and Kales, H. C. 2004. Age-related modifiers of clinical presentation and health service use among veterans with bipolar disorder. *Psychiatr Serv, 55,* 1014–21.

Sajatovic, M., et al. 2015. A report on older-age bipolar disorder from the International Society for Bipolar Disorders Task Force. *Bipolar Disord, 17,* 689–704.

Scott, J., Greenwald, B. S., Kramer, E., and Shuwall, M. 2011. Atypical (second generation) antipsychotic treatment response in very late-onset schizophrenia-like psychosis. *Int Psychogeriatr, 23,* 742–8.

Sheeran, T., Greenberg, R. L., Davan, L. A., Dealy, J. A., Young, R. C., and Bruce, M. L. 2012. A descriptive study of older bipolar disorder residents living in New York City's adult congregate facilities. *Bipolar Disord, 14,* 756–63.

Shores, M. M., Kivlahan, D. R., Sadak, T. I., Li, E. J., and Matsumoto, A. M. 2009. A randomized, double-blind, placebo-controlled study of testosterone treatment in hypogonadal older men with subthreshold depression (dysthymia or minor depression). *J Clin Psychiatry, 70,* 1009–16.

Snowdon, J., and Baume, P. 2002. A study of suicides of older people in Sydney. *Int J Geriatr Psychiatry, 17,* 261–269.

Snowdon, J., Draper, B., and Wyder, M. 2011. Age variation in the prevalence of DSM-IV disorders in cases of suicide of middle-aged and older persons in Sydney. *Suicide Life Threat Behav*, 41, 465–70.

Snyder, P. J. et al. 2016. Effects of testosterone treatment in older men. *N Engl J Med*, 374, 611–24.

Stringhini, S. et al. 2017. Socioeconomic status and the 25 × 25 risk factors as determinants of premature mortality: a multicohort study and meta-analysis of 1.7 million men and women. *Lancet*, 389, 1229–37.

Taylor, M. H., and Grossberg, G. T. 2012. The growing problem of illicit substance abuse in the elderly: a review. *Prim Care Companion CNS Disord*, 14.

Tham, A., Jonsson, U., Andersson, G., Soderlund, A., Allard, P., and Bertilsson, G. 2016. Efficacy and tolerability of antidepressants in people aged 65 years or older with major depressive disorder – a systematic review and a meta-analysis. *J Affect Disord*, 205, 1–12.

United Nations. 2015. Department of Economic and Social Affairs. Population Division. World population ageing 2015. New York: United Nations, Dept. of Economic and Social Affairs, Population Division.

United Nations. 2017. Department of Economic and Social Affairs. Population Division. World Population Prospects: The 2017 Revision – Key Findings and Advance Tables. Working Paper No. ESA/P/WP/248. New York: United Nations, Dept. of Economic and Social Affairs, Population Division.

van Grootheest, D. S., Beekman, A. T., Broese van Groenou, M. I., and Deeg, D. J. 1999. Sex differences in depression after widowhood. Do men suffer more? *Soc Psychiatry Psychiatr Epidemiol*, 34, 391–8.

West, N. A., Severtson, S. G., Green, J. L., and Dart, R. C. 2015. Trends in abuse and misuse of prescription opioids among older adults. *Drug Alcohol Depend*, 149, 117–21.

Wolitzky-Taylor, K. B., Castriotta, N., Lenze, E. J., Stanley, M. A., and Craske, M. G. 2010. Anxiety disorders in older adults: a comprehensive review. *Depress Anxiety*, 27, 190–211.

Xu, L., Freeman, G., Cowling, B. J., and Schooling, C. M. 2013. Testosterone therapy and cardiovascular events among men: a systematic review and meta-analysis of placebo-controlled randomized trials. *BMC Med*, 11, 108.

Young, R. C. et al. 2017. GERI-BD: a randomized double-blind controlled trial of lithium and divalproex in the treatment of mania in older patients with bipolar disorder. *Am J Psychiatry*, 174, 1086 93.